HANDBOOK ON DIGITAL HEALTH MONITORING

Handbook on Digital Health Monitoring

Oscar Dunhum
Chinedu Nwosu

Kruger Brentt
Publishers
2026

Kruger Brentt Publishers UK. LTD.
Company Number 9728962

Regd. Office: 68 St Margarets Road, Edgware, Middlesex HA8 9UU

ISBN: 978-1-78715-614-2

For information on all our publications visit our website at http://krugerbrentt.com/

PREFACE

The advent of digital technologies has transformed healthcare, enabling continuous, real-time monitoring of patients and populations. Digital health monitoring encompasses the use of wearable devices, sensors, mobile applications, and remote monitoring systems to track physiological, behavioral, and environmental data, thereby enhancing preventive care, diagnosis, and treatment outcomes.

Handbook on Digital Health Monitoring provides a comprehensive exploration of the principles, technologies, and applications that define this rapidly evolving field. The book integrates insights from biomedical engineering, computer science, healthcare, and data analytics to present a holistic understanding of digital health systems. It examines the design, deployment, and evaluation of digital health monitoring tools, emphasizing accuracy, reliability, privacy, and ethical considerations.

This handbook is intended for healthcare professionals, biomedical engineers, researchers, students, and technology developers who are involved in designing, implementing, or studying digital health solutions. By combining theoretical foundations with practical examples and case studies, the book equips readers with the knowledge required to leverage digital monitoring technologies for improved health outcomes and patient care.

Oscar Dunhum

Chinedu Nwosu

CONTENTS

1 Chapter INTRODUCTION TO DIGITAL HEALTH MONITORING

1.0 DEFINING DIGITAL HEALTH MONITORING

Digital health monitoring uses wearable devices, apps, and connected systems to track vital health data in real time, empowering individuals and improving healthcare efficiency. It plays a crucial role in managing chronic diseases and promoting preventive care by encouraging healthier lifestyles. Technologies like AI and sensors enable continuous data collection and intelligent insights, supporting remote patient monitoring, especially in underserved areas. This approach reduces hospital visits and enhances early detection of health issues. However, challenges such as data privacy, cybersecurity, and equitable access must be addressed. Overall, digital health monitoring is transforming healthcare into a more personalized, proactive, and accessible system.

In the modern era, the integration of technology into healthcare has revolutionized the way health is monitored, managed and delivered. One of the most transformative aspects of this evolution is digital health monitoring, a field that leverages digital tools, wearable devices, mobile apps and connected systems to track and manage an individual's health in real time. This approach is not only enhancing the efficiency of healthcare systems but also empowering individuals to take a more active role in managing their well-being. Digital health monitoring refers to the continuous or periodic tracking of vital signs, physical activity, mental health status and other physiological parameters using digital devices and platforms. These include smartwatches, fitness trackers, smartphone applications, biosensors and remote patient monitoring systems. Such tools collect health-related data, which can be analyzed to detect abnormalities, support diagnosis, guide treatment decisions and alert both users and healthcare providers when necessary. A key driver behind this transformation is the rapid advancement in sensor technology, data analytics, artificial intelligence (AI) and wireless communication. These innovations allow for seamless data collection, real-time feedback and intelligent insights based on individual health patterns. For example, a smartwatch can now monitor heart rate, blood oxygen levels and sleep quality, while specialized devices can track glucose levels or detect arrhythmias, often without the need for invasive procedures. The adoption of digital health monitoring is particularly valuable in chronic disease management. Conditions such as diabetes, hypertension, asthma and cardiovascular diseases require ongoing monitoring and timely interventions.

With digital tools, patients can receive reminders for medication, visualize their health trends and communicate with healthcare professionals remotely, reducing the need for frequent in-person visits. Moreover, digital health monitoring is essential in preventive care and wellness promotion. By tracking lifestyle factors such as diet, exercise and sleep, individuals are encouraged to make healthier choices. Gamification and personalized feedback in health apps further motivate users to stick to fitness goals and adopt sustainable habits. Another critical benefit of digital monitoring lies in its potential to support healthcare systems through remote patient monitoring (RPM), especially in rural or underserved areas. This enables clinicians to monitor patients at home, detect complications early and reduce hospital readmissions. During public health crises like the COVID-19 pandemic, such technology proved vital for managing patient loads and maintaining continuity of care without exposing vulnerable populations to infection.

Despite its advantages, digital health monitoring also presents challenges. Concerns around data privacy, cybersecurity, user compliance and the digital divide must be addressed to ensure equitable and secure implementation. Regulatory frameworks and ethical standards are evolving to govern the use of digital health data and ensure user trust. Digital health monitoring represents a paradigm shift in healthcare delivery. It fosters a more proactive, personalized and data-driven approach to health, with the potential to improve outcomes, increase accessibility and reduce costs. As technology continues to evolve, the integration of digital monitoring into everyday healthcare will likely become not just a complement, but a cornerstone of modern medicine. Fig. 1 depicted the digital health care- a new era of innovation.

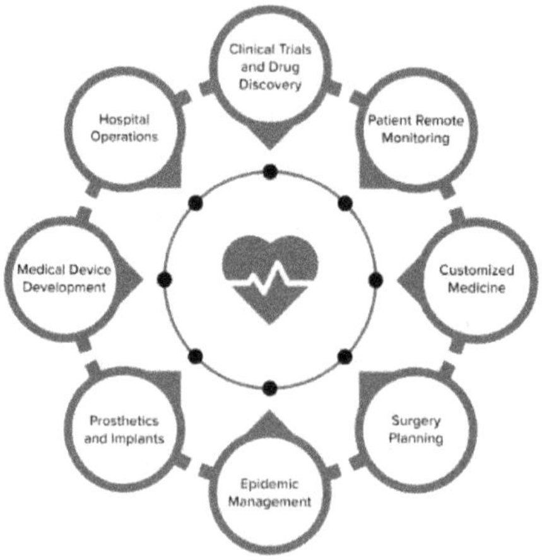

Fig.1 Digital Healthcare – A New Era of Innovation

Digital Health Monitoring is the use of digital technologies to observe, track and manage an individual's health remotely and continuously. It combines data from wearable devices, mobile health apps, smart sensors and other digital tools to monitor health parameters such as heart rate, blood pressure, glucose levels, sleep patterns and physical activity. This approach allows both patients and healthcare professionals to gain real-time or near real-time insights into a person's health status.

The system works by collecting data through connected devices that transmit health metrics to centralized platforms or cloud-based systems. These platforms often use artificial intelligence and machine learning algorithms to analyze data, detect patterns and provide alerts or recommendations. For example, an abnormal heart rhythm detected by a smartwatch can automatically notify a healthcare provider, prompting early intervention before a condition worsens.

Digital health monitoring plays a vital role in managing chronic conditions such as diabetes, cardiovascular diseases and respiratory disorders. It also supports preventive care by helping individuals recognize early warning signs and modify behaviors accordingly. Additionally, the integration of telemedicine services enhances patient-doctor communication, making healthcare more accessible, especially for those in remote or underserved areas.

Despite its benefits, digital health monitoring faces challenges such as ensuring data privacy, maintaining device accuracy and achieving interoperability across platforms. Regulatory compliance and patient trust are also essential for its widespread adoption. Nonetheless, as technology continues to evolve, digital health monitoring is becoming a cornerstone of modern, proactive and personalized healthcare delivery.

Here are several definitions of Digital Health Monitoring, phrased in different ways to suit academic, technical and general contexts:

- **General Definition:** Digital Health Monitoring refers to the use of electronic devices and software to continuously or periodically track an individual's health status. It enables real-time data collection and sharing with healthcare providers to support early detection, diagnosis and management of diseases.
- **Technical/Scientific Definition:** Digital Health Monitoring is a system-based approach that utilizes digital tools such as wearable sensors, mobile health applications and cloud-connected devices to capture physiological and behavioral health data. These data are processed using algorithms and analytics to provide feedback, detect anomalies and inform clinical decisions.
- **Healthcare Industry Definition:** Digital Health Monitoring involves integrating digital technologies into patient care to remotely monitor vital signs, symptoms and treatment responses. This approach enhances

patient engagement, supports chronic disease management and reduces the burden on traditional healthcare systems.

- **Academic/Research-Oriented Definition:** Digital Health Monitoring is the application of information and communication technologies (ICT) in healthcare to observe and analyze health indicators over time. It supports data-driven care models through the collection, transmission and analysis of biometric and behavioral data, aiming to improve clinical outcomes and promote preventive healthcare.

1.1 EVOLUTION FROM TRADITIONAL TO DIGITAL HEALTH SYSTEMS

The evolution from traditional to digital health systems marks one of the most significant transformations in modern healthcare. Historically, healthcare was centered around reactive treatment, where patients sought medical attention only after symptoms became evident. Medical records were handwritten, stored in paper files and often inaccessible across different departments or providers, leading to inefficiencies, duplication and limited continuity of care. Communication between patients and doctors occurred solely during physical visits and follow-up care was minimal unless patients proactively returned. Over time, the growing complexity of healthcare needs, rising patient expectations and global health challenges highlighted the limitations of this approach. The first wave of digital transformation began with the adoption of Electronic Health Records (EHRs), which improved documentation, reduced errors and enabled better coordination among healthcare providers. This transition laid the groundwork for digitization but still largely kept care within the clinical setting. As internet access and mobile technology became widespread, patients began using online portals, mobile apps and search engines to learn about their health and engage more actively in their care. This era introduced the concept of patient empowerment and self-management. Further advancements came with the integration of wearable devices and remote monitoring tools, which enabled continuous tracking of health data such as heart rate, blood pressure and glucose levels. Healthcare shifted from episodic treatment to proactive monitoring, especially for chronic diseases. Artificial Intelligence (AI) and big data analytics later enhanced digital health by allowing personalized, predictive and data-driven decision-making. Today, digital health systems have grown into interconnected ecosystems that support remote care, telemedicine, real-time monitoring and population health management. This shift from traditional to digital healthcare has fundamentally redefined how care is delivered, accessed and experienced. It brings numerous benefits including increased accessibility, early diagnosis, cost savings and better patient outcomes. However, it also introduces challenges like data security, technological literacy and equitable access. Understanding this evolution is key to navigating the future of global healthcare. Fig. 2 represents the medical innovation in the era of digital health.

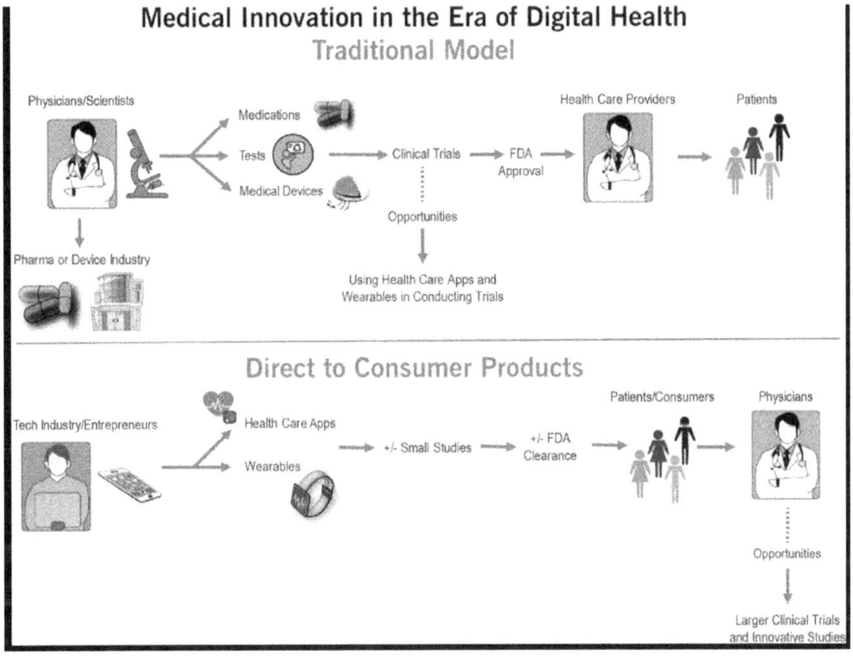

Fig. 2 Medical Innovation in the Era of Digital Health

The evolution from traditional to digital health systems can be summarized as follows:

1.1.1 Traditional Health Systems

Reactive and Paper-Based: Traditional health systems were largely reactive, operating on the principle of treating illness only after symptoms appeared. Healthcare interactions were limited to physical visits to clinics or hospitals and patient records were maintained manually in paper files. These records were often fragmented, stored in different departments and lacked continuity across providers. Communication between patients and healthcare professionals was face-to-face and follow-up was minimal unless patients returned on their own. This model, while foundational, was time-consuming, resource-intensive and often inaccessible to people in rural or underserved areas.

1.1.2 Emergence of Electronic Health Records (EHRs)

The initial shift toward digital healthcare began with the adoption of Electronic Health Records (EHRs) and Electronic Medical Records (EMRs). These digital systems replaced paper files with structured, searchable and more accessible formats. EHRs enabled better documentation, improved coordination between healthcare providers and reduced errors due to illegible handwriting or lost files. Although this was a major step forward, these systems were still mostly used within healthcare facilities and did not significantly empower patients or support remote care.

1.1.3 Rise of Internet and Mobile Technology in Healthcare

With the rise of the internet and smartphones, healthcare entered a more interactive and accessible era. Patients began using online platforms to schedule appointments, access test results and communicate with doctors. The introduction of mobile health (mHealth) apps allowed users to track basic health metrics like steps, sleep and diet. These innovations shifted some control from providers to patients, encouraging more active participation in health management. This period also saw the emergence of telemedicine, allowing remote consultations—especially beneficial during emergencies or in remote regions.

1.1.4 Integration of Wearables and Remote Monitoring Tools

The next evolution came with the integration of wearables (e.g., smartwatches, fitness trackers) and remote monitoring devices like blood pressure cuffs, glucose meters and ECG patches. These devices collect continuous or periodic health data and transmit it to healthcare providers in real time or at regular intervals. This marked a shift from episodic care to continuous, preventive care, where health problems could be detected and addressed earlier. These tools made chronic disease management more efficient and reduced hospital readmissions and emergency visits.

1.1.5 Artificial Intelligence and Big Data Analytics in Digital Health

As digital health data grew in volume and complexity, the role of artificial intelligence (AI) and big data analytics became central. AI-driven algorithms now analyze vast amounts of health data to predict disease risk, personalize treatment plans and support clinical decision-making. Machine learning models can detect patterns from medical images, genetic profiles and real-time sensor data, offering insights far beyond traditional diagnostic methods. This transition signifies a move toward predictive and precision medicine, enabled by digital platforms.

1.1.6 The Connected Digital Health Ecosystem

Today, health systems are evolving into fully connected ecosystems that integrate patients, providers, insurers, devices and data platforms. Cloud computing, 5G networks and interoperability standards allow for seamless data sharing and coordination. Digital health monitoring has become a core part of remote patient management, telehealth, mental health support and even public health surveillance (e.g., during pandemics). Digital platforms not only improve care quality but also increase accessibility and cost-efficiency across the healthcare spectrum.

1.1.7 Challenges and the Path Ahead

Despite the advancements, the digital transformation of healthcare faces challenges. Data privacy, regulatory compliance, technology literacy and system interoperability are major concerns. There is also a risk of digital inequality, where vulnerable populations lack access to devices or internet connectivity. Going forward, health systems must focus on inclusive design, strong cybersecurity and policy support to ensure that the benefits of digital health reach everyone. The future lies in hybrid care models—a blend of digital and in-person services tailored to each patient's needs. The evolution from traditional to digital health systems are summarised in Table-1.

Table 1: The evolution from traditional to digital health systems

Aspect	Traditional Health Systems	Digital Health Systems
Approach to Care	Reactive – treatment after symptoms appear	Proactive and preventive – early detection and continuous monitoring
Patient Role	Passive recipient of care	Active participant and self-manager of health
Medical Records	Paper-based, fragmented, often inaccessible	Electronic Health Records (EHRs), integrated and easily shareable
Doctor-Patient Interaction	In-person visits only	In-person and remote (telemedicine, video consultations, chat)
Data Collection	Manual during visits	Continuous via wearables, sensors and mobile apps
Diagnosis and Treatment	Based on periodic clinical assessments	Enhanced with AI, real-time data and predictive analytics
Monitoring	Episodic check-ups	Continuous remote monitoring (e.g., RPM – Remote Patient Monitoring)
Access to Care	Limited by geography and availability	Accessible from anywhere via digital platforms
Information Flow	Siloed between departments or providers	Interoperable systems with real-time data sharing
Cost and Efficiency	High cost due to hospital-centric model	Cost-effective with reduced hospital visits and early interventions
Patient Engagement	Minimal – dependent on provider	High – patients track and manage their health using digital tools
Technology Use	Minimal technology in daily care	Advanced tech: AI, cloud, IoT, mobile health, big data
Health Education	Dependent on doctors and printed materials	On-demand via apps, portals, online content
Chronic Disease Management	Infrequent visits, hard to track progress	Continuous tracking and alerts for personalized care
Response Time	Slow – dependent on appointment availability	Fast – real-time alerts and digital communication
Health System Structure	Institution-centric (hospital, clinic)	Patient-centric, decentralized and mobile
Data Security	Physical files, vulnerable to loss/damage	Digital security protocols, encryption and access controls

Aspect	Traditional Health Systems	Digital Health Systems
Public Health Surveillance	Manual reporting, delayed data collection	Real-time digital reporting and analytics
Clinical Decision Making	Based on physician judgment and limited data	AI-assisted decisions using large-scale health data
Scalability	Limited scalability	Highly scalable through cloud and mobile platforms

1.2 BENEFITS AND CHALLENGES OF DIGITAL MONITORING

Digital monitoring refers to the use of digital technologies to observe, track and collect data on systems, individuals or environments in real time or over a specified period. It is used across many sectors — including healthcare, education, workplaces, environmental science, security and IT infrastructure — to enhance efficiency, safety and decision-making.

1.2.1 Benefits of Digital Monitoring

1. Improved Efficiency and Performance

- **Automation of Data Collection:** Automation of data collection significantly reduces the need for manual labor, which not only saves time but also minimizes human errors. Traditionally, gathering data involved repetitive tasks such as recording measurements or entering information by hand, which could be both tedious and error-prone. With automation, sensors, software and devices continuously collect data without human intervention. This not only speeds up the data acquisition process but also ensures that the data is consistent and accurate. Automated systems can operate around the clock, capturing data in real-time, which is essential for environments that require constant monitoring, such as manufacturing plants, environmental studies or healthcare. Additionally, automation enables large volumes of data to be collected swiftly, which would be impractical with manual methods. This wealth of data can then be analyzed to uncover trends, anomalies or opportunities for improvement. Furthermore, freeing employees from repetitive data collection allows them to focus on higher-value tasks like data analysis and decision-making. Overall, automating data collection enhances operational efficiency by improving the speed, accuracy and volume of data gathered.
- **Real-Time Feedback:** Real-time feedback systems are critical in optimizing performance by providing immediate insights and responses to changing conditions. Unlike traditional reporting methods, which may delay information by hours or days, real-time feedback delivers instant alerts, enabling quick corrective actions. This immediacy is particularly valuable

in dynamic environments where delays can lead to lost productivity or increased risks, such as in manufacturing lines, customer service or logistics operations. For example, sensors on a production line can detect faults or inefficiencies as they occur, allowing operators to address problems before they escalate. In software and online services, real-time user feedback helps improve user experience by identifying bugs or usability issues promptly. Additionally, real-time feedback fosters a proactive rather than reactive approach, enabling continuous improvement and adaptation to new challenges or market conditions. By quickly responding to deviations or unexpected events organizations can reduce downtime, enhance product quality and improve customer satisfaction. In essence, real-time feedback creates a feedback loop that accelerates learning and optimization across processes.

- **Resource Management:** Effective resource management is essential for optimizing the use of energy, water, time and other valuable assets, thereby reducing waste and costs. By implementing data-driven strategies organizations can monitor consumption patterns and identify areas where resources are being underutilized or wasted. For example, smart energy systems can adjust lighting and heating based on occupancy or natural light, reducing unnecessary electricity usage. Similarly, automated irrigation systems in agriculture use soil moisture sensors to optimize water use, ensuring crops receive only what they need. Time management also benefits from resource optimization by scheduling tasks efficiently, preventing bottlenecks and ensuring that personnel and machinery are used to their fullest potential. Advanced analytics can forecast demand and allocate resources accordingly, avoiding shortages or surpluses. Resource management tools also contribute to sustainability goals by minimizing environmental impact and promoting responsible usage. Ultimately, efficient resource management leads to cost savings, improved productivity and a smaller ecological footprint, making it a vital aspect of modern operations.

Example: In manufacturing, digital monitoring systems can detect machinery inefficiencies early, reducing downtime.

2. Enhanced Decision-Making

- **Data-Driven Insights:** Data-driven insights form the backbone of intelligent decision-making in today's fast-paced business environment. Instead of relying solely on intuition or outdated methods organizations now leverage accurate and comprehensive data to guide their strategies. These insights are gathered from a variety of sources, such as customer behavior, market trends, operational metrics and financial records, providing a full picture of the current state of the business. By analyzing this data, decision-makers can identify inefficiencies, recognize opportunities and assess the impact of previous actions. For instance, customer data can reveal purchasing habits and preferences, helping businesses tailor their marketing efforts or product offerings. Operational data might highlight underperforming departments or supply chain bottlenecks. Because the information is factual and measurable, data-driven decisions are often more effective and less biased than those made purely from experience. Moreover, having access to real-time and historical data improves the agility of an organization, allowing it to quickly pivot in response to new challenges or opportunities. In essence, data-driven insights bring clarity and confidence to complex decision-making processes.

- **Predictive Analytics:** Predictive analytics uses historical data, statistical algorithms and machine learning techniques to forecast future outcomes and trends. It helps organizations move from reactive to proactive decision-making. By understanding patterns in past data, predictive models can identify potential issues before they arise or highlight trends that can be leveraged for competitive advantage. For example, in retail, predictive analytics can forecast customer demand, helping companies optimize inventory and reduce overstock or stockouts. In finance, it can predict credit risk or market shifts, allowing for smarter investment strategies. In healthcare, it can anticipate patient readmissions or the spread of disease. These forecasts are not just guesses—they are calculated projections based on data. The use of predictive analytics allows businesses to plan more effectively, allocate resources efficiently and mitigate risks early. As these models are refined with more data, their accuracy improves over time. Thus, predictive analytics not only enhances current decision-making but also builds a framework for sustainable, forward-thinking strategies that keep businesses ahead of the curve.
- **Custom Reporting:** Custom reporting allows organizations to create personalized dashboards and reports tailored to specific business needs, departments or stakeholders. Instead of being overwhelmed by irrelevant or excessive data, managers can focus on the metrics that matter most to their objectives. These reports consolidate complex data into visual and easy-to-understand formats such as graphs, charts and KPIs, facilitating quicker comprehension and action. For example, a sales manager might receive weekly reports highlighting conversion rates, customer acquisition costs and top-performing products, while an HR manager might monitor

employee engagement, turnover rates and recruitment timelines. Custom reporting tools also enable real-time updates, ensuring decisions are based on the most current data available. They can be automated and scheduled, reducing the workload on staff and improving consistency. Additionally, reports can be shared easily across teams, fostering collaboration and transparency. By making data accessible, relevant and understandable, custom reporting empowers stakeholders at all levels to make informed, confident decisions that align with organizational goals.

Example: In healthcare, wearable devices monitor patient vitals and help doctors detect health issues before they become critical.

3. Increased Safety and Security

- **Surveillance and Alerts:** Surveillance and alert systems are essential components in ensuring physical security and monitoring safety across various environments, from workplaces to public spaces. Advanced surveillance technologies, such as CCTV cameras, motion detectors and AI-enabled video analytics, continuously scan for unauthorized access, suspicious behavior or potential safety hazards. These systems are capable of issuing real-time alerts when anomalies are detected, allowing security personnel or management to take immediate action. For instance, if someone attempts to enter a restricted area, the system can notify security teams instantly or trigger an automatic lockdown. Similarly, abnormal patterns like loitering in sensitive zones or leaving packages unattended in public areas can prompt alerts. In industrial settings, surveillance may include thermal cameras or gas leak detectors to identify environmental hazards before they escalate. Automated alert systems reduce reliance on human observation, minimizing errors or delays in response. Moreover, digital surveillance offers recorded evidence, which is valuable for investigations or compliance with regulations. Overall, surveillance and alert mechanisms create a proactive safety net, preventing incidents before they cause harm.
- **Employee Safety:** Employee safety is a top priority, especially in high-risk industries such as construction, mining, oil and gas and manufacturing. Technology plays a vital role in monitoring working conditions and ensuring that employees operate in a safe environment. Sensors and wearable devices can track environmental parameters such as temperature, humidity, gas levels or vibrations—alerting workers and supervisors if thresholds are exceeded. For example, in a chemical plant, sensors can detect toxic gas leaks, triggering alarms and evacuation procedures. Wearable health monitors can also keep track of workers' vitals, such as heart rate or fatigue levels, helping prevent accidents due to exhaustion or medical issues. Real-

time location tracking through GPS or RFID ensures workers are accounted for and can be quickly located in case of emergencies. Additionally, automated systems can shut down machines if unsafe conditions are detected, preventing accidents. Data collected from these technologies can also be analyzed to identify recurring risks, allowing for long-term safety improvements. Ultimately, by integrating smart monitoring tools organizations not only comply with safety regulations but also foster a culture of care and responsibility.

- **Cybersecurity:** Cybersecurity is a crucial pillar of safety in the digital age, where data breaches and cyberattacks can result in severe financial and reputational damage. Modern cybersecurity systems utilize network monitoring tools, firewalls and artificial intelligence to detect suspicious activities and prevent intrusions. These systems continuously scan for unusual traffic patterns, unauthorized login attempts, malware or phishing schemes—flagging or blocking threats in real time. For instance, AI-based cybersecurity can learn the normal behaviour of a system and alert administrators the moment a deviation occurs, such as unexpected data access or massive file transfers. Encryption protocols and multi-factor authentication further enhance protection against unauthorized access. In addition to preventing external attacks, cybersecurity measures help detect insider threats and accidental data leaks by monitoring user behaviour. With increasing cloud usage and remote work environments, the attack surface has expanded, making robust cybersecurity more important than ever. A well-monitored and secure network not only protects intellectual property and customer data but also builds trust with clients and partners. In summary, cybersecurity is an indispensable part of any organization's overall safety and risk management strategy.

Example: Smart home systems can alert homeowners of smoke, carbon monoxide or break-ins remotely.

4. Compliance and Accountability

- **Regulatory Compliance:** Regulatory compliance refers to an organization's adherence to laws, guidelines and specifications relevant to its operations. In highly regulated industries—such as healthcare, finance, energy and manufacturing—failure to comply with standards can result in heavy fines, legal action and damage to reputation. Digital systems play a critical role in helping businesses meet these requirements by automating documentation, monitoring activities and ensuring that necessary protocols are followed. For example, compliance management software can track changes in regulations and ensure that processes are updated accordingly. Real-time alerts notify managers when activities deviate from legal standards, reducing the risk of violations. Furthermore, digital records make it easier to prove compliance during inspections or certifications. For instance, in the pharmaceutical industry, every step of drug manufacturing must be documented and traceable. Similarly, in financial institutions, data handling must meet strict privacy and anti-fraud laws. By embedding compliance checks directly into business operations organizations can operate more confidently and transparently. Ultimately, regulatory compliance isn't just about avoiding penalties—it's about building trust with customers, stakeholders and regulators.

- **Audit Trails:** Audit trails are digital records that chronologically document every action taken within a system, creating a transparent and traceable history of activities. These logs are invaluable for accountability, security and compliance purposes. Each log entry typically includes details such as who performed the action, what was done, when it occurred and where it happened. For example, in a financial system, an audit trail might record who approved a transaction, the time it was authorized and any changes made to the amount. In the event of fraud, data breaches or errors, these logs provide a reliable source of truth that investigators or auditors can review to trace the root cause. Audit trails are also crucial for internal reviews, ensuring that company policies and procedures are being followed. In healthcare, they help track access to sensitive patient records to prevent unauthorized disclosure. Moreover, automated logging reduces the risk of manipulation or human oversight. Overall, audit trails strengthen transparency, support legal compliance and reinforce a culture of accountability by ensuring that all actions can be traced and verified.
- **Employee Monitoring:** Employee monitoring systems are designed to ensure productivity, enforce company policies and protect organizational assets. These systems can track various activities such as computer usage, login times, website visits, email communications and location data. In office environments, monitoring tools can provide insights into how employees spend their time, helping managers identify patterns of inefficiency or time theft. For example, excessive idle time on workstations or frequent access to non-work-related websites may indicate a need for intervention or training. In field-based or remote work scenarios, GPS tracking ensures that employees are where they need to be and are completing assigned tasks. Beyond productivity, monitoring also enforces compliance with workplace policies—such as data handling protocols, communication standards and acceptable software use. Importantly, modern monitoring systems often come with analytics and dashboards that summarize trends without micromanaging employees. While transparency and ethical use

of monitoring are essential, when implemented appropriately, these tools help maintain performance standards, protect sensitive data and create a more accountable work environment. Ultimately, employee monitoring supports both operational efficiency and organizational integrity.

Example: Financial institutions use digital monitoring to ensure compliance with anti-money laundering laws.

5. Remote Monitoring Capability

- **Access Anywhere:** Remote monitoring offers the ability to access and control systems from virtually anywhere, breaking the limitations of physical presence and enhancing operational flexibility. With the help of cloud-based platforms, IoT devices and secure network connections, users can observe, manage and adjust processes in real time using computers, tablets or smartphones. This capability is especially valuable for industries that require continuous monitoring, such as manufacturing, utilities, agriculture and healthcare. For instance, a plant manager can monitor equipment performance, receive alerts about faults or even initiate shutdowns without being on-site. In the medical field, doctors can remotely monitor patients' vitals and intervene when necessary. This not only saves time and travel costs but also improves response time to critical issues. Additionally, remote access ensures that business continuity is maintained even during emergencies such as natural disasters or pandemics. Security features like multi-factor authentication, encrypted connections and access controls help protect sensitive systems from unauthorized intrusion. Overall, the ability to access systems from anywhere empowers faster decision-making, enhances efficiency and ensures operational resilience in a rapidly changing world.
- **Global Operations:** In today's globalized business environment, many organizations operate across multiple cities, countries or continents. Remote monitoring enables centralized oversight of these dispersed operations, offering a unified view of activities regardless of location. This centralized control improves consistency, standardization and coordination across different sites. For example, a logistics company can track fleet performance worldwide from a single dashboard, ensuring deliveries stay on schedule and vehicles are maintained properly. Similarly, an international manufacturing firm can monitor production lines across several plants to ensure uniform quality and detect issues in real time. Centralized monitoring also allows corporate leadership to make informed, enterprise-wide decisions based on integrated data from all branches. This approach reduces the reliance on fragmented, location-specific reports and

eliminates data silos. Moreover, global remote monitoring facilitates faster troubleshooting—experts can analyse issues at distant sites without needing to travel. It also simplifies compliance by applying consistent monitoring standards across borders. Ultimately, remote monitoring strengthens control, improves communication and enhances operational efficiency on a global scale, making it a powerful tool for organizations with widespread operations.

Example: IT administrators can monitor server health from anywhere in the world.

1.2.2 Challenges of Digital Monitoring

1. Privacy Concerns

- **Surveillance Overreach:** One of the most pressing challenges of digital monitoring is the potential for surveillance overreach, especially in workplaces, schools or public areas. While the intent of monitoring is often to enhance security, productivity or operational efficiency, excessive or intrusive surveillance can cross ethical boundaries. For instance, constant video or digital tracking in the workplace can lead employees to feel distrusted or dehumanized, creating a climate of stress and anxiety. In public spaces, facial recognition systems and location tracking may be used without adequate public consultation or regulation, raising civil liberties concerns. Overreach occurs when surveillance captures more information than necessary or monitors individuals outside the scope of legitimate purposes. This can violate fundamental rights to privacy and personal freedom. There's also a risk of creating a "chilling effect," where people alter their behaviour out of fear of being constantly watched. Without strict legal frameworks, oversight and ethical guidelines, digital monitoring can easily shift from protective to invasive. Thus organizations and governments must strike a careful balance between safety and privacy when implementing surveillance technologies.
- **Data Misuse:** Another significant privacy concern in digital monitoring is the misuse of collected data. Monitoring systems gather vast amounts of sensitive information—ranging from user behaviour, biometric data, to location and communication logs. If not properly safeguarded, this data can be accessed by unauthorized individuals, sold to third parties or used for purposes beyond the original intent. For example, an employer may collect data to monitor productivity but could later use it in hiring or disciplinary decisions without consent. In worse cases, this data might be exposed in a cyberattack or data breach, putting individuals at risk of identity theft or blackmail. Additionally, companies that store and process this data may

share it with advertisers, insurance providers or other entities without informing the individuals involved. The lack of strict data protection policies and insufficient encryption methods increases the chances of such misuse. To address these issues, strong data governance practices must be in place, including access controls, transparency policies and regular audits. Ultimately, ensuring ethical data use is critical to maintaining public trust and safeguarding individual rights.

- **Lack of Transparency:** Lack of transparency is a major concern when it comes to digital monitoring systems. Many individuals are unaware that they are being monitored, what type of data is being collected, how long it is stored or how it will be used. This lack of disclosure undermines informed consent, which is a cornerstone of ethical data practices. In workplace settings, employees may not be fully informed about surveillance policies or the extent to which their digital activity is being tracked. In public spaces, technologies like facial recognition or mobile tracking may operate in the background without any visible signs or public notifications. This secrecy leads to mistrust and potential backlash, especially if the data collected is later used in ways that affect individuals' rights or freedoms. Transparent practices—such as clear policies, opt-in mechanisms, regular disclosures and user controls—are essential to mitigate these issues. When people understand what is being monitored and why, they are more likely to support the use of such technologies. Transparency not only protects individual rights but also enhances the credibility and accountability of the organization implementing the monitoring.

Example: Employees may feel uncomfortable or distrusted if every action is tracked.

2. Security Risks

- **Cyberattacks:** Digital monitoring systems, while designed to improve oversight and security, themselves become attractive targets for cyberattacks. Because these systems often collect and store large volumes of sensitive information—ranging from personal data to proprietary business insights—hackers see them as valuable sources of data to exploit. Cybercriminals use techniques like malware, ransomware, phishing and denial-of-service attacks to breach these monitoring platforms. Once compromised, attackers can manipulate system controls, disable alarms or falsify records, undermining the very security the monitoring was intended to provide. Additionally, breaches can lead to widespread disruption of business operations, financial losses and damage to an organization's reputation. The interconnected nature of digital monitoring systems, often integrated with other IT infrastructure, means that a successful attack on one part can cascade into broader vulnerabilities. Defending against cyberattacks requires continuous investment in advanced security technologies, regular system updates and employee training to recognize potential threats. Without robust defences, the risks associated with cyberattacks on monitoring systems can be severe and far-reaching.

- **Unauthorized Access:** A critical security risk in digital monitoring is unauthorized access caused by weak or insufficient authentication protocols. If access controls are not stringent, attackers or even insiders with malicious intent can gain entry to critical monitoring systems or sensitive data. Weak passwords, lack of multi-factor authentication (MFA) and poorly managed user privileges create opportunities for unauthorized users to infiltrate these systems. Once inside, they might steal confidential information, alter surveillance footage or disable monitoring devices without detection. Insider threats also pose a significant challenge, as employees with legitimate access may misuse their privileges. Furthermore, systems exposed to the internet without adequate protections are particularly vulnerable to brute force attacks or exploitation of software vulnerabilities. Preventing unauthorized access demands implementing best practices such as MFA, role-based access controls, regular audits of user permissions and secure password policies. Ensuring that only authorized individuals can access sensitive systems helps maintain the integrity and confidentiality of monitored data and reduces the risk of security breaches.
- **Data Breaches:** Data breaches pose a significant risk when sensitive information collected by digital monitoring systems is not properly encrypted or securely stored and transmitted. Without encryption, data in transit can be intercepted by attackers using man-in-the-middle attacks, while data at rest is vulnerable to unauthorized access if storage systems lack adequate protections. A breach can expose personal information, business secrets or critical operational data, leading to financial penalties, legal liabilities and loss of customer trust. Many data breaches occur due to misconfigured databases, outdated software or failure to apply security patches promptly. In some cases, data breaches are the result of insider negligence or malicious insiders intentionally leaking information. Organizations must adopt comprehensive encryption protocols, both for data at rest and in motion, to safeguard sensitive data. Additionally, secure backup strategies and incident response plans are necessary to mitigate the impact of breaches if they occur. Protecting data from breaches is essential to maintaining the confidentiality, integrity and availability of digital monitoring systems and the sensitive information they handle.

Example: Hackers accessing surveillance camera feeds due to weak passwords.

3. High Costs and Technical Complexity

- **Installation and Maintenance:** Installing and maintaining advanced technological systems involves significant costs, primarily due to the need for specialized hardware components. These components often come at a premium price, especially if they incorporate cutting-edge technology or require high durability. Beyond the initial purchase, installation itself demands meticulous planning to ensure compatibility with existing infrastructure, which can involve rewiring, structural changes or even upgrades to supporting systems like power and cooling. Software installation also adds layers of complexity, requiring careful configuration and integration with current platforms and databases. Often, the deployment involves collaboration between multiple vendors and specialists, making coordination challenging and time-consuming. Once installed, ongoing maintenance is crucial to keep systems running smoothly and to prevent unexpected downtime. This maintenance includes routine checks, hardware repairs or replacements and software updates, all of which necessitate dedicated resources and budget allocation. Maintenance teams must be equipped to troubleshoot a variety of issues that may arise due to hardware failures, software bugs or network interruptions. The complexity is further heightened when systems span multiple locations, requiring synchronized management and remote monitoring tools. The financial burden of continuous maintenance, combined with the operational disruption it may cause, underscores the high costs and complexity involved in installing and maintaining such systems.
- **Staff Training:** Advanced systems require highly trained personnel to operate them effectively and extract meaningful insights from the data generated. The complexity of the technology often means that operators need a strong foundational knowledge of both the hardware and software components involved. This necessitates comprehensive training programs, which can be lengthy and costly. Employees must understand not only how to use the system but also how to recognize and troubleshoot potential issues that could impact performance or data accuracy. Interpreting the data output demands specialized analytical skills as well. Data from sophisticated systems can be voluminous, complex and sometimes ambiguous, requiring expertise in data science, statistical analysis or domain-specific knowledge to draw accurate conclusions. Without properly trained staff, the risk of misinterpreting data or missing critical insights increases, which can lead to poor decision-making or operational inefficiencies. Continuous training is also necessary to keep staff updated with system upgrades or changes in protocols. This ongoing education ensures that personnel remain competent

and confident in managing evolving technologies. Overall, investing in staff training is essential but adds to the overall cost and complexity of deploying such systems.

- **Upgrades and Compatibility:** Technological systems require regular upgrades to stay current with evolving standards, security requirements and performance expectations. Software components often need periodic patches to fix bugs, close security vulnerabilities and enhance functionality. These updates, while essential, can disrupt operations and require careful scheduling to minimize downtime. Moreover, upgrades may necessitate retraining staff or even adapting workflows to new features or interface changes. Hardware, too, can become obsolete over time, demanding replacements or enhancements to maintain compatibility with new software versions or other system components. This cycle of upgrades and replacements can be financially demanding, especially for organizations that rely on cutting-edge or proprietary technology. Incompatibility issues may arise when integrating newer components with legacy systems, causing operational challenges and requiring additional customization or middleware solutions. The complexity of maintaining compatibility extends to third-party software and external devices that interact with the system. As these external elements evolve, ensuring seamless interoperability requires ongoing testing, adjustments and sometimes negotiation with vendors. All these factors contribute to a continuous cycle of maintenance and improvement that adds complexity and cost to managing advanced technological systems.

Example: A small business might struggle to afford comprehensive digital monitoring tools.

4. Data Overload

- **Too Much Information:** One of the major challenges in modern data-driven systems is the sheer volume of data collected. When organizations gather excessive information without clearly defined goals, they risk overwhelming their analytical capabilities. This phenomenon, often referred to as analysis paralysis, occurs when decision-makers are flooded with too much data, making it difficult to prioritize what to analyse or act upon. Instead of facilitating insight, the abundance of data can slow down the decision-making process, causing delays or indecision. Collecting data indiscriminately can also lead to wasted resources, as storing, processing and managing unnecessary data consumes time and money. Without targeted objectives, analysts may spend excessive effort sifting through irrelevant data, reducing overall efficiency. Moreover, the presence of redundant or low-quality data can obscure meaningful trends or patterns, further complicating the extraction of actionable intelligence. To avoid data overload organizations must establish clear data collection strategies aligned with specific business goals. This helps ensure that only relevant, high-quality data is gathered and analysed. Defining priorities enables teams to focus on meaningful metrics and make informed decisions faster. Thus, setting clear objectives and maintaining disciplined data management practices are crucial to preventing the negative impacts of too much information.

- **Noise vs. Signal:** Another significant challenge within data overload is separating meaningful signals from background noise. In many systems, vast quantities of data generate numerous alerts, notifications or readings—only a small portion of which may indicate critical issues or opportunities. Distinguishing these important alerts from irrelevant or false alarms requires sophisticated filtering, prioritization and context-aware analysis. If the noise overwhelms the signal, users may become desensitized to alerts, leading to important warnings being ignored or missed entirely. This problem is often referred to as "alert fatigue," where users receive so many notifications that they start dismissing them without proper evaluation. Such behaviour increases the risk of overlooking significant events, which can result in operational failures, security breaches or missed opportunities. Effective approaches to managing noise versus signal include implementing advanced algorithms, machine learning models and rule-based filtering systems. These methods help highlight anomalies or high-priority alerts while suppressing irrelevant data. Additionally, contextual information and user customization allow alert systems to better match organizational needs and reduce distractions. Proper noise management is essential for ensuring that data overload does not hinder timely and effective responses.
- **Storage Issues:** Handling the massive volume of data generated by modern systems presents substantial storage challenges. Organizations need scalable, reliable and cost-effective storage infrastructures to accommodate growing datasets. Traditional storage solutions may quickly become inadequate as data accumulates, forcing companies to invest in advanced technologies such as cloud storage, distributed databases or data lakes. Besides capacity, storage systems must ensure data integrity, availability and security. Data loss or corruption can have severe consequences, making backup and disaster recovery mechanisms indispensable. Regular backups, replication strategies and off-site storage help protect valuable information against hardware failures, cyberattacks or natural disasters. The cost of

maintaining large-scale storage systems includes not only hardware and software but also energy consumption, cooling and ongoing management. Organizations must carefully balance storage costs against the value of the data retained, often implementing data retention policies that archive or delete less critical data over time. Furthermore, rapid data access and retrieval speeds are vital for timely analysis and operational efficiency. Storage architectures must be optimized for performance, supporting quick querying and processing. In summary, managing the storage of large datasets requires robust, flexible solutions combined with strategic policies to mitigate costs and risks associated with data overload.

Example: Environmental monitoring systems might generate terabytes of data that require significant storage and filtering.

5. Ethical and Legal Implications

- **Consent Issues:** One of the foremost ethical and legal challenges in data monitoring is obtaining proper consent from individuals whose data is being collected. Failing to secure explicit, informed consent can violate privacy laws and regulations, exposing organizations to legal penalties and reputational damage. Many jurisdictions have strict rules requiring clear communication about what data is collected, how it will be used and who will have access. Without transparency, individuals may feel their privacy is being infringed upon, leading to mistrust and resistance. Proper consent mechanisms not only protect legal compliance but also help build trust between organizations and stakeholders. Ignoring these requirements can result in lawsuits, fines and even bans on data collection practices, highlighting the critical need to prioritize consent.
- **Bias and Discrimination:** Algorithms used to analyse monitored data are not immune to biases, which can inadvertently perpetuate discrimination or unfair treatment. These biases often stem from biased training data, flawed model assumptions or lack of diversity in development teams. As a result, decisions made by automated systems—such as hiring, loan approvals or law enforcement actions—may unfairly disadvantage certain groups based on race, gender or socioeconomic status. Such outcomes raise serious ethical concerns and can violate anti-discrimination laws. Addressing algorithmic bias requires ongoing auditing, transparency and the implementation of fairness frameworks. Without these efforts, reliance on biased algorithms risks reinforcing social inequalities and eroding public confidence in technology.
- **Overreliance on Technology:** Overdependence on technology for monitoring and decision-making can undermine the role of human

judgment, which is essential for interpreting complex or ambiguous situations. Blindly trusting automated systems may lead to errors being overlooked, especially when the technology is flawed or unable to account for nuances. This over trust can reduce critical thinking and the willingness to question system outputs, increasing the risk of costly mistakes. Human oversight remains vital to validate findings, handle exceptions and ensure ethical considerations are addressed. Striking a balance between leveraging technology and maintaining human control is necessary to avoid harmful consequences stemming from excessive reliance on automated systems.

Example: Facial recognition systems have been criticized for racial and gender biases.

1.3 TECHNOLOGIES ENABLING DIGITAL HEALTH

Digital health is a rapidly evolving field powered by a diverse range of technologies. These tools enhance healthcare delivery, improve outcomes, and empower patients. However, each comes with its own set of challenges that require careful consideration in implementation and governance. The future of healthcare lies in effectively integrating these technologies while ensuring equity, privacy, and security.

Digital health represents a revolutionary shift in the way healthcare is delivered, managed and experienced. At its core, it leverages innovative technologies to enhance clinical outcomes, personalize patient care and make healthcare systems more efficient and accessible. From the use of mobile apps that monitor vital signs to AI-powered diagnostic tools, digital health solutions are reshaping every touchpoint in the patient journey. The global healthcare ecosystem is witnessing unprecedented advancements as technology bridges gaps in access, quality and cost. Virtual consultations, wearable devices and health information systems now enable real-time care, even in the most remote areas. Machine learning algorithms can detect anomalies in medical images with remarkable accuracy, while big data analytics provides actionable insights into disease trends and treatment efficacy. Robotics and automation are redefining surgery and rehabilitation. Meanwhile, cloud computing ensures seamless sharing and storage of patient data across institutions. Cybersecurity protocols safeguard this sensitive data, fostering trust and compliance. The Internet of Medical Things (IoMT) creates interconnected networks of health devices that enhance monitoring and preventive care. Genomics and precision medicine are tailoring treatments to individual genetic profiles, promising better health outcomes. Blockchain technology is improving data integrity and traceability. Augmented and virtual reality tools are transforming medical training and therapy. With all these advances, patients are becoming active participants in their own care. As these technologies mature, they promise to democratize healthcare, making it smarter, faster and more equitable.

Understanding the key technologies that enable this transformation is essential for navigating the future of medicine. The Changing Needs of Care Team of the Future is depicted in Fig.3

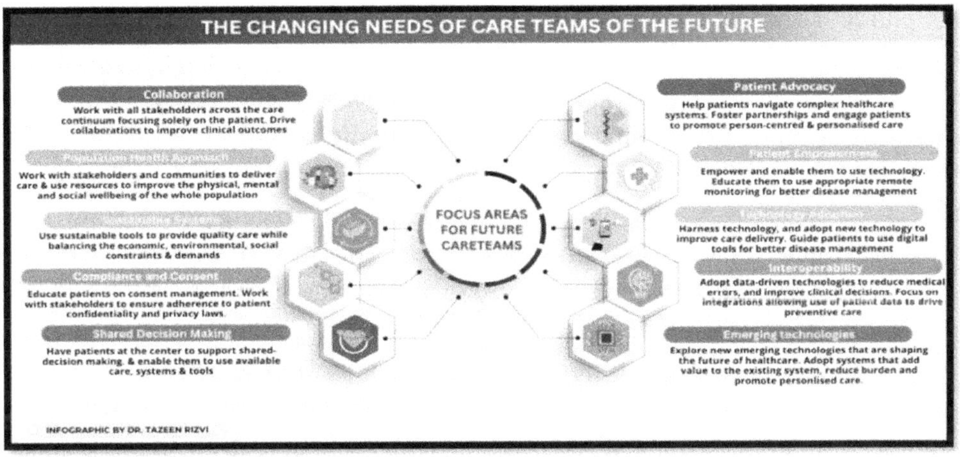

Fig. 3 The Changing Needs of Care Team of the Future

Below is a detailed overview of the most important ones:

1.3.1 Electronic Health Records (EHRs)

Electronic Health Records (EHRs) are a cornerstone of digital health, transforming traditional paper charts into dynamic, digital records that provide real-time, patient-centered information. Accessible to authorized healthcare providers, EHRs consolidate a patient's complete medical history—including lab results, diagnoses, medications and treatment plans—into a single, centralized system. This comprehensive access enhances the quality and continuity of care by allowing clinicians to make better-informed decisions. EHRs play a vital role in supporting coordinated care among multiple providers and reducing medical errors through timely and accurate information sharing. They also improve efficiency by minimizing redundant tests and streamlining administrative processes. Patients benefit from increased transparency, as many systems allow individuals to view their own records, improving engagement and self-management. Despite these advantages, EHR implementation faces several challenges. Interoperability remains a major hurdle, as systems often struggle to exchange data across different platforms. Additionally, the cost of implementing and maintaining EHR systems can be prohibitive, especially for smaller practices. Data security and patient privacy are also critical concerns, requiring robust cybersecurity measures. Technical issues, workflow disruptions and resistance to change among staff can further complicate adoption. Nevertheless, when effectively integrated, EHRs serve as a foundational technology in digital health, fostering safer, more connected and more efficient healthcare delivery.

1.3.2 Telemedicine and Telehealth

Telemedicine and telehealth are pivotal components of digital health, enabling healthcare delivery through remote communication technologies such as video calls, phone consultations and secure messaging platforms. These solutions bridge geographical gaps, providing critical access to medical care for patients in rural, remote or underserved areas where healthcare resources may be limited. By reducing the need for in-person visits, telemedicine not only saves time and travel costs but also helps alleviate pressure on healthcare facilities. It promotes continuity of care, especially for chronic disease management, mental health support and follow-up consultations. Patients benefit from improved convenience, quicker access to specialists and the ability to receive care from the comfort of their homes. For providers, it enhances scheduling flexibility and expands patient reach. However, several challenges hinder widespread adoption. Licensing restrictions across state or national borders can limit service availability, while inconsistent reimbursement policies may discourage provider participation. Dependence on reliable internet infrastructure poses a significant barrier, particularly in low-connectivity regions. Data privacy, digital literacy and integration with other health systems also remain concerns. Despite these obstacles, telemedicine continues to gain momentum as a scalable, patient-centered approach to modern healthcare, playing a crucial role in expanding access and optimizing resource use within the digital health ecosystem.

1.3.3 Mobile Health (mHealth)

Mobile Health (mHealth) is a key enabler of digital health, utilizing mobile devices like smartphones, tablets and wearables to deliver healthcare services and information. Through health apps, SMS reminders and sensor-enabled wearables, mHealth allows users to track vital signs, medication adherence, fitness goals and more. It fosters greater patient engagement by encouraging individuals to take an active role in monitoring and managing their health. mHealth also supports preventive care by delivering timely reminders and educational content, helping reduce the risk of illness progression. For patients with chronic conditions, it offers real-time monitoring and remote support, enhancing disease management and improving outcomes. Its accessibility makes healthcare more convenient and inclusive, especially in underserved areas. However, challenges persist. Concerns about the accuracy and reliability of health data collected via mobile devices can affect clinical decisions. Ensuring user privacy and securing sensitive health information is critical, especially as many apps lack robust data protection measures. Additionally, the regulatory oversight of mobile health apps is still evolving, raising questions about quality control and clinical validity. Despite these issues, mHealth remains a transformative force in personalizing care and extending the reach of healthcare services globally.

1.3.4 Wearable Devices and Remote Monitoring

Wearable devices and remote monitoring technologies are integral to digital health, providing continuous, real-time tracking of physiological parameters through tools like fitness trackers, smartwatches and biosensors. These devices collect valuable health metrics such as heart rate, blood pressure, glucose levels, sleep patterns and physical activity, offering both patients and healthcare providers a detailed picture of one's health status over time. By enabling proactive monitoring, wearables facilitate early detection of potential health issues, allowing for timely intervention and more personalized treatment plans. They are especially beneficial for managing chronic conditions, promoting healthier lifestyles and supporting remote patient care without the need for frequent clinical visits. These technologies also empower individuals to engage more actively in their own health management. However, challenges remain, including the accuracy and reliability of the collected data, which can vary depending on device quality and user behaviour. Calibration issues and inconsistencies between different brands or models may impact clinical decision-making. Additionally, maintaining long-term user engagement can be difficult, as interest may decline over time without clear incentives or visible health improvements. Despite these hurdles, wearable technology continues to evolve, playing a pivotal role in transforming preventive care and supporting a more connected, data-driven healthcare system.

1.3.5 Artificial Intelligence (AI) and Machine Learning (ML)

Artificial Intelligence (AI) and Machine Learning (ML) are transformative technologies in digital health, enabling the analysis of vast and complex medical datasets to uncover patterns, make predictions and support clinical decision-making. These tools are widely used in diagnostics—especially in fields like radiology, pathology and dermatology—where they can detect anomalies in images with remarkable speed and accuracy. AI also powers personalized medicine by analysing genetic, lifestyle and clinical data to tailor treatment plans to individual patients. In addition, ML algorithms assist in risk assessment, predicting disease onset or progression and optimizing resource allocation in healthcare settings. Virtual health assistants, chatbots and automated triage systems are further applications that enhance patient engagement and provider efficiency. The benefits of AI and ML include improved diagnostic precision, streamlined workflows, reduced clinician workload and the ability to forecast health trends through predictive analytics. However, challenges remain. Algorithmic bias can result in unequal care outcomes, especially if training data lacks diversity. The opaque nature of some AI systems, often referred to as "black-box" models, raises concerns about transparency and accountability. Regulatory hurdles also slow adoption, as rigorous validation is needed to ensure patient safety. Despite these issues, AI and ML are rapidly advancing, offering immense potential to reshape modern healthcare delivery.

1.3.6 Blockchain Technology

Blockchain technology is emerging as a powerful tool in digital health, offering a decentralized and secure framework for recording, storing and sharing sensitive health data. By utilizing cryptographic techniques and distributed ledger systems, blockchain ensures that medical records are tamper-proof, transparent and traceable. It plays a significant role in enhancing the security and integrity of patient data, particularly in areas such as electronic health records (EHRs), clinical trials and supply chain tracking. Blockchain also promotes interoperability by enabling different healthcare systems to access and exchange standardized data without compromising privacy or trust. A key advantage is that it gives patients greater control over their personal health information, allowing them to manage access permissions across providers. Furthermore, in clinical research, blockchain can improve transparency and accountability by securely documenting trial protocols, data entries and consent processes. However, the technology faces several challenges that hinder widespread adoption. These include scalability issues, as blockchain networks may struggle to handle the volume and speed of healthcare data. Technical complexity, high implementation costs and the difficulty of integrating blockchain with existing legacy systems are additional obstacles. Despite these challenges, blockchain holds significant potential to reinforce trust, efficiency and security in the digital health landscape.

1.3.7 Cloud Computing

Cloud computing is a foundational technology in digital health, offering a flexible and scalable way to store, manage and access healthcare data and applications over the internet. It allows healthcare providers to retrieve patient information in real time from virtually anywhere, facilitating improved decision-making and seamless collaboration among care teams. Cloud platforms support the integration of electronic health records, telehealth services, mobile health apps and AI-driven analytics, creating a more connected and efficient healthcare environment. One of the key benefits is the reduction of infrastructure and maintenance costs, as providers no longer need to invest heavily in on-site servers and IT systems. Additionally, cloud computing enables the processing of large datasets for predictive analytics, population health management and personalized medicine. It also powers telehealth platforms by providing secure, high-performance environments for video consultations and remote monitoring tools. However, the widespread adoption of cloud technology comes with important challenges. Ensuring data privacy and security is paramount, especially when relying on third-party providers. Healthcare organizations must also navigate complex regulatory requirements such as HIPAA in the U.S. or GDPR in Europe, which govern data protection and patient rights. Despite these concerns, cloud computing continues to drive innovation and agility in healthcare delivery, playing a vital role in the digital transformation of the sector.

1.3.8 Internet of Medical Things (IoMT)

The Internet of Medical Things (IoMT) is a vital component of digital health, comprising a network of connected medical devices, sensors and applications that communicate through the internet to collect, transmit and analyse health data. These devices range from wearable fitness trackers and smart inhalers to remote patient monitoring systems and connected imaging equipment. IoMT enables continuous, real-time monitoring of patients, allowing healthcare providers to receive timely alerts and intervene proactively when health metrics deviate from normal ranges. This capability is especially beneficial for managing chronic conditions such as diabetes, heart disease and respiratory illnesses, helping to reduce hospital admissions and improve long-term outcomes. IoMT also facilitates more efficient use of healthcare resources by enabling virtual care and early intervention, thus lowering operational costs. However, the rapid expansion of connected devices introduces several challenges. Cybersecurity is a major concern, as sensitive health data transmitted over networks is vulnerable to breaches and unauthorized access. Ensuring reliable connectivity is critical for maintaining uninterrupted monitoring, especially in remote or underserved areas. Additionally, lack of standardization across devices can hinder interoperability, making it difficult to integrate data into existing health systems. Despite these issues, IoMT continues to advance, offering powerful tools to enhance care delivery, patient engagement and overall healthcare efficiency.

1.3.9 Virtual Reality (VR) and Augmented Reality (AR)

Virtual Reality (VR) and Augmented Reality (AR) are immersive technologies that either simulate fully virtual environments (VR) or overlay digital information onto the real world (AR), playing an increasingly important role in digital health. These technologies are widely used in medical education, allowing students and professionals to practice procedures in a risk-free, controlled environment, which significantly improves learning retention and skill acquisition. In surgical planning, VR and AR provide detailed 3D visualizations of patient anatomy, enhancing precision and outcomes during complex operations. For patient care, these tools support rehabilitation by creating engaging, interactive exercises that motivate recovery and improve motor skills. They are also effective in pain management by distracting patients during painful procedures or chronic pain episodes. Despite their benefits, VR and AR face challenges including high development and equipment costs, which limit accessibility for some healthcare providers. User acceptance varies, as some patients and clinicians may find the technology unfamiliar or uncomfortable. Additionally, current limitations in the realism and responsiveness of VR/AR systems can affect their effectiveness and user experience. Nonetheless, as these technologies evolve, they hold great promise for transforming medical training, treatment and patient engagement across healthcare settings.

1.4 THE ROLE OF DIGITAL HEALTH IN PRECISION AND PREVENTIVE MEDICINE

- Digital health technologies, such as wearable devices, mobile health apps and electronic health records, have transformed healthcare by enabling more personalized and data-driven approaches. These tools collect vast amounts of real-time health data, which can be used to tailor medical treatments to individual patients, forming the foundation of precision medicine.
- In precision medicine, digital health facilitates the integration of genetic, environmental and lifestyle information. By combining these diverse data sources, healthcare providers can predict disease risks more accurately and design interventions that target the unique biological makeup of each patient, improving treatment outcomes.
- Preventive medicine also greatly benefits from digital health innovations. Wearables and mobile apps empower individuals to monitor their health continuously, encouraging proactive management of chronic conditions and early detection of potential health issues before they become severe. Fig. 4 describes the methods of changing the future of precision medicine.

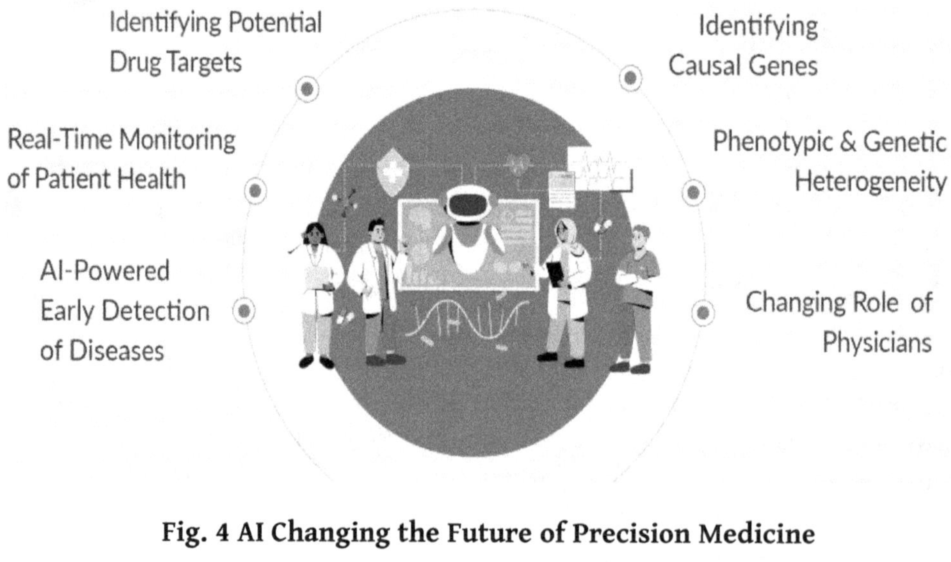

Fig. 4 AI Changing the Future of Precision Medicine

- Digital health platforms support population health management by enabling remote monitoring and telemedicine services. These platforms help reduce healthcare disparities by providing access to care in underserved or remote areas, promoting early intervention and reducing hospital admissions.
- Moreover, artificial intelligence and machine learning algorithms applied to digital health data enhance predictive analytics, enabling clinicians to identify at-risk patients and recommend preventive measures more efficiently. This shift from reactive to proactive healthcare optimizes resource use and improves overall public health.
- Despite its promise, the integration of digital health in precision and preventive medicine faces challenges such as data privacy concerns, interoperability issues and the need for rigorous clinical validation. Addressing these obstacles is essential to fully realize the benefits of digital health in transforming patient care.

Role of digital health in precision and preventive medicine is given in Table -2.

Table 2 : Role of Digital Health in Precision and Preventive Medicine

Digital Health Component	Function	Role in Precision Medicine	Role in Preventive Medicine
Electronic Health Records (EHRs)	Centralized access to patient history, lab results and medications	Supports tailored treatment by providing comprehensive medical context	Identifies risk factors and tracks early signs of disease
Wearable Devices	Monitor real-time vitals (e.g., heart rate, activity, sleep)	Enables individualized health profiling	Detects early physiological changes; encourages healthy behavior
Genomic Data Analysis	Interprets DNA sequences and genetic predispositions	Drives personalized drug selection and targeted therapy	Assesses hereditary risk and enables early intervention
AI and Machine Learning	Pattern recognition, risk prediction, clinical decision support	Develops precision diagnostics and treatment models	Predicts disease onset and guides preventive strategies
Mobile Health (mHealth) Apps	Deliver health coaching, reminders and symptom tracking	Customizes user interactions based on personal data	Promotes adherence to lifestyle changes and medication

Digital Health Component	Function	Role in Precision Medicine	Role in Preventive Medicine
Telemedicine	Remote consultation and continuous care delivery	Ensures precision follow-ups and data-driven adjustments	Provides access to preventive care in underserved regions
Digital Imaging & Diagnostics	High-resolution scans, analyzed using AI	Aids in accurate diagnosis and treatment planning	Enables early detection of conditions like cancer or stroke
Clinical Decision Support Systems (CDSS)	Provides evidence-based recommendations during care	Offers personalized treatment options	Flags preventive screenings and vaccinations
Patient Portals & Engagement Tools	Allow patients to access and manage their health data	Enhances patient involvement in care decisions	Educates on risk prevention and lifestyle changes
Population Health Analytics	Aggregates and analyzes data across patient groups	Identifies sub-populations for precision targeting	Monitors trends for outbreak prevention and community interventions

2 Chapter
CORE TECHNOLOGIES AND TOOLS

2.0 INTRODUCTION: AN OVERVIEW

The core technologies and tools that underpin digital health monitoring create a sophisticated and interconnected framework, aimed at delivering continuous, personalized, and proactive healthcare solutions. At the heart of this ecosystem lie advanced sensors capable of capturing a wide range of physiological and biochemical data with remarkable precision. These sensors, embedded in wearables, implantable, and even environmental devices, continuously gather critical health metrics. Complementing these are robust wireless communication protocols—such as Bluetooth Low Energy, 5G, and Near Field Communication—which ensure seamless, real-time transmission of data between devices, patients, and healthcare providers. This connectivity is vital for enabling remote monitoring and timely interventions. Cloud computing platforms form the backbone of data storage and processing, offering scalable infrastructure to manage the vast influx of health data while providing secure access across multiple healthcare stakeholders. Within this digital infrastructure, artificial intelligence and machine learning algorithms analyse complex datasets, identifying patterns, predicting health risks, and enabling personalized treatment recommendations. These intelligent systems enhance diagnostic accuracy and streamline clinical workflows by automating routine analyses and generating actionable insights.

Digital health monitoring represents a transformative frontier in modern healthcare, leveraging advanced technologies and innovative tools to enhance patient care, improve health outcomes and enable proactive disease management. At its core, digital health monitoring integrates a wide array of hardware and software solutions designed to continuously track, collect and analyse vital health data in real time. The evolution of digital health has been driven by the rapid advancements in sensor technologies, wireless communication, cloud computing, artificial intelligence and data analytics, all of which converge to create a seamless ecosystem for personalized health management. One of the foundational technologies in digital health monitoring is wearable devices, including smartwatches, fitness trackers and biosensors. These devices are equipped with multiple sensors such as accelerometers, gyroscopes, photoplethysmography (PPG) sensors and electrocardiogram (ECG) monitors that enable continuous measurement of physiological parameters like heart rate, blood oxygen levels, activity, sleep patterns and more. Wearables empower users with real-time feedback and allow healthcare providers to remotely monitor patients outside clinical settings, facilitating early detection of abnormalities and timely intervention. In addition to wearables, implantable devices have gained prominence in the digital health landscape. Devices such as glucose monitors for diabetic patients, pacemakers and neurostimulators provide continuous monitoring of critical health indicators from within the body. These implantable solutions communicate wirelessly with external readers or smartphones, enhancing patient convenience and adherence to treatment plans. Wireless communication technologies form the backbone of digital health monitoring systems by enabling seamless data transmission. Bluetooth Low Energy (BLE), Near Field Communication (NFC), Zigbee and 5G networks allow for efficient, secure and real-time communication between devices, mobile applications and cloud platforms. This connectivity ensures that health data is continuously uploaded and accessible for analysis, facilitating remote monitoring and telehealth services (Fig. 1).

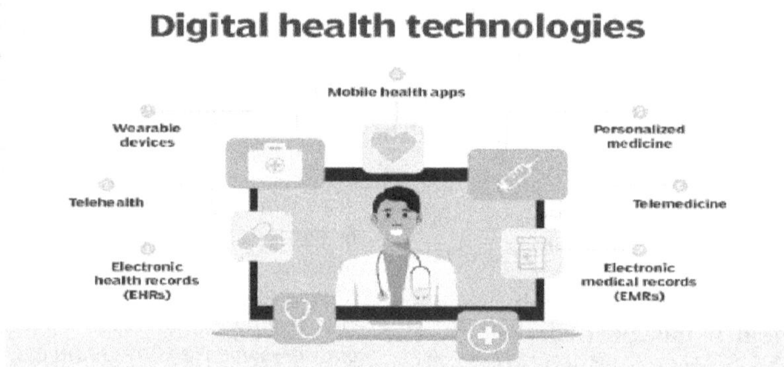
Digital health technologies
Mobile health apps
Wearable devices
Personalized medicine
Telehealth
Telemedicine
Electronic health records (EHRs)
Electronic medical records (EMRs)

Fig. 1 Digital Health Technologies

Cloud computing plays a pivotal role in managing the vast amount of data generated by digital health devices. It offers scalable storage, powerful processing capabilities and ubiquitous access to health information. Cloud platforms enable healthcare professionals to aggregate data from multiple sources, perform complex analytics and derive actionable insights. Moreover, cloud infrastructure supports integration with electronic health records (EHRs), fostering a holistic view of patient health and improving care coordination. Artificial intelligence (AI) and machine learning (ML) are revolutionizing digital health monitoring by enhancing the accuracy and efficiency of data interpretation. AI algorithms analyse patterns within the collected data to predict potential health risks, detect early signs of disease and personalize treatment plans. These technologies also facilitate the automation of routine tasks such as anomaly detection, alert generation and patient triaging, thereby reducing the burden on healthcare providers. Mobile health applications (mHealth apps) serve as the user interface for digital health monitoring systems, enabling individuals to track their health metrics, receive reminders and communicate with healthcare professionals. These apps often integrate with wearable and implantable devices, presenting users with intuitive dashboards, trend analyses and educational resources to support health management. Telemedicine platforms, integrated with digital health monitoring tools, have redefined patient-provider interactions by enabling remote consultations and continuous patient engagement. This combination enhances access to care, particularly in underserved or rural areas and supports chronic disease management through consistent monitoring and timely adjustments to treatment. Security and privacy are critical considerations in digital health monitoring. Technologies such as data encryption, multi-factor authentication and blockchain are employed to safeguard sensitive health information against breaches and unauthorized access. Compliance with regulations like HIPAA (Health Insurance Portability and Accountability Act) and GDPR (General Data Protection Regulation) ensures that patient data is handled responsibly and ethically.

Emerging technologies such as the Internet of Medical Things (IoMT) and edge computing further enhance digital health monitoring by connecting a network of medical devices and processing data closer to the source. This reduces latency, improves response times and supports real-time decision-making in critical scenarios.

2.1 WEARABLE DEVICES

Wearable devices have emerged as one of the most transformative innovations in modern healthcare, fundamentally reshaping the way individuals and professionals monitor, manage and understand health. These compact, body-worn technologies—such as smartwatches, fitness bands, biosensors, smart clothing and even wearable patches—are designed to continuously collect real-time physiological and behavioural data from users. The integration of miniaturized sensors, advanced microprocessors, wireless connectivity (e.g., Bluetooth, Wi-Fi) and AI algorithms enables wearables to track a wide array of vital signs including heart rate, respiratory rate, sleep quality, physical activity, blood oxygen saturation (SpO_2), skin temperature and stress levels. The portability, convenience and non-invasive nature of wearable devices make them particularly well-suited for preventive healthcare, chronic disease management, fitness tracking and remote patient monitoring (Fig. 2). By offering continuous and passive data collection, wearables help detect subtle changes in health that might otherwise go unnoticed until they develop into more serious conditions. They enable early warning systems and predictive analytics, giving both users and healthcare providers the ability to intervene sooner and more effectively. A major advantage of wearables is their seamless integration with mobile apps and cloud platforms, which allows real-time synchronization and long-term storage of health data. Advanced platforms can leverage machine learning to generate personalized health insights, trend visualizations and actionable recommendations. Some wearables also support integration with electronic health records (EHRs), creating a more holistic view of patient health and enhancing clinical decision-making. These devices are increasingly adopted in diverse domains such as corporate wellness programs, sports science, elder care, rehabilitation and military fitness. In workplaces, they support wellness initiatives by promoting movement, stress reduction and healthy sleep habits. In athletics, wearable sensors monitor performance metrics, injury risks and recovery status. Among the elderly and those with cognitive impairments, devices with GPS and fall detection features enhance safety and independence.

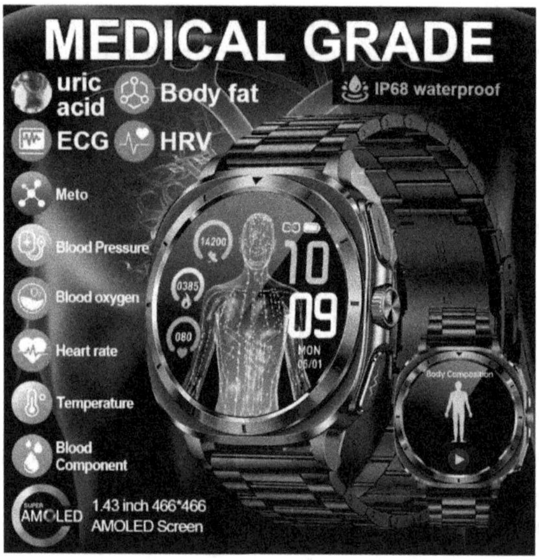

Fig. 2 Wearable devices

Recent advancements in wearable technology have greatly improved biometric accuracy, battery life and form factor. Flexible electronics and smart textiles have further enabled the creation of ultra-light, comfortable and even washable wearables that fit naturally into daily life. The inclusion of features like real-time alerts, medication reminders, emergency SOS calls and remote communication with doctors makes them indispensable in-home healthcare and telemedicine. Regulatory bodies such as the FDA and CE are increasingly certifying medical-grade wearables, boosting their credibility and adoption in clinical settings. These approvals have enabled wearables to be used in managing conditions like atrial fibrillation, diabetes, hypertension and sleep apnea. Furthermore, anonymized data from wearable devices can support large-scale epidemiological research, enhance public health surveillance and contribute to the development of population-level health models. Wearable devices are rapidly evolving from consumer gadgets into essential healthcare tools that support proactive, personalized and participatory medicine. Their scalability, accessibility and ability to empower individuals to take charge of their health position them as a foundational element in the future of digital health ecosystems.

2.1.1 Smartwatches, Fitness Bands, Biosensors

Smartwatches, fitness bands and biosensors represent a diverse yet interconnected ecosystem within wearable health technology, each offering unique features tailored to different aspects of health and activity monitoring. These devices have rapidly evolved from basic step counters and notification tools into intelligent health companions capable of delivering clinically relevant data. Smartwatches are the most multifunctional among wearables, combining traditional timekeeping and smartphone integration with advanced health features such as continuous heart rate monitoring, sleep quality analysis, oxygen saturation (SpO_2) tracking, ECG recording, stress detection and even fall detection. With high-resolution touchscreens, customizable health apps and voice assistant integration, smartwatches are now sophisticated health hubs that fit seamlessly into users' daily routines. Smartwatches are ideal for users who want a blend of lifestyle convenience and comprehensive health tracking. Many models now include GPS, temperature sensors and even skin conductance sensors for monitoring emotional or stress responses. Athletes and fitness enthusiasts use them to measure VO_2 max, recovery time and training load, while patients with chronic illnesses can benefit from real-time symptom tracking and medication reminders. The ability to sync data across health apps and cloud storage further enhances long-term monitoring and personalized recommendations. Fitness bands, while typically more compact and focused in function, are highly efficient tools for tracking core physical activities. They are designed for users who prioritize step counting, calorie tracking, sleep monitoring and heart rate measurement in a lightweight, distraction-free format. Fitness bands are valued for their long battery life, water resistance and affordability, making them widely accessible to users of all ages. Many are optimized for everyday activity tracking and have started to incorporate basic features like blood oxygen monitoring, guided breathing and menstrual cycle tracking. Their simplified user interface and minimalist design make them ideal for people seeking low-maintenance but effective health feedback.

In contrast, biosensors represent the most specialized and medically oriented segment of wearables. These devices are designed to detect and measure specific physiological biomarkers with a high degree of accuracy. Examples include continuous glucose monitors (CGMs), hydration sensors, respiratory rate trackers, skin temperature monitors and wearable electrochemical or optical sensors. Biosensors can be embedded in patches, adhesive strips, textiles or even semi-implantable devices, allowing for continuous, non-invasive or minimally invasive health monitoring. They are especially critical for individuals managing chronic conditions such as diabetes, heart disease, respiratory illnesses and neurological disorders. Biosensors often provide real-time alerts when physiological parameters cross safe thresholds, enabling prompt intervention. Integration with mobile apps and healthcare platforms allows users to share their data with clinicians, caregivers or family members. For example, a biosensor detecting abnormal glucose trends can automatically alert a caregiver or adjust insulin delivery in connected insulin pumps. Beyond physical health, biosensors are also increasingly being developed for mental health monitoring—using parameters like galvanic skin response, heart rate variability and cortisol levels to estimate stress and emotional states. Innovations in AI, machine learning, flexible electronics and nanotechnology are accelerating the capabilities and precision of biosensors and other wearable technologies. Material science advancements have enabled biosensors to become thinner, more flexible, skin-friendly and even biodegradable in some research applications. Enhanced data encryption and compliance with privacy regulations (like HIPAA or GDPR) ensure that users' sensitive health information is securely transmitted and stored. Together, smartwatches, fitness bands and biosensors form a comprehensive suite of tools that support preventive health, lifestyle optimization, chronic disease management and personalized medicine. They empower users to make informed decisions about their health, bridge the gap between patient and provider and foster a proactive approach to well-being. As these technologies continue to advance, they will play a critical role in the broader movement toward connected, data-driven and user-centered healthcare systems.

2.1.2 ECG, PPG, Blood Pressure Monitoring

Electrocardiogram (ECG), Photoplethysmography (PPG) and blood pressure monitoring are foundational technologies in the development of modern wearable health devices, significantly enhancing personal health tracking and remote diagnostics. These sensor technologies, when embedded in smartwatches, fitness trackers and biosensors, enable continuous, non-invasive monitoring of cardiovascular health and vital signs—paving the way for early detection, chronic disease management and personalized healthcare interventions.

- Electrocardiogram (ECG) technology is a medical-grade tool traditionally used in clinical settings to measure the electrical activity of the heart. When integrated into wearables, ECG allows users to capture on-demand, single-lead readings by placing fingers on metal contact sensors, often embedded in the bezel or crown of a smartwatch. This capability enables the detection of arrhythmias, particularly atrial fibrillation (AFib), with high accuracy. Many consumer-grade wearables have received FDA clearance for their ECG features, demonstrating their growing reliability and utility in both personal and clinical environments. By recording heart rhythm and waveform data, wearable ECG devices provide valuable information for cardiologists and can significantly reduce the time between symptom onset and diagnosis.

- Photoplethysmography (PPG), in contrast, is an optical sensing method used to estimate physiological parameters such as heart rate, heart rate variability, blood oxygen saturation (SpO_2) and respiratory rate. PPG operates by emitting a light—usually green, red or infrared—into the skin and measuring the amount of light absorbed or reflected by blood vessels. As blood volume changes with each heartbeat, the amount of reflected light fluctuates, allowing the device to interpret cardiovascular metrics. Though less precise than ECG for diagnosing heart rhythm disorders, PPG is invaluable for continuous and passive health tracking, particularly in fitness and wellness applications. It also contributes to stress analysis by evaluating heart rate variability and pulse patterns.
- Blood pressure monitoring in wearable technology has advanced considerably in recent years. Traditional cuff-based methods, while accurate, are bulky and not suitable for continuous use. Wearables now offer cuffless blood pressure monitoring, primarily using PPG signals combined with machine learning algorithms or pulse transit time (PTT) measurements derived from ECG and PPG sensors. Though the clinical accuracy of these cuffless systems is still being refined, recent studies and device validations indicate promising results. Continuous blood pressure monitoring could revolutionize hypertension management by offering real-time insights into fluctuations related to stress, diet, sleep or medication adherence.

The combination of ECG and PPG in a single wearable device enhances diagnostic capabilities significantly. These dual-sensor systems can analyze arterial stiffness, estimate pulse wave velocity and derive other advanced hemodynamic indicators that go beyond traditional heart rate metrics. Such comprehensive cardiovascular profiling is particularly beneficial for patients with chronic conditions like hypertension, heart failure and diabetes, offering insights that support timely medical intervention and reduce the risk of complications or hospitalization. The adoption of these sensing technologies is also accelerating due to increasing regulatory approvals and clinical validations, signaling a broader acceptance within mainstream healthcare. Wearable devices featuring ECG and PPG are now being prescribed or recommended by healthcare providers, particularly for remote monitoring programs and post-discharge patient care. The real-time alerts generated by these sensors allow users to respond promptly to abnormal readings, thereby supporting healthier lifestyles and improving self-management of chronic conditions. Moreover, these technologies are expanding into mental health and wellness monitoring, where indicators like heart rate variability (from PPG) and stress-related rhythm changes (from ECG) are used to assess emotional well-being. With data visualizations, cloud-based analytics and seamless app integrations, users gain a clearer understanding of their cardiovascular trends and overall health trajectory. The convergence of ECG, PPG and blood pressure monitoring in wearable devices is transforming how health data is collected, analyzed and acted upon. These innovations not only offer convenience and early intervention but also signal a major step toward data-driven, predictive and personalized healthcare—where real-time biometric insights can lead to better outcomes and a higher quality of life.

2.2 MOBILE HEALTH (MHEALTH) APPLICATIONS

Mobile Health, commonly known as mHealth, refers to the use of mobile devices such as smartphones, tablets and wearable technology to support medical and public health practices. Over the past decade, mHealth applications have emerged as a vital component of digital health, transforming the way healthcare services are delivered and accessed globally. These applications enable users to monitor their health, manage chronic diseases, communicate with healthcare providers and access medical information anytime and anywhere, breaking down traditional barriers to healthcare access. The widespread adoption of smartphones and the expansion of mobile internet networks have fueled the rapid growth of mHealth apps. These applications range from simple fitness trackers and diet planners to complex platforms that offer remote patient monitoring, medication management, mental health support and teleconsultations. Their portability, ease of use and affordability make them especially valuable in remote or underserved areas where healthcare infrastructure may be limited.

mHealth apps leverage various technologies, including sensors embedded in mobile devices, GPS tracking and real-time data synchronization with cloud services, to provide personalized health insights. They empower individuals by promoting health awareness, encouraging preventive behaviors and facilitating early detection of potential health issues. For patients with chronic conditions such as diabetes, hypertension or asthma, mHealth applications offer tools to record symptoms, track medication adherence and receive alerts and reminders, thereby improving disease management and reducing hospital visits. In addition to patient-centered features, mHealth apps also serve healthcare professionals by providing decision support systems, clinical guidelines and access to patient data remotely. This supports timely diagnosis and intervention, improves clinical workflows and enhances communication between care teams. Integration with electronic health records (EHR) and other health information systems further strengthens the continuity of care.

Security and privacy are critical considerations in mHealth app development. Ensuring compliance with regulations such as HIPAA and GDPR, implementing encryption and safeguarding user data are essential to building trust and protecting sensitive health information from cyber threats.

The growing field of mHealth is also leveraging artificial intelligence and machine learning to provide advanced analytics, personalized recommendations and predictive insights. These capabilities enhance the effectiveness of mHealth solutions and contribute to precision medicine. Moreover, gamification, social networking and behavioral science techniques are increasingly incorporated to boost user engagement and motivation. Overall, mobile health applications represent a dynamic and rapidly evolving sector within digital health. They hold great promise for improving healthcare accessibility, quality and outcomes, while empowering individuals to take an active role in managing their health. As technology continues to advance and regulatory frameworks mature, the potential of mHealth apps to transform healthcare on a global scale will only continue to grow.

2.2.1 Health Tracking Apps and Interfaces

Mobile health (mHealth) applications have revolutionized the way individuals monitor and manage their health. Among the most popular are health tracking apps, which enable users to track a variety of personal health metrics such as physical activity, heart rate, sleep quality, caloric intake, hydration levels, blood pressure, menstrual cycles and more (Fig. 3). These apps often work in conjunction with wearable devices such as fitness bands or smartwatches to automatically collect and analyze data, providing users with real-time feedback and personalized insights into their health and wellness behaviors. Health tracking apps are designed with user-friendly interfaces to ensure accessibility for people of all ages and tech literacy levels. Through intuitive dashboards, visual graphs, notifications and reminders, users are encouraged to make healthier lifestyle choices and stick to long-term health goals. For instance, an app may send a reminder to drink water every hour or notify the user when they've been sedentary for too long. Many apps also offer goal-setting features, allowing users to track progress toward targets like step counts, calorie burn or weight loss. Beyond personal use, health tracking apps are becoming valuable tools for healthcare professionals. With user consent, data collected by these apps can be shared with doctors or caregivers to assist in monitoring chronic conditions such as diabetes, hypertension or obesity. Some advanced apps include features for mood tracking, medication reminders, symptom diaries and telehealth integrations, making them vital tools in preventive care and remote patient monitoring.

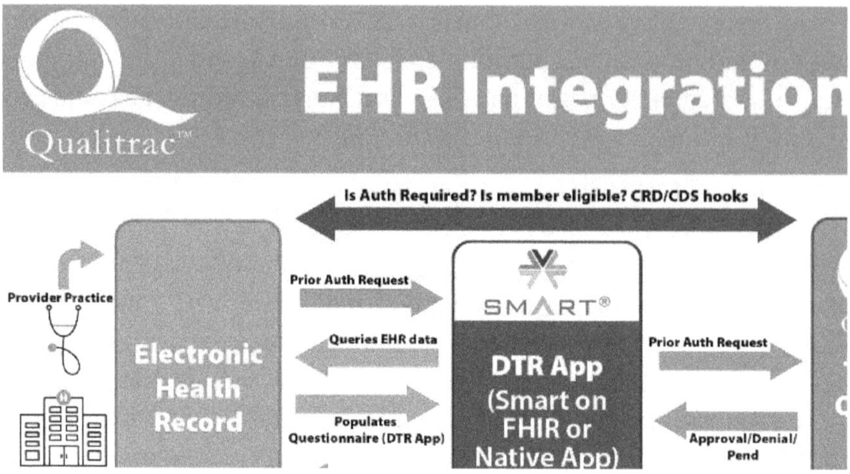

Fig. 3 Mobile health (mHealth)

A key advantage of these apps is their potential to identify early warning signs of health issues. For example, irregular heart rate trends or patterns in sleep disruption can prompt timely medical evaluation. Furthermore, many apps now incorporate artificial intelligence (AI) to offer smart recommendations, detect anomalies and adapt to user behavior over time. Some platforms even support community features, offering social support, health challenges or forums where users can engage with others pursuing similar health goals. However, there are notable challenges. Data privacy and security remain top concerns, especially as health data is highly sensitive. Unauthorized access or misuse of this information can have serious consequences. Additionally, the accuracy of self-reported data or sensor-based measurements can vary significantly, affecting the reliability of the insights derived. Despite these challenges, the increasing sophistication of health tracking apps is transforming how individuals engage with their health and empowering proactive healthcare management.

2.2.2 Integration with Electronic Health Records (EHRs)

One of the most transformative developments in mobile health (mHealth) is the integration of health applications with Electronic Health Records (EHRs). This integration bridges the gap between patient-generated health data and clinically managed health information, allowing for a more comprehensive, real-time understanding of a patient's overall health status. EHRs are digital versions of patients' paper charts, containing complete medical history, diagnoses, medications, treatment plans, lab results and more. When connected to mHealth applications, they provide clinicians with up-to-date patient data beyond the clinical setting. Integration enables seamless data sharing between patients and healthcare providers. For example, a patient using a mobile app to monitor their blood glucose levels can automatically sync this data to their EHR, where the physician can access it during follow-ups. This leads to better-informed clinical decisions and more personalized care plans. It also reduces the burden on patients who previously had to manually track and report such data. Moreover, EHR integration helps reduce redundant tests, prevents medication errors and enhances care coordination across different healthcare providers (Fig. 4).

From a technological perspective, this integration is made possible through APIs (Application Programming Interfaces) and FHIR (Fast Healthcare Interoperability Resources) standards, which ensure that different systems can communicate and exchange data efficiently. Many healthcare institutions and app developers are adopting these interoperability standards to facilitate smoother data exchange, enabling a more connected health ecosystem.

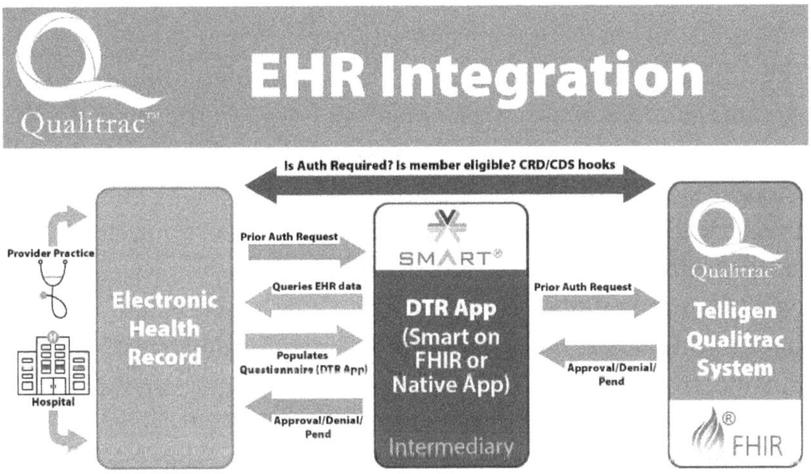

Fig. 4 Integration with Electronic Health Records (EHRs)

For patients with chronic conditions, integrated EHR systems can provide alerts and recommendations based on real-time data from mHealth apps. For instance, if a hypertensive patient's blood pressure readings spike, the EHR system might trigger an alert to the physician, prompting early intervention. Integration also supports telemedicine services, where a doctor can review patient vitals collected at home before or during virtual consultations, enhancing diagnostic accuracy and continuity of care.

However, achieving seamless EHR-mHealth integration comes with significant challenges. Data standardization across different platforms, privacy regulations like HIPAA (Health Insurance Portability and Accountability Act) and varying levels of digital infrastructure in healthcare facilities can hinder smooth adoption. Additionally, concerns about cybersecurity, data ownership and consent management need to be addressed to build trust among users and providers. Despite these hurdles, the integration of mHealth apps with EHRs holds immense promise. It empowers patients to take an active role in managing their health while enabling providers to deliver more efficient, data-driven and proactive care. As healthcare continues its digital transformation, integrated systems are expected to become the cornerstone of a truly patient-centered and technology-enabled healthcare model.

2.3 REMOTE PATIENT MONITORING (RPM) SYSTEMS

Remote Patient Monitoring (RPM) systems are a pivotal advancement in healthcare technology that allow for the continuous tracking and management of patients' health outside traditional clinical settings. By leveraging digital devices and communication networks, RPM enables healthcare providers to monitor vital signs, symptoms and treatment adherence remotely, facilitating timely interventions and reducing the need for frequent hospital visits. This technology is especially valuable for managing chronic diseases such as diabetes, hypertension, heart failure and respiratory conditions, where ongoing monitoring is crucial for preventing complications and hospital readmissions. At the core of RPM systems are connected medical devices, including wearable sensors, implantable devices and home monitoring equipment, which collect a variety of health metrics such as blood pressure, glucose levels, heart rate, oxygen saturation and weight. These devices transmit real-time data to centralized platforms via wireless technologies like Bluetooth, Wi-Fi or cellular networks, ensuring that clinicians have continuous access to patient information regardless of geographical location. The integration of RPM with electronic health records (EHR) provides a comprehensive view of patient health, enhancing care coordination and clinical decision-making. RPM systems not only improve patient outcomes but also empower individuals by involving them actively in their own care. Patients receive feedback, alerts and personalized recommendations through mobile apps or web portals, fostering greater engagement and adherence to treatment plans. The ability to monitor health in real-time helps detect early warning signs of deterioration, enabling healthcare providers to intervene promptly and often avoid emergency hospitalizations. Beyond clinical benefits, RPM offers economic advantages by lowering healthcare costs through reduced inpatient stays, fewer emergency visits and optimized resource utilization. This has made RPM a key component in value-based care models aimed at improving quality while controlling expenses. The COVID-19 pandemic further accelerated the adoption of RPM by highlighting the need for remote healthcare solutions that minimize physical contact while maintaining continuous care. Remote Patient Monitoring App is given in Fig. 5.

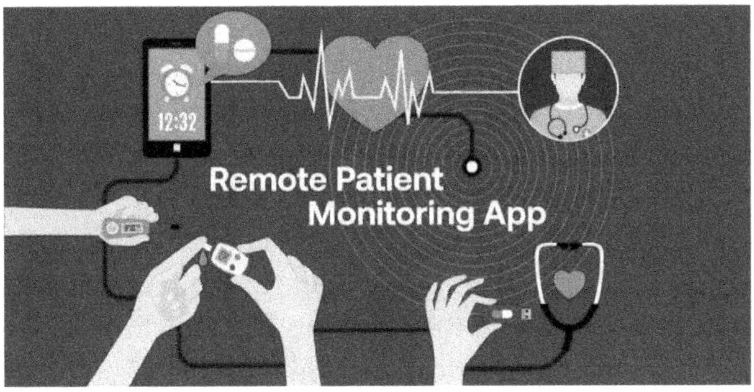

Fig. 5 Remote Patient Monitoring

Advanced analytics, artificial intelligence (AI) and machine learning enhance RPM by analyzing large volumes of patient data to identify trends, predict adverse events and tailor treatments to individual needs. These intelligent systems support clinicians in making data-driven decisions, improving diagnostic accuracy and personalized care delivery. However, the successful implementation of RPM systems requires addressing challenges related to data security, patient privacy, interoperability and user training. Ensuring compliance with healthcare regulations such as HIPAA and GDPR is essential to protect sensitive health information and build trust among users. Remote Patient Monitoring systems represent a transformative shift in healthcare delivery, blending technology with clinical practice to provide continuous, patient-centered care beyond hospital walls. By enabling early detection of health issues, fostering patient engagement and supporting efficient healthcare management, RPM is redefining chronic disease management and setting new standards for quality care in the digital age.

2.3.1 Devices for Home-Based Health Surveillance

Remote Patient Monitoring (RPM) systems are an essential component of modern healthcare delivery, especially in enabling home-based health surveillance. These systems utilize digital technologies and specialized devices to collect medical and health data from individuals in their homes and transmit that information securely to healthcare providers. This approach significantly reduces the need for frequent in-person visits while maintaining continuous oversight of the patient's health status. There are a wide variety of RPM devices designed for home use, each tailored to monitor specific health parameters. Some of the most commonly used devices include digital blood pressure monitors, glucometers, pulse oximeters, electronic thermometers, weight scales, ECG monitors and smart inhalers. For patients with heart conditions, wearable ECG patches can continuously record heart activity, while those with respiratory issues may use spirometers to measure lung function. More advanced devices such as implantable sensors can provide minute-by-minute data on internal body functions.

These devices often feature wireless connectivity options like Bluetooth, Wi-Fi or cellular networks, which enable them to transmit data to cloud platforms or EHR systems in real-time. Many RPM devices are integrated with mobile applications or web dashboards that allow both patients and healthcare providers to view trends, set thresholds and receive alerts when abnormal readings are detected. For example, a patient with high blood pressure might receive an immediate notification if their readings exceed a safe range, prompting them to contact a healthcare provider or adjust medication. Home-based RPM devices are typically designed to be user-friendly, even for older adults or those unfamiliar with digital technology. Many systems incorporate voice assistance, automated guidance or even telehealth support, making it easier for patients to use the equipment correctly. They also improve adherence to care plans by providing regular reminders to measure vital signs or take medications. One of the major advantages of home-based health surveillance is that it promotes early detection of health deterioration. Instead of waiting for symptoms to become severe, continuous monitoring can catch subtle changes, leading to faster interventions and potentially reducing the risk of hospitalization. For healthcare systems, this model also eases the burden on hospitals and clinics, enabling providers to manage more patients effectively from a distance. However, challenges remain, including concerns about data privacy, device accuracy, internet connectivity in rural or underserved areas and the need for patient education. Ensuring that devices are certified, secure and integrated with clinical workflows is critical for effective implementation. Despite these barriers, RPM devices for home-based monitoring represent a pivotal shift toward patient-centered, technology-driven and preventive healthcare.

2.3.2 Use Cases in Chronic Disease Management

Remote Patient Monitoring (RPM) plays a transformative role in the management of chronic diseases, which require consistent oversight and long-term care. By enabling continuous health tracking from home, RPM systems enhance patient engagement, improve disease control and reduce emergency visits or hospital readmissions. This is especially beneficial for patients suffering from chronic conditions such as diabetes, hypertension, heart failure, COPD (Chronic Obstructive Pulmonary Disease) and chronic kidney disease. For instance, in diabetes management, RPM systems allow patients to use connected glucometers to track blood glucose levels multiple times a day. These readings can be instantly shared with healthcare teams, who can adjust insulin doses or dietary plans accordingly. Over time, trend analysis through RPM platforms helps detect patterns that may indicate the risk of complications, such as hypoglycemia or hyperglycemia, enabling timely interventions. In the case of hypertension, patients use smart blood pressure monitors to track readings at home. Regular monitoring helps identify whether medications are effective or if lifestyle modifications are needed. Some systems are programmed to send alerts to providers when readings fall outside of predefined safe limits, prompting early clinical responses before the situation escalates.

Heart failure is another area where RPM has shown measurable impact. Patients can use weight scales, pulse oximeters and ECG devices to monitor signs of fluid retention and cardiac stress. An unexpected weight gain, for example, can be an early sign of fluid buildup, signaling the need for medication adjustment. Such proactive monitoring helps reduce hospitalizations and improves quality of life. For COPD and other respiratory conditions, RPM tools like connected spirometers and pulse oximeters enable monitoring of lung function and oxygen saturation. These metrics help clinicians determine whether the patient's condition is stable or worsening. Some systems also offer tele-coaching for smoking cessation or pulmonary rehab, further supporting long-term disease control.

RPM also supports patients with chronic kidney disease by tracking blood pressure, fluid intake and weight to manage symptoms and slow disease progression. In advanced cases, it may assist with dialysis monitoring from home, ensuring adherence to treatment schedules and timely follow-ups.

Beyond physical health, RPM systems are increasingly used for managing mental health and neurological conditions, using wearable devices that track sleep, heart rate variability and behavioral patterns. This data is analyzed to detect changes that may indicate depression, anxiety or cognitive decline. Despite these benefits, successful RPM implementation in chronic disease management requires collaboration between patients, caregivers and clinicians. Challenges include ensuring device usability, maintaining patient motivation, securing funding or insurance coverage and integrating RPM data into EHR systems. Nevertheless, the ability to provide real-time, continuous and personalized care makes RPM an indispensable tool in chronic disease management and a cornerstone of the future of healthcare.

2.4 INTERNET OF MEDICAL THINGS (IOMT)

The Internet of Medical Things (IoMT) represents a revolutionary convergence of medical devices and internet connectivity, creating a vast network of interconnected health technologies designed to improve patient care, enhance operational efficiency and enable real-time health monitoring. As a specialized segment of the broader Internet of Things (IoT), IoMT encompasses a wide variety of medical devices—ranging from wearable sensors and implantable gadgets to remote monitoring tools and hospital equipment—all connected via wireless networks. This interconnected ecosystem facilitates the seamless collection, transmission and analysis of critical health data, empowering healthcare providers to deliver more informed, timely and personalized care (Fig. 6).

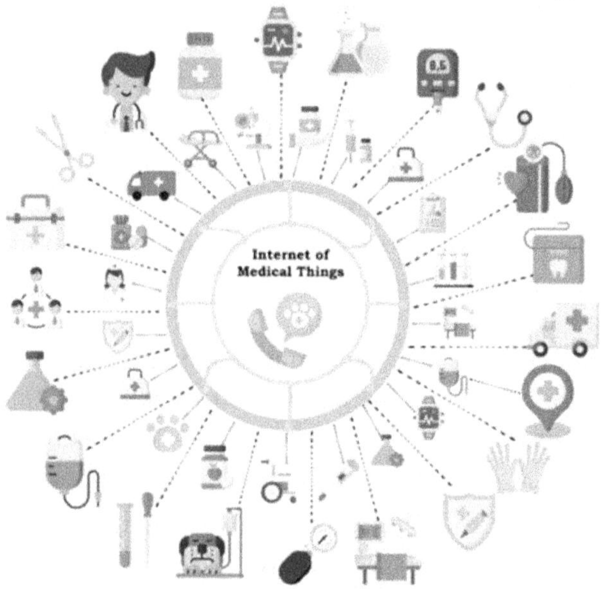

Fig. 6 IoMT-Internet of Medical Things

IoMT devices continuously capture vital health parameters such as heart rate, blood glucose, blood pressure, respiratory rate and body temperature, transmitting this information to cloud-based platforms or centralized healthcare databases. By integrating with electronic health records (EHR) systems, IoMT supports comprehensive patient profiles that enhance clinical decision-making and improve the coordination of care across multidisciplinary teams. This real-time data flow also enables proactive interventions, helping prevent complications and hospital readmissions. One of the core strengths of IoMT lies in its ability to support remote patient monitoring, telemedicine and chronic disease management on an unprecedented scale. Patients can be monitored continuously outside clinical environments, allowing for early detection of anomalies and swift medical responses. This is particularly valuable for managing conditions such as diabetes, cardiovascular diseases and respiratory illnesses, where ongoing monitoring can significantly impact outcomes.

The rapid advancement of wireless communication technologies—including 5G, Bluetooth Low Energy (BLE) and Wi-Fi—has been instrumental in expanding IoMT capabilities. These technologies enable secure, low-latency data transmission, critical for applications requiring real-time feedback, such as emergency alert systems or wearable defibrillators. Furthermore, edge computing has enhanced IoMT by processing data closer to the source, reducing latency and bandwidth usage and enabling faster decision-making.

Artificial intelligence (AI) and machine learning (ML) play a pivotal role within the IoMT ecosystem by analyzing the enormous volumes of data generated to identify patterns, predict health risks and optimize treatment plans. AI-driven analytics facilitate early diagnosis, personalized care and improved resource allocation, helping clinicians focus on high-risk patients and tailor interventions accordingly. Despite its transformative potential, IoMT also faces significant challenges, including data security, privacy concerns and interoperability issues. Protecting sensitive medical information from cyber threats requires robust encryption, authentication protocols and adherence to regulatory standards such as HIPAA and GDPR. Interoperability between diverse devices and healthcare systems remains critical to ensure smooth data exchange and comprehensive patient care. IoMT also contributes to healthcare efficiency by enabling smart hospital management systems that optimize equipment utilization, automate routine tasks and monitor environmental conditions to maintain patient safety. In emergency settings, IoMT devices provide rapid, accurate diagnostics and facilitate timely communication between healthcare teams, enhancing patient outcomes. Overall, the Internet of Medical Things is reshaping the healthcare landscape by creating a connected, data-driven environment that supports continuous, personalized and proactive medical care. As IoMT technologies evolve and mature, they promise to drive innovation, improve patient experiences, reduce healthcare costs and ultimately transform global health systems for the better. Internet of Medical Things Examples is predicted in Fig. 7.

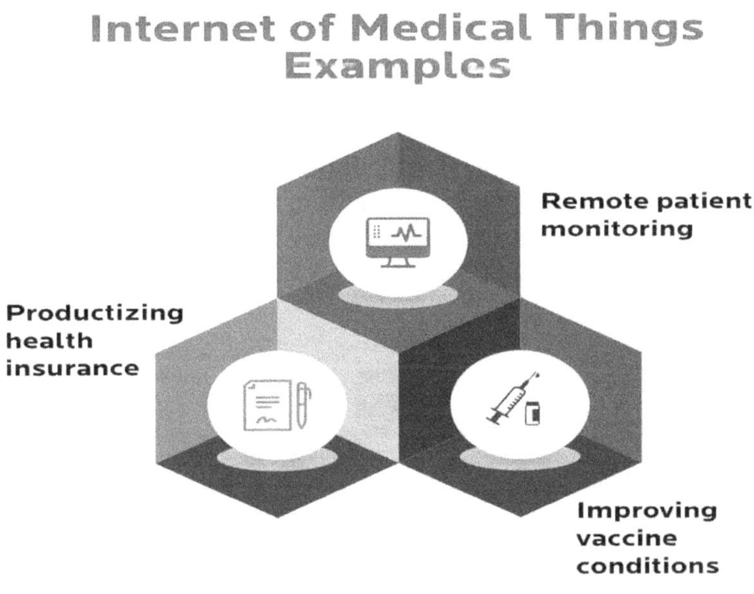

Fig.7 Internet of Medical Things Examples

2.4.1 Networked Health Devices and Sensors

The Internet of Medical Things (IoMT) refers to the vast network of interconnected medical devices, software applications, sensors and systems that collect, transmit and analyze health data through the internet. These technologies play a transformative role in modern healthcare by enabling real-time monitoring, diagnostics and treatment, often without the need for physical clinical visits. The core idea of IoMT is to integrate smart, sensor-enabled devices into the healthcare ecosystem, forming a connected infrastructure that supports data-driven and patient-centered care. IoMT encompasses a broad range of networked health devices and sensors, including wearable fitness trackers, ECG monitors, connected inhalers, smart implants, insulin pens and even robotic surgical systems. These devices collect biometric and physiological data such as heart rate, oxygen saturation, glucose levels, body temperature and movement patterns. The collected data is then transmitted via wireless networks—such as Wi-Fi, Bluetooth or cellular—to cloud platforms or electronic health records (EHRs), where it can be accessed by healthcare providers for diagnosis, monitoring and decision-making. One of the most common examples of IoMT in action is a smart wearable device, like a smartwatch with ECG capability, that continuously monitors heart rhythm and detects arrhythmias. Another example is a smart pill—a tiny ingestible sensor that sends data after ingestion to confirm medication adherence (Fig. 8). In hospital settings, networked infusion pumps and connected ventilators are used to precisely control and monitor patient treatment while minimizing human error. Some devices even incorporate AI and machine learning to generate predictive insights, such as warning signs of sepsis or cardiac arrest. These connected health technologies enable better disease management, early detection of health deterioration, remote patient monitoring and personalized care delivery. For patients with chronic illnesses, IoMT can significantly improve quality of life by reducing the need for hospital visits and enabling 24/7 monitoring from home. In surgical or critical care settings, IoMT systems streamline workflows by automating routine measurements, alerts and logs.

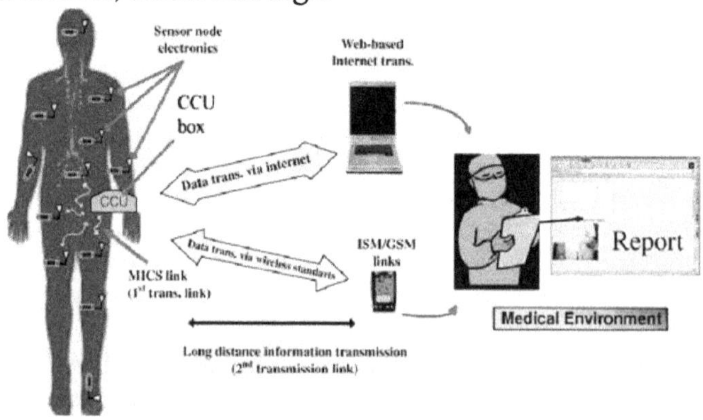

Fig. 8 A medical sensor network application

The benefits of IoMT are particularly evident in large-scale public health initiatives. For example, during pandemics, connected thermometers or pulse oximeters can support remote screening and epidemiological tracking. In rural or underserved areas, IoMT devices combined with telemedicine platforms help close healthcare access gaps. Despite its promise, the deployment of networked medical devices must be carefully managed to ensure interoperability, reliability and data accuracy. The growing number of devices in the ecosystem also increases complexity, requiring standardized communication protocols and centralized data platforms. Nonetheless, IoMT is rapidly becoming a foundational pillar of smart healthcare systems, capable of delivering proactive, scalable and efficient medical services.

2.4.2 Security, Connectivity and Power Management

While the Internet of Medical Things (IoMT) offers immense benefits, it also presents critical challenges, especially in the areas of security, connectivity and power management. These technical and operational concerns must be addressed to ensure safe, reliable and sustainable use of IoMT technologies in both clinical and home settings. Security is a primary concern in IoMT, given that these devices handle highly sensitive patient health data and often have direct influence over medical treatment. Cyberattacks or data breaches can compromise patient privacy, disrupt care or even endanger lives if a device is manipulated. Many IoMT devices have limited computational power and may not support strong encryption or advanced security protocols, making them vulnerable to threats. Common risks include unauthorized data access, malware infections and device hijacking. For example, a compromised infusion pump could result in an incorrect dosage of medication. To mitigate these threats, healthcare organizations must implement robust cybersecurity frameworks, including encryption, authentication protocols, regular software updates and network segmentation. Connectivity is another essential element of IoMT, as devices must communicate reliably over wireless or wired networks to transmit real-time data. Poor network infrastructure, signal interference or bandwidth limitations can lead to data loss, delays or device malfunctions. In hospital environments, dozens or even hundreds of devices may compete for the same network resources, increasing the risk of congestion and latency. Additionally, in rural or remote locations, limited internet coverage can hinder device performance and reduce the reliability of telehealth or remote monitoring services. To address this, advanced networking technologies like 5G, edge computing and mesh networks are being explored to provide low-latency, high-bandwidth connectivity and reduce dependence on centralized servers.

Power management is also a critical factor, especially for portable or implantable medical devices. Many IoMT devices are battery-powered and expected to operate for extended periods without recharging. This requires efficient power consumption strategies, such as low-power hardware design, adaptive data transmission schedules and energy-efficient communication protocols. For wearable sensors, battery life directly impacts usability and patient adherence—frequent recharging can be inconvenient and reduce overall effectiveness. In more advanced applications like pacemakers or neurostimulators, power failure is not just inconvenient but potentially life-threatening. Innovations like energy harvesting, wireless charging and ultra-low-power chipsets are being developed to extend device lifespan and reliability. Regulatory compliance adds another layer of complexity. IoMT devices must meet stringent standards from agencies like the FDA, CE or ISO, especially regarding patient safety, data security and interoperability. Additionally, privacy regulations such as HIPAA in the U.S. and GDPR in the EU must be considered when designing systems that collect and transmit personal health information. The long-term success of IoMT depends not only on technological innovation but also on solving the practical challenges of security, connectivity and power efficiency. By investing in secure infrastructure, resilient communication systems and sustainable energy solutions, healthcare systems can fully harness the potential of IoMT to deliver intelligent, continuous and accessible care across a wide range of settings (Fig. 9).

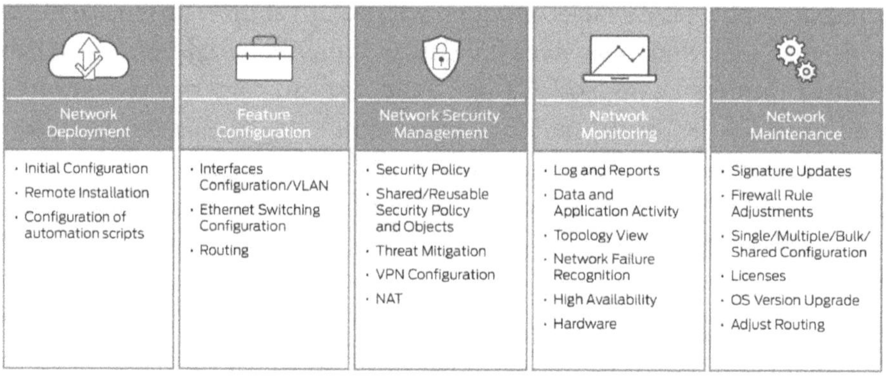

Fig.9 Network Security Management

2.5 ARTIFICIAL INTELLIGENCE AND MACHINE LEARNING

The integration of Artificial Intelligence (AI) and Machine Learning (ML) into health monitoring represents a revolutionary shift in modern healthcare. These technologies have redefined how medical data is collected, analyzed and acted upon, enabling faster, more accurate and personalized health interventions. As global healthcare systems face increasing pressure from rising chronic disease rates, aging populations and resource constraints, AI and ML have emerged as essential tools in supporting both preventative care and ongoing disease management. AI encompasses a broad range of computer-based techniques that mimic human intelligence, while ML, a subset of AI, allows systems to learn and improve from data without being explicitly programmed. Together, they offer the capability to analyze vast amounts of complex medical data—ranging from wearable sensor readings and medical imaging to genetic information and electronic health records (EHRs). Through pattern recognition and predictive modeling, ML algorithms can identify subtle indicators of disease progression, recommend personalized treatment plans and detect anomalies that may go unnoticed by human clinicians. One of the most significant contributions of AI and ML in health monitoring lies in their ability to support real-time data analysis. With the rise of wearable technologies—like smartwatches, fitness bands and implantable biosensors—health monitoring has become continuous, non-invasive and highly data-driven. These devices generate streams of physiological data, such as heart rate, oxygen saturation, blood glucose levels and sleep patterns, which can be automatically analyzed by ML models to detect early signs of health deterioration. This empowers patients and healthcare providers to act proactively rather than reactively. Moreover, AI-driven health monitoring systems enhance diagnostic accuracy. For instance, AI algorithms can analyze medical images (e.g., X-rays, MRIs and CT scans) with a level of precision that often rivals or exceeds human experts. ML models trained on large datasets of annotated images can rapidly detect abnormalities like tumors, fractures or neurological issues, thus supporting radiologists and reducing diagnostic errors. Similarly, natural language processing (NLP)—another AI domain—enables machines to interpret and summarize clinical notes, facilitating easier access to relevant patient history.

In chronic disease management, ML algorithms predict potential complications before they arise. For example, diabetic patients can benefit from AI systems that predict glucose fluctuations based on diet, activity and historical trends, enabling timely insulin adjustments. Cardiovascular patients may use AI-powered ECG monitors that detect arrhythmias or predict cardiac events with minimal patient intervention. This predictive capability not only improves patient outcomes but also reduces hospital admissions and healthcare costs. AI and ML also play a critical role in remote health monitoring, a field that gained prominence during the COVID-19 pandemic. Telehealth platforms integrated with intelligent analytics enable clinicians to remotely track patient conditions, provide timely consultations and adjust treatments as needed. This approach is particularly valuable in rural or underserved areas where access to healthcare providers may be limited. However, the adoption of AI and ML in health monitoring is not without challenges. Concerns about data privacy, algorithmic bias, regulatory compliance and the need for explainable AI remain critical issues. Ensuring that AI systems are transparent, ethical and equitable is essential to gaining public trust and achieving widespread adoption. Additionally, healthcare professionals must be adequately trained to interpret and interact with AI-driven insights, making interdisciplinary collaboration a key component of successful implementation. AI and ML are transforming health monitoring from a reactive, episodic process to a proactive, continuous and personalized approach. By enhancing early diagnosis, improving chronic disease management and facilitating remote care, these technologies are paving the way for a more efficient, responsive and patient-centered healthcare system. As innovation continues and regulatory frameworks evolve, AI and ML will undoubtedly play an increasingly vital role in shaping the future of global health.

2.5.1 Predictive Analytics and Risk Scoring

Predictive analytics and risk scoring are two transformative components of Artificial Intelligence (AI) and Machine Learning (ML) in modern healthcare. They involve analysing historical and real-time patient data to forecast future health events and assess an individual's risk for specific medical conditions. Using large datasets from electronic health records (EHRs), wearable devices, lab tests and imaging systems, ML models can detect hidden patterns and correlations. These insights help predict the likelihood of diseases such as diabetes, heart disease, cancer and more. Risk scoring assigns a numerical value to a patient's likelihood of developing a condition or facing complications, helping clinicians prioritize care. For example, a patient with a high-risk score for stroke may be monitored more closely and receive preventative treatment. Predictive analytics plays a critical role in chronic disease management. In diabetes, for instance, AI can predict dangerous blood glucose fluctuations, prompting timely adjustments in insulin or diet. In cardiovascular care, AI models can forecast the risk of heart attacks or arrhythmias using ECG and lifestyle data. Hospitals use risk scoring to predict which patients are likely to be readmitted within 30 days. This supports discharge planning and targeted follow-ups, improving outcomes and reducing healthcare costs. Common machine learning techniques include logistic regression, decision trees, random forests, support vector machines and deep learning, especially when handling complex data like images or real-time vitals. Natural Language Processing (NLP) helps extract useful information from unstructured data such as doctors' notes, enhancing model accuracy. The benefits of predictive analytics are vast: early disease detection, timely intervention, personalized treatment, reduced hospitalizations and better patient outcomes. However, challenges remain. These include data quality issues, potential algorithmic bias, lack of explainability and privacy concerns. Ethical implementation and regulatory compliance are essential.

Predictive analytics and risk scoring are enabling healthcare providers to move from reactive to proactive care. As AI and ML technologies evolve, they will continue to enhance risk prediction and revolutionize the future of health monitoring.

Definition and Overview: Predictive Analytics refers to the use of historical and real-time data, statistical algorithms and machine learning techniques to identify the likelihood of future outcomes. Risk Scoring involves assigning a numerical value to a patient based on their risk level for specific health conditions or adverse events such as hospitalization, readmission or disease onset. Together, these methods enable early interventions and informed decision-making in clinical practice.

Data Sources for Predictive Modeling

Predictive analytics relies on diverse datasets, including:

- **Electronic Health Records (EHRs):** Electronic Health Records (EHRs) are comprehensive digital records of a patient's medical history, offering a rich source of structured and unstructured health data. They include demographics, diagnoses, prescriptions, allergies, immunizations, lab test results, radiology reports and physician notes. AI algorithms can mine EHRs to identify risk patterns, predict disease onset and track treatment effectiveness. For instance, trends in blood pressure or cholesterol over time can help forecast the likelihood of cardiovascular issues. Clinical notes, though unstructured, can be processed using Natural Language Processing (NLP) to extract critical insights. By integrating EHR data across different visits and departments, predictive models gain a holistic view of a patient's health. EHRs also enable longitudinal analysis, helping to detect subtle but significant changes in health over time. Risk scoring tools often use EHR inputs to stratify patients based on their medical history. EHRs can also be updated in real-time, ensuring that AI predictions are current and relevant. Their accessibility across healthcare systems supports continuity of care and collaborative decision-making.
- **Wearable Devices:** Wearable devices such as fitness trackers, smartwatches and biosensors continuously monitor physiological parameters like heart rate, blood pressure, respiratory rate, glucose levels, sleep cycles and physical activity. These devices generate real-time, high-frequency data that AI models can analyze for early warning signs of disease. For example, a sudden drop in heart rate variability might indicate a cardiac issue or impending illness. Machine learning algorithms use this data to create personalized baselines and detect deviations that may signal health risks. Wearables are especially useful in remote health monitoring and chronic disease management, allowing patients to stay connected to their care teams without frequent hospital visits. They empower users with actionable insights, promoting preventive care and lifestyle improvements. Data from wearables also enrich traditional datasets, making predictive models more dynamic and accurate. Their integration with mobile apps provides user-friendly interfaces for health tracking. As technology advances, wearables

are becoming more accurate and less invasive. They play a critical role in shifting healthcare from reactive treatment to proactive prevention.

- **Medical Imaging:** Medical imaging—such as X-rays, MRIs, CT scans and ultrasounds—provides detailed visual information about the body's internal structures. AI, especially deep learning, has shown exceptional ability in analyzing these images to detect abnormalities like tumors, fractures and organ damage. By training on large datasets of annotated images, AI models can match or even exceed the accuracy of human radiologists in certain tasks. Early detection of conditions like cancer, Alzheimer's or pneumonia is possible through subtle image pattern recognition that may be missed by the human eye. Medical imaging data also allows for the staging of diseases and monitoring of treatment progress. AI-enhanced imaging supports precision medicine by customizing diagnostics and treatments based on the individual's imaging profile. Integration with predictive analytics allows the combination of image data with other inputs, like lab results and patient history, for more comprehensive risk assessment. Cloud-based platforms enable real-time image sharing and analysis, especially in rural or under-resourced areas. Medical imaging is a cornerstone of modern diagnostics and a powerful input for predictive modeling. As image recognition algorithms evolve, their impact on clinical decision-making will only grow.
- **Genomic Data:** Genomic data refers to information derived from a person's DNA, including gene sequences, mutations and expression patterns. It holds tremendous potential for predicting hereditary diseases such as cancer, diabetes and cardiovascular conditions. AI algorithms can sift through millions of genetic variants to identify those associated with disease risk, drug response or adverse reactions. This enables personalized treatment plans—also known as pharmacogenomics—where medications and dosages are tailored based on a person's genetic profile. Genomic risk scoring helps identify individuals who may develop conditions years before symptoms appear, allowing for early interventions. Integration of genomic data with EHRs and lifestyle data creates a fuller picture for precision medicine. Machine learning models are essential in handling the complexity and volume of genomic data. These models can discover gene-disease associations and predict outcomes more accurately than traditional statistical tools. AI also supports the automation of genome sequencing analysis, reducing costs and turnaround times. As genomic testing becomes more accessible, it will play a growing role in population-level screening and individualized care.
- **Patient-Reported Outcomes (PROs):** Patient-reported outcomes (PROs) are data directly provided by patients about their health, symptoms,

lifestyle and quality of life—often through surveys, mobile apps or digital diaries. These inputs offer valuable insight into areas that clinical tests might overlook, such as pain severity, fatigue, mood fluctuations or treatment side effects. AI can analyze PROs alongside physiological and clinical data to improve risk prediction and personalize care strategies. For example, daily reports of breathlessness from a patient with heart failure could indicate decompensation and prompt early intervention. Sentiment analysis tools assess emotional well-being from text or voice inputs, supporting mental health monitoring. PROs enhance patient engagement by giving individuals an active role in their care. Machine learning models can detect patterns in PROs to forecast disease exacerbations or identify non-adherence to treatment. These outcomes are also used in clinical trials and research to measure treatment effectiveness from the patient's perspective. Incorporating PROs into predictive analytics creates a more patient-centered approach. As digital health tools evolve, the quantity and quality of PROs will continue to improve, strengthening AI-driven health monitoring systems.

Machine Learning Techniques Used

Several ML techniques are employed for predictive analytics and risk scoring:

- **Supervised Learning:** Supervised learning is a machine learning approach where algorithms are trained on labeled datasets—meaning the input data is paired with known outcomes. In healthcare, these labels might indicate the presence or absence of a disease, patient readmission status or treatment success. Algorithms such as logistic regression, decision trees, support vector machines (SVM) and random forests are commonly used. These models learn from historical health data to predict future events like disease onset, treatment response or complications. For instance, a supervised model can predict the risk of developing diabetes based on age, BMI and blood glucose levels. The accuracy of these predictions improves as more quality-labeled data is available. These models can be evaluated and validated using metrics such as precision, recall and AUC-ROC curves. Supervised learning forms the foundation for many risk scoring systems in clinical practice. It allows for transparent, data-driven decision-making and can be easily integrated into electronic health systems. With continuous training on new data, these models evolve and remain relevant over time.
- **Unsupervised Learning:** Unsupervised learning deals with data that has no predefined labels or outcomes. Instead, it identifies hidden patterns, trends or groupings within the data. Clustering algorithms like k-means, DBSCAN or hierarchical clustering are often used in healthcare to discover patient

subgroups or disease phenotypes. For example, unsupervised models might reveal that patients with similar symptoms and biomarkers form a unique subtype of asthma requiring specialized treatment. This can lead to more targeted and effective care strategies. Dimensionality reduction techniques such as PCA (Principal Component Analysis) also help simplify complex datasets for visualization and analysis. These models are especially useful in early-stage research and exploratory data analysis. Unsupervised learning contributes to identifying unknown correlations between variables, generating hypotheses for further study. It also helps in patient segmentation, resource allocation and population health management. While predictions are not directly generated, the insights extracted often inform the development of supervised models. Unsupervised learning is key to uncovering new knowledge from large-scale health data.

- **Deep Learning:** Deep learning is a subset of machine learning based on artificial neural networks with multiple layers (hence "deep"). It is particularly effective in handling large, complex and unstructured data, such as medical images, ECG signals and wearable time-series data. Convolutional Neural Networks (CNNs) are used for image recognition tasks like identifying tumors in radiology scans, while Recurrent Neural Networks (RNNs) or Long Short-Term Memory (LSTM) networks are ideal for analyzing sequential data like heart rate over time. Deep learning models can automatically extract features from raw data, eliminating the need for manual feature engineering. Their high accuracy and ability to capture non-linear relationships make them invaluable in precision diagnostics and risk forecasting. However, they often require large amounts of labeled data and significant computational power. One challenge is their "black box" nature, making it difficult to interpret how decisions are made. Despite this, advances in explainable AI are helping bridge that gap. Deep learning continues to push the boundaries of what's possible in healthcare analytics.
- **Natural Language Processing (NLP):** Natural Language Processing (NLP) enables machines to understand, interpret and analyze human language, particularly unstructured text data. In healthcare, NLP is used to extract insights from clinical notes, discharge summaries, radiology reports and even patient feedback. For example, NLP can identify mentions of symptoms, disease history or medication adherence in doctor's notes, which structured data might miss. It can also detect social determinants of health like housing instability or substance use, often buried in free-text records. Sentiment analysis and named entity recognition (NER) help pinpoint relevant information for risk scoring and predictive modeling.

NLP models can transform qualitative data into quantitative inputs for AI systems, enhancing the completeness of health profiles. Advanced NLP models, such as those built on transformer architectures like BERT, can understand medical context with high accuracy. NLP also supports clinical coding automation, reducing administrative burden. When combined with machine learning, NLP expands the scope of data-driven healthcare by tapping into the vast, untapped resource of text-based health data.

Clinical Applications

Predictive analytics and risk scoring are applied across multiple health domains:

- **Cardiovascular Risk Prediction:** AI and machine learning models are increasingly used to predict cardiovascular events such as heart attacks, strokes and arrhythmias. These models analyze a combination of EHR data, including blood pressure, cholesterol levels, lifestyle factors and medication history, alongside ECG signals and other diagnostic tests. By identifying subtle patterns and risk factors, they provide earlier and more accurate risk assessments than traditional methods. Classic tools like the Framingham Risk Score are being enhanced with real-time data from wearable devices, offering continuous monitoring of heart rate variability, oxygen saturation and physical activity. This integration allows for dynamic, personalized risk scoring and early warnings, leading to timely medical intervention. AI based prediction models also assist physicians in selecting appropriate treatments and prioritizing high-risk patients. As a result, these systems contribute to reduced mortality, fewer emergency hospital visits and more efficient cardiac care.
- **Diabetes Management:** In diabetes care, predictive analytics plays a vital role in maintaining blood glucose control and preventing complications. AI systems monitor real-time data from continuous glucose monitors (CGMs), wearable sensors, meal logs and insulin usage to detect trends and forecast dangerous highs or lows in blood sugar levels. These systems can predict events like hypoglycemia hours in advance, enabling proactive adjustments to medication or diet. For patients using insulin, predictive tools provide dose recommendations based on individual patterns and history. AI also identifies risk factors for long-term complications such as diabetic retinopathy, nephropathy and neuropathy. Mobile apps integrated with ML algorithms give patients personalized alerts and feedback, encouraging better self-care. Doctors benefit from dashboard summaries that highlight patients most at risk. Overall, AI-driven diabetes management supports safer, more efficient and more personalized treatment plans.

- **Hospital Readmission Risk:** Hospital readmissions place a significant financial and clinical burden on healthcare systems. Predictive models use machine learning algorithms to analyze patient data—such as previous admissions, diagnoses, treatment adherence and social determinants of health—to assess the likelihood of readmission within 30 days of discharge. These insights help care teams identify high-risk individuals and develop targeted follow-up strategies, such as more frequent check-ins or community health support. AI also highlights modifiable risk factors, allowing for tailored discharge planning and education. Hospitals can allocate resources more effectively and reduce penalties associated with excessive readmissions. Real-time scoring tools integrated into EHRs provide clinicians with actionable alerts before the patient leaves the hospital. This approach not only reduces avoidable readmissions but also improves patient satisfaction and long-term health outcomes.
- **Sepsis Detection:** Sepsis is a life-threatening response to infection that can rapidly progress to organ failure if not treated promptly. Early diagnosis is critical, but traditional methods often detect sepsis too late. AI-powered models can predict the onset of sepsis several hours before clinical signs become apparent. By continuously analyzing vital signs, lab results (e.g., white blood cell count, lactate levels) and EHR data, these systems identify patterns suggestive of sepsis risk. Real-time alerts allow medical staff to intervene sooner, administering fluids, antibiotics or other treatments quickly. Predictive analytics thus plays a vital role in reducing mortality rates and intensive care unit (ICU) admissions. These models are especially valuable in emergency departments and high-dependency wards where rapid decision-making is essential. As model accuracy improves, sepsis detection tools are becoming a standard part of hospital monitoring systems.
- **Mental Health Risk Scoring:** Mental health is often underdiagnosed, but predictive analytics is opening new avenues for early detection and intervention. ML models analyze a variety of data sources—including speech patterns, text input from messaging apps, sleep habits, smartphone usage and even social media activity—to detect signs of mental distress. For example, reduced sleep, changes in communication style or increased isolation can signal depression or suicidal ideation. These non-invasive indicators are especially useful for populations reluctant to seek help. AI-powered mental health tools are also integrated into chatbots and mobile apps that assess mood and deliver real-time support or referrals. For clinicians, risk scores generated from such data help prioritize care for those most in need. Predictive analytics enhances the ability to offer

personalized and timely mental health support, reducing the risk of crisis situations and promoting long-term well-being.

Benefits of Predictive Analytics and Risk Scoring

- **Early Intervention:** Predictive analytics enables early identification of patients at risk of developing serious health issues—even before symptoms manifest. By analyzing historical data, real-time vitals and behavioral patterns, AI models can flag warning signs such as irregular heart rhythms, rising glucose levels or subtle respiratory changes. Early detection allows healthcare providers to intervene proactively rather than wait for conditions to worsen. For instance, catching signs of sepsis or heart failure in early stages can prevent life-threatening outcomes. This approach not only saves lives but also improves patient confidence and long-term health. Early intervention also reduces the need for emergency room visits and intensive treatments, making care more manageable and less disruptive.
- **Personalized Care:** AI-driven risk scoring enables healthcare professionals to move away from a one-size-fits-all model and instead tailor treatment plans to individual needs. By considering a person's unique genetic makeup, lifestyle, clinical history and risk profile, personalized care becomes both precise and effective. For example, two diabetic patients may have very different glucose patterns and therefore require different treatment strategies. Machine learning can adjust recommendations in real time, based on changing health data. This personalization improves treatment adherence, enhances patient satisfaction and boosts overall health outcomes. It also helps clinicians prioritize interventions for those who will benefit the most. Personalized care is a core principle of modern, data-driven medicine.
- **Resource Optimization:** Predictive analytics helps healthcare organizations allocate resources more effectively by identifying which patients need immediate attention and which can be managed with routine care. Hospitals can use risk scores to prioritize ICU beds, discharge planning and follow-up schedules. This targeted approach prevents overuse of emergency services and underuse of preventive care. AI can also forecast demand for services, staffing needs or medication supplies based on population-level trends. By optimizing the use of staff, time and medical equipment, healthcare systems can improve operational efficiency. This ensures better service delivery without overwhelming the system, especially in times of crisis or high patient volumes.
- **Improved Outcomes:** One of the most impactful benefits of predictive analytics is the overall improvement in clinical outcomes. By detecting

conditions early, guiding accurate diagnoses and informing targeted treatments, predictive models contribute to fewer complications, quicker recoveries and lower mortality rates. For chronic illnesses, predictive systems help patients maintain better control of their conditions through continuous monitoring and timely alerts. Hospitals using AI-assisted risk scoring have reported reductions in readmission rates and adverse events. These improvements reflect a shift from reactive care to a more proactive, patient-centered approach. Better outcomes also foster trust in the healthcare system and strengthen provider-patient relationships.

- **Cost Reduction:** Preventive and predictive healthcare significantly reduces overall medical costs—for both patients and providers. By catching diseases early and preventing hospitalizations or emergency interventions, predictive models decrease the need for expensive treatments and prolonged hospital stays. For example, identifying patients at high risk of heart failure before a crisis can avoid costly ER visits and ICU admissions. Efficient resource utilization also cuts operational costs for hospitals and insurance providers. Additionally, patients benefit from fewer missed workdays, reduced out-of-pocket expenses and improved quality of life. In the long run, AI-enabled cost reduction contributes to a more sustainable and accessible healthcare system.

Implementation Challenges

Despite their promise, several challenges exist:

- **Data Quality and Integration:** The effectiveness of predictive analytics relies heavily on the quality and completeness of the data used. In healthcare, data is often fragmented across various systems, such as electronic health records (EHRs), lab reports, imaging archives and wearable devices. Inconsistencies, missing values, outdated entries or incorrect coding can significantly impact the accuracy of AI predictions. Furthermore, integrating diverse data sources—structured and unstructured—poses technical and interoperability challenges. If the input data is not harmonized or standardized, models may produce unreliable or misleading results. High-quality, well-curated data is essential for training accurate and trustworthy predictive models that can support real-world clinical decisions.
- **Bias and Fairness:** Machine learning models are only as fair as the data they are trained on. If the training datasets reflect historical disparities or underrepresent certain populations (e.g., based on race, gender, age or socioeconomic status), the resulting models may perpetuate or even amplify these biases. This can lead to unequal risk assessments and care recommendations, putting vulnerable groups at greater risk. For

example, a model trained predominantly on data from urban hospitals may perform poorly for rural populations. Ensuring fairness requires diverse, representative datasets and continuous monitoring of model performance across demographic subgroups. Ethical AI development must prioritize equity, transparency and accountability to avoid reinforcing systemic biases in healthcare.

- **Interpretability:** While many machine learning models offer high predictive accuracy, they often lack transparency in how they arrive at their conclusions—especially complex models like deep learning networks. This "black box" nature creates a barrier for clinicians, who need to understand and trust the model's reasoning before acting on its predictions. Interpretability is critical for clinical acceptance and decision-making. Tools such as SHAP (SHapley Additive exPlanations), LIME (Local Interpretable Model-agnostic Explanations) and rule-based AI help explain how specific inputs contribute to a prediction. Balancing performance with interpretability is a key design challenge in deploying AI in real-world healthcare settings, where life-impacting decisions are at stake.
- **Privacy and Security:** Healthcare data is highly sensitive and the use of AI introduces new concerns about privacy and cybersecurity. Predictive analytics systems require access to large volumes of personal health information, which must be stored, processed and shared securely. Any data breach or unauthorized use can lead to serious consequences for patients and institutions. Compliance with data protection regulations such as HIPAA (Health Insurance Portability and Accountability Act) in the U.S. and GDPR (General Data Protection Regulation) in Europe is mandatory. Techniques like data anonymization, encryption and federated learning are being explored to protect patient identities while enabling effective analytics. Building secure, privacy-conscious AI systems is essential for public trust and ethical healthcare innovation.
- **Clinical Validation:** Before predictive models can be deployed in clinical practice, they must undergo rigorous testing and validation to ensure safety, reliability and effectiveness. A model that performs well in development may not maintain the same accuracy in different patient populations or healthcare settings. Clinical validation involves prospective trials, peer-reviewed studies and regulatory review—similar to the approval process for new drugs or devices. Without this validation, there's a risk of false predictions leading to inappropriate treatment decisions. Additionally, models must be continuously monitored and updated to adapt to changes in clinical practice and population health trends. Only through proper

validation can AI tools gain the trust of clinicians, patients and regulatory bodies.

Future Directions

- **Real-Time Risk Scoring Systems:** Real-time risk scoring systems are set to transform healthcare by integrating AI with wearable and Internet of Things (IoT) devices for continuous health monitoring. These systems collect vital signs such as heart rate, oxygen saturation, glucose levels and movement data 24/7. Using AI algorithms, they analyze this stream of information in real time to detect deviations from normal patterns and generate instant alerts for patients and providers. This enables early intervention before a condition worsens, especially in chronic disease management and post-discharge monitoring. Real-time systems reduce dependency on in-person visits, lower hospitalization rates and promote proactive care. They offer immense potential in managing elderly care, cardiac monitoring and emergency response situations.
- **Federated Learning:** Federated Learning is a cutting-edge AI approach that allows models to be trained across multiple decentralized data sources—such as hospitals, clinics and research institutions—without the need to share raw patient data. This technique enhances patient privacy and data security, as sensitive health data remains on local devices or servers. Instead, only model updates (not personal information) are shared and aggregated centrally. Federated learning enables the development of robust, generalizable predictive models using diverse datasets from different populations and healthcare environments. It also addresses regulatory challenges related to data sharing across regions or countries. As privacy concerns grow, federated learning represents a sustainable way to scale AI in healthcare.
- **Explainable AI (XAI):** Explainable AI (XAI) focuses on making AI model decisions transparent, understandable and interpretable by humans—especially clinicians. Unlike traditional "black box" models, XAI provides insights into which features or inputs influenced a specific prediction and how. This builds clinician trust, supports ethical decision-making and ensures accountability in high-stakes environments like healthcare. For example, a risk score predicting a heart attack might highlight high cholesterol, irregular ECG patterns and lifestyle factors as key contributors. Tools like SHAP values, LIME and attention mechanisms are commonly used in XAI. As regulatory and clinical standards evolve, explainability will become essential for the adoption and approval of AI tools in medical practice.

- **Integration with Telehealth:** The rise of telehealth has created new opportunities for integrating AI-driven risk scoring into virtual care platforms. By embedding predictive analytics tools into telemedicine systems, healthcare providers can prioritize patient outreach, monitor chronic conditions remotely and deliver personalized care without needing face-to-face visits. For instance, a telehealth platform could flag patients at high risk of COPD exacerbation based on self-reported symptoms and wearable data, prompting timely video consultations or medication adjustments. This integration enhances care continuity, reduces emergency visits and supports rural or underserved populations with limited access to physical clinics. As virtual healthcare becomes more mainstream, risk scoring will be central to optimizing remote patient management and improving digital health outcomes.

Predictive analytics and risk scoring represent a paradigm shift in health monitoring by moving from reactive care to proactive and preventive healthcare. With the help of AI and ML, healthcare systems can identify health risks early, tailor interventions to individual needs and ultimately improve outcomes for patients across the globe. However, careful consideration of ethical, technical and practical issues is essential to maximize their potential and ensure equitable healthcare delivery.

2.5.2 Pattern Recognition in Health Data

Pattern recognition is a foundational capability of artificial intelligence (AI) systems, referring to their ability to automatically identify and interpret regularities, anomalies, trends and clusters within complex and often large-scale datasets. In the context of healthcare, this capability has tremendous value because medical data is inherently multifaceted, heterogeneous and continuously generated from a variety of sources such as electronic health records (EHRs), wearable devices, medical imaging and genomic sequencing. Traditional methods of data analysis rely heavily on manual review or straightforward statistical techniques, which can be time-consuming, subjective and limited in detecting subtle or complex patterns. AI-powered pattern recognition, by contrast, uses advanced machine learning algorithms that can learn from vast amounts of historical and real-time data, uncovering hidden relationships that may not be evident even to experienced clinicians. Through this process, AI can detect early warning signs of diseases before clinical symptoms become apparent, enabling earlier interventions and improving patient outcomes. For example, subtle variations in electrocardiogram (ECG) waveforms can signal an impending cardiac event, while changes in retinal imaging can reveal early diabetic complications. Moreover, pattern recognition allows the identification of disease signatures—unique combinations of biomarkers, imaging features or physiological signals—that can differentiate between various types or stages of illness. This leads to more accurate diagnoses and helps clinicians personalize treatment plans according to the specific needs of each patient.In addition to diagnosing diseases, AI can monitor treatment responses over time by recognizing how a patient's data evolves, highlighting whether therapies are effective or if adjustments are needed. It can also identify clusters of patients with similar characteristics or disease trajectories, which is invaluable for understanding disease progression and for clinical trial recruitment. The ability to analyze real-time streaming data from wearable devices and Internet of Things (IoT) sensors further enhances continuous health monitoring, offering dynamic insights and timely alerts. The speed at which AI-powered systems analyze complex datasets far surpasses human capabilities, enabling quicker clinical decisions that can be lifesaving in critical situations such as sepsis or stroke. Furthermore, pattern recognition supports population health management by identifying epidemiological trends and emerging health threats, guiding public health interventions more effectively. However, the success of these systems depends on the quality and integration of data, as well as ensuring algorithms are transparent, interpretable and free from bias. Overall, pattern recognition is transforming healthcare by enabling proactive, precise and personalized medicine, shifting the paradigm from reactive treatment to prevention and early intervention. It empowers clinicians with powerful tools to navigate vast data landscapes, uncovering meaningful patterns that improve diagnosis, monitoring and treatment—ultimately enhancing patient care and health outcomes across diverse populations.

Pattern recognition in health data involves using machine learning and statistical algorithms to identify recurring structures or behaviors in medical data. This includes detecting abnormal heart rhythms, cancerous lesions in imaging or blood glucose patterns over time. Recognizing such patterns helps predict disease onset, recommend personalized treatments and monitor patient progress. Unlike rule-based systems, AI models learn from data, improving their recognition capabilities over time.

Types of Health Data for Pattern Recognition

AI systems work with various types of health-related data, including:

- **Time-series Data:** Time-series data in healthcare refers to sequences of measurements recorded over time, such as electrocardiograms (ECG), blood pressure readings, oxygen saturation levels and respiratory rates. These data streams capture dynamic physiological changes and provide rich information about a patient's current health status and trends. AI algorithms analyze this temporal data to detect abnormal patterns, like arrhythmias in ECG or sudden drops in oxygen levels, that could signal impending medical events. The continuous nature of time-series data enables real-time monitoring and early warning systems, which are critical for managing chronic diseases and acute conditions. Advanced models such as recurrent neural networks (RNNs) and long short-term memory networks (LSTMs) are particularly suited for extracting meaningful patterns from time-dependent health signals. This continuous analysis improves timely interventions and patient outcomes by alerting healthcare providers promptly.

- **Medical Imaging:** Medical imaging includes techniques such as X-rays, magnetic resonance imaging (MRI) and computed tomography (CT) scans, which produce detailed visual representations of the body's internal structures. Pattern recognition in medical imaging allows AI to identify abnormalities like tumors, fractures or lesions with high accuracy and speed. Deep learning models, especially convolutional neural networks (CNNs), excel at detecting subtle image features that might be overlooked by human eyes. For instance, AI can highlight suspicious nodules in lung scans or early signs of stroke in brain imaging. This automation supports radiologists by reducing diagnostic errors and workload and enhances early diagnosis and treatment planning. Additionally, pattern recognition aids in monitoring disease progression by comparing imaging results over time, providing quantitative insights into therapy effectiveness.
- **Genomic Data:** Genomic data consists of DNA sequences and their variations, which provide insights into inherited conditions and disease susceptibility. AI analyzes patterns in genomic data to identify mutations or gene expressions linked to diseases like cancer, rare genetic disorders or cardiovascular conditions. By recognizing these genetic signatures, clinicians can predict risks, tailor treatments and guide personalized medicine strategies. Machine learning models handle the high dimensionality and complexity of genomic datasets, detecting associations that may be missed by traditional methods. Moreover, pattern recognition helps in understanding gene-environment interactions and pharmacogenomics—how patients respond to medications based on their genetic makeup. This empowers precision health approaches, improving preventive care and targeted therapies.
- **Electronic Health Record (EHR) Data:** EHR data includes patient demographics, clinical notes, diagnoses, lab results, medication histories and treatment plans recorded over time. Pattern recognition in EHR data helps identify recurring trends or risk factors, such as frequent hospital admissions, medication non-adherence or worsening lab markers. Natural language processing (NLP) techniques extract useful information from

unstructured text like physician notes or discharge summaries. This enables AI to generate comprehensive risk profiles and predict disease progression or hospital readmission. Analyzing EHR data supports clinical decision-making by highlighting critical changes in a patient's condition, facilitating timely interventions. Integration of longitudinal data enhances understanding of complex, chronic conditions and guides personalized treatment pathways.

- **Wearable Device Data:** Wearable devices, such as fitness trackers and smartwatches, continuously collect health-related data including daily physical activity, sleep quality, heart rate variability and stress indicators. Pattern recognition applied to this data enables real-time health monitoring outside clinical settings. AI algorithms detect deviations from normal patterns, such as irregular heartbeats or disrupted sleep cycles, alerting users and clinicians to potential health issues. This continuous data stream supports chronic disease management, fitness optimization and early detection of conditions like atrial fibrillation or sleep apnea. Wearables empower individuals with personalized feedback and encourage healthier behaviors, while also providing valuable longitudinal data for clinical research. The integration of wearable data with other health records enhances holistic patient care and remote monitoring capabilities.

These diverse sources offer rich datasets for discovering both normal and abnormal health trends.

Algorithms Used in Pattern Recognition

Several ML and AI techniques are employed to identify patterns in health data:

- **Convolutional Neural Networks (CNNs):** Convolutional Neural Networks (CNNs) are a class of deep learning models specifically designed for processing grid-like data such as images. In healthcare, CNNs are extensively used for medical image analysis, including tumor detection, identifying fractures and diagnosing diseases from X-rays, MRIs and CT scans. CNNs automatically learn spatial hierarchies of features, from edges and textures to complex shapes, enabling them to detect subtle abnormalities that might escape human eyes. Their ability to process high-dimensional imaging data with minimal preprocessing has revolutionized radiology and pathology workflows. By improving the speed and accuracy of image interpretation, CNNs help reduce diagnostic errors and support early intervention. Moreover, CNNs can segment organs and lesions precisely, aiding treatment planning and monitoring.
- **Recurrent Neural Networks (RNNs) and LSTMs:** Recurrent Neural Networks (RNNs) and their advanced variant, Long Short-Term Memory

networks (LSTMs), are well-suited for analyzing sequential or time-series data, making them ideal for healthcare applications like ECG signal analysis and glucose monitoring. These models have memory cells that capture temporal dependencies, allowing them to understand how current data points relate to previous ones. This enables the detection of irregular heartbeats, blood sugar trends or respiratory patterns over time. LSTMs address the vanishing gradient problem of standard RNNs, allowing them to learn long-range dependencies critical in clinical time-series data. Their application facilitates continuous patient monitoring, early warning of adverse events and improved chronic disease management through accurate prediction of future physiological states.

- **Clustering Algorithms (e.g., k-means):** Clustering algorithms, such as k-means, group similar data points without requiring labeled outcomes, making them valuable for discovering patient subgroups or disease phenotypes in healthcare data. These unsupervised learning methods analyze features like symptoms, genetic markers or treatment responses to identify natural groupings within patient populations. For example, clustering can reveal different types of diabetes or cancer subtypes based on clinical and molecular data. This stratification helps tailor treatment plans to specific patient groups, improving personalized medicine. Clustering also supports epidemiological studies by uncovering patterns in population health and identifying risk factors. The simplicity and scalability of algorithms like k-means make them practical for exploratory data analysis in large healthcare datasets.
- **Principal Component Analysis (PCA):** Principal Component Analysis (PCA) is a statistical technique used to reduce the dimensionality of complex healthcare datasets while preserving the most important variation related to patterns. By transforming original correlated variables into a smaller set of uncorrelated components, PCA simplifies data visualization and analysis. This is especially useful in genomics, imaging and multi-parameter clinical data where thousands of features can overwhelm traditional models. PCA helps eliminate noise and redundancy, improving the efficiency and accuracy of subsequent machine learning tasks. It also facilitates the discovery of underlying patterns, such as gene expression profiles associated with disease or imaging features correlated with outcomes. PCA remains a foundational tool for pre-processing and exploratory analysis in healthcare AI.
- **Anomaly Detection Algorithms:** Anomaly detection algorithms are designed to identify rare or unusual patterns that deviate significantly

from normal health data, such as sudden spikes in blood pressure or unexpected changes in heart rhythms. These methods are critical for early detection of acute medical events like sepsis, stroke or arrhythmias. By continuously monitoring patient data from EHRs, wearables or ICU sensors, anomaly detection models can trigger alerts for clinicians before conditions deteriorate. Techniques include statistical methods, clustering-based approaches and neural network models tailored to detect outliers. Effective anomaly detection improves patient safety, reduces emergency admissions and supports proactive interventions. Its ability to handle streaming data in real time makes it indispensable in critical care and remote health monitoring.

Each algorithm is chosen based on the nature of the data and the clinical objective.

Clinical Applications of Pattern Recognition

Anomaly detection algorithms are designed to identify rare or unusual patterns that deviate significantly from normal health data, such as sudden spikes in blood pressure or unexpected changes in heart rhythms. These methods are critical for early detection of acute medical events like sepsis, stroke or arrhythmias. By continuously monitoring patient data from EHRs, wearables or ICU sensors, anomaly detection models can trigger alerts for clinicians before conditions deteriorate. Techniques include statistical methods, clustering-based approaches and neural network models tailored to detect outliers. Effective anomaly detection improves patient safety, reduces emergency admissions and supports proactive interventions. Its ability to handle streaming data in real time makes it indispensable in critical care and remote health monitoring.

- **Early Disease Detection:** AI-based pattern recognition enables the identification of diseases at their earliest stages—often before noticeable symptoms arise. By analyzing subtle physiological or imaging changes, AI can detect signs of illness that may go undetected during routine checkups. For instance, in ophthalmology, AI can identify microaneurysms or minor hemorrhages in retinal scans, which are early indicators of diabetic retinopathy. Similarly, AI models trained on time-series data can find unusual trends in heart rate, oxygen saturation or lab results that precede acute conditions like sepsis or heart attacks. Early detection allows for timely interventions, improved prognoses and reduced treatment costs. It shifts the focus of healthcare from reactive to proactive, fundamentally transforming patient care. This approach is especially impactful in chronic and lifestyle-related diseases, where early management can prevent long-term complications.

- **Cancer Diagnosis:** Pattern recognition through AI plays a significant role in improving the speed and accuracy of cancer diagnosis. AI systems can process and interpret medical imaging—such as mammograms, CT scans and MRIs—to detect irregularities like abnormal tissue density, unusual cell growth or early tumor formations. Convolutional Neural Networks (CNNs) excel at identifying these subtle patterns, often surpassing human accuracy, especially in complex or borderline cases. These tools assist radiologists by highlighting suspicious regions, reducing oversight and diagnostic variability. AI can also compare current imaging with previous scans to track tumor progression or regression. Furthermore, AI algorithms can analyze biopsy slides for histological patterns, helping pathologists classify cancer types and grades. Ultimately, AI augments diagnostic confidence, speeds up decision-making and contributes to better treatment planning.
- **Arrhythmia Detection:** AI and pattern recognition techniques are widely used in analyzing electrocardiogram (ECG) signals to detect arrhythmias—abnormal heart rhythms that may lead to serious complications if left unnoticed. Recurrent Neural Networks (RNNs) and LSTMs are particularly effective at processing the sequential nature of ECG data. These models learn from large datasets to identify deviations such as premature beats, tachycardia, bradycardia or atrial fibrillation. While some arrhythmias are transient and difficult to catch in clinical settings, AI can monitor continuous ECG data from wearable devices and flag irregularities in real time. This aids in early diagnosis and timely treatment of heart rhythm disorders, reducing the risk of strokes or cardiac arrest. AI-enhanced ECG monitoring also enables remote cardiac care, improving access for at-risk patients in rural or underserved areas.
- **Chronic Disease Monitoring:** Chronic conditions like asthma, diabetes and chronic obstructive pulmonary disease (COPD) require continuous and long-term monitoring, which AI can efficiently facilitate through pattern recognition. By analyzing time-series data from wearables, EHRs and patient-reported outcomes, AI systems detect patterns in symptoms, medication adherence and environmental factors (e.g., pollution or allergens). For example, an AI model may identify a correlation between air quality and asthma flare-ups, prompting preventive alerts. These insights help clinicians personalize treatment and make real-time adjustments to care plans. Moreover, predictive algorithms can warn patients of potential exacerbations before they occur, minimizing emergency visits. Chronic disease management becomes more proactive, efficient and patient-centered through intelligent monitoring and early intervention tools.

- **Mental Health Monitoring:** Pattern recognition is increasingly being applied to monitor mental health conditions such as depression, anxiety and bipolar disorder. AI analyzes linguistic patterns from speech, chat messages or social media posts, detecting changes in tone, word choice or sentence structure associated with mental distress. Additionally, wearable and smartphone data—such as changes in sleep patterns, physical activity, phone usage and social interactions—can reveal behavioral changes linked to mood disorders. Machine learning models identify these subtle deviations from personal baselines, enabling early detection of mental health deterioration. This non-invasive approach supports continuous monitoring and allows for timely mental health interventions. It also helps clinicians track treatment effectiveness and adjust strategies accordingly, improving long-term outcomes and patient well-being.

Advantages of Pattern Recognition in Healthcare

- **Speed and Efficiency:** One of the key advantages of AI in healthcare is its unparalleled speed and efficiency. AI systems can rapidly analyze vast amounts of complex and multi-dimensional health data, such as electronic health records, medical images and real-time sensor outputs. Tasks that would take healthcare professionals hours or even days—like reviewing patient histories or detecting abnormalities in scans—can be completed in seconds with AI. This rapid processing capability supports faster diagnoses, quicker decision-making and more efficient clinical workflows. It also reduces administrative burden, freeing up time for doctors and nurses to focus more on direct patient care. Overall, AI helps streamline healthcare delivery, especially in high-volume settings like emergency rooms and large hospitals.
- **Accuracy:** AI algorithms, when properly trained and validated, can significantly reduce human error in medical analysis and decision-making. By identifying subtle patterns and correlations that may not be apparent to clinicians, AI systems can enhance diagnostic precision. For example, AI models have shown high accuracy in detecting cancers from radiology scans, identifying cardiac arrhythmias from ECGs and predicting disease risks from EHRs. These systems are also consistent—they don't suffer from fatigue or cognitive bias like human observers. Improved accuracy means fewer missed diagnoses, better treatment planning and reduced risk of complications. This contributes directly to better patient outcomes and increased confidence in healthcare processes.
- **Real-Time Analysis:** AI-powered real-time analysis allows for the continuous monitoring of patients using data from wearables, IoT devices

and bedside monitors. By evaluating health metrics such as heart rate, oxygen saturation, glucose levels and sleep patterns in real time, AI can detect critical changes as they occur. This capability is particularly important for managing patients with chronic illnesses, those in critical care or individuals recovering at home. Immediate alerts can be sent to healthcare providers or caregivers if anomalies are detected, allowing for timely interventions. Real-time monitoring also empowers patients with up-to-date insights into their own health, promoting self-care and early response to health concerns.

- **Scalability:** AI systems are inherently scalable, making them well-suited for deployment across large healthcare networks, national screening programs or global research initiatives. Once developed and trained, an AI model can be deployed to analyze millions of patient records, scans or wearable outputs with minimal additional cost or labor. This scalability allows healthcare providers to extend high-quality services to more people, even in resource-limited settings. AI also enables centralized analysis of distributed data, which is especially useful in telemedicine and remote health monitoring. As health systems deal with growing patient loads and limited staff, scalable AI solutions offer a sustainable way to meet demand without compromising care quality.
- **Personalization:** AI excels at identifying individual patterns in a patient's health data, paving the way for truly personalized medicine. By analyzing genetic profiles, lifestyle behaviors, historical health records and physiological responses, AI can tailor treatment plans to each patient's unique characteristics. For instance, two patients with the same diagnosis may receive different drug recommendations based on how their bodies metabolize medications. Similarly, AI can predict which lifestyle changes are most likely to benefit a specific individual. Personalized care improves treatment efficacy, reduces side effects and enhances patient engagement. As precision medicine advances, AI will continue to be a vital tool in customizing healthcare delivery at an individual level.

Challenges and Limitations

- **Data Noise and Quality:** The accuracy of AI-driven pattern recognition heavily depends on the quality of the input data. In healthcare, data is often incomplete, inconsistent or collected using different standards across institutions. Noise in the data—such as errors in medical records, faulty sensor readings or transcription mistakes—can lead to incorrect pattern identification. For instance, mislabeling a disease diagnosis or inconsistent use of medical terminology can mislead machine learning models. Cleaning and standardizing healthcare data is time-consuming and requires domain expertise. Without high-quality data, even the most sophisticated algorithms can produce unreliable results. Ensuring data integrity is essential for building trustworthy and accurate AI systems in healthcare.

- **Overfitting:** Overfitting occurs when an AI model becomes too tailored to the training dataset, learning even the random noise instead of generalizable patterns. In healthcare, this can be particularly dangerous, as the model may perform well on test data but fail to identify patterns correctly in real-world, unseen cases. For example, a model trained on a specific hospital's imaging data might struggle with images from a different facility due to slight variations in equipment or population demographics. Overfitting often results from small datasets, overly complex models or insufficient validation. Mitigating overfitting requires careful model tuning, diverse training data and rigorous cross-validation techniques.
- **Interpretability Issues:** Many AI models, especially deep learning systems, function as "black boxes," offering little insight into how specific predictions or pattern recognitions are made. This lack of interpretability can hinder clinical adoption, as healthcare providers need to understand and trust the rationale behind AI-driven decisions. For example, if an AI model flags a patient as high risk for stroke, clinicians need to know which features or patterns led to that conclusion. Without transparency, it's difficult to validate the model's reasoning or identify errors. Tools like Explainable AI (XAI) and feature attribution methods aim to bridge this gap, but explainability remains a major challenge in clinical environments.
- **Bias in Training Data:** AI models learn patterns based on the data they are trained on, so if the training data contains bias or lacks representation, the resulting model can produce skewed outcomes. In healthcare, bias may stem from underrepresentation of certain ethnicities, genders, age groups or socioeconomic backgrounds. For example, a model trained primarily on data from urban hospitals might not perform well in rural or minority populations. This can lead to unequal healthcare outcomes, reinforcing existing disparities. Addressing bias requires deliberate inclusion of diverse datasets and ongoing fairness audits throughout model development and deployment. Ethical AI demands that pattern recognition tools be equitable and inclusive.
- **Computational Requirements:** Training and deploying AI models for pattern recognition—especially those using deep learning—requires significant computational power, memory and storage. Medical data, such as 3D imaging or high-frequency wearable sensor streams, can be extremely

large and complex. Running real-time analytics or processing data across large hospital networks often demands high-performance GPUs, specialized software and scalable infrastructure. These requirements can pose barriers for smaller healthcare facilities or developing regions with limited IT resources. Additionally, the cost of maintaining and updating these systems may be prohibitive. Balancing computational needs with accessibility is a key consideration in scaling AI solutions across the healthcare system.

Future Directions

- **Multimodal Pattern Recognition:** Multimodal pattern recognition involves combining various types of healthcare data—such as medical imaging, genomic profiles, clinical records and wearable sensor outputs—to gain a comprehensive understanding of a patient's condition. By integrating these diverse data streams, AI can uncover complex relationships and improve diagnostic accuracy. For instance, combining imaging data with genetic markers can help detect cancer subtypes more precisely. This holistic approach enables better risk stratification, more accurate predictions and personalized treatment recommendations. Multimodal AI systems reflect the real-world complexity of patient health, enhancing both clinical and research applications. As data interoperability improves, this integrated analysis will become increasingly practical and powerful in clinical decision-making.
- **Real-Time Decision Support:** Real-time decision support refers to the integration of AI-powered pattern recognition tools directly into clinical workflows to assist healthcare professionals during patient care. These systems provide immediate feedback and suggestions based on continuously updated data, such as alerts for abnormal vitals, drug interaction risks or potential diagnoses. For example, in emergency departments, AI can analyze a patient's symptoms and history in real-time to suggest likely causes or recommend urgent interventions. This instant support reduces response time, enhances accuracy and helps clinicians make better-informed decisions under pressure. Real-time tools can also prioritize high-risk patients, optimize resource use and reduce medical errors.
- **Edge Computing in Wearables:** Edge computing refers to processing data locally on the device (such as a smartwatch or fitness tracker) rather than sending it to centralized servers. In healthcare, this enables real-time pattern recognition directly on wearable devices, allowing for faster detection of anomalies such as irregular heart rhythms or falls. By eliminating delays caused by data transmission to the cloud, edge computing ensures immediate alerts and actions, which is critical for managing conditions

like epilepsy, diabetes or cardiovascular issues. It also reduces bandwidth usage and enhances data privacy since sensitive information doesn't need to leave the device. As wearable technology advances, edge AI will become central to continuous, responsive and patient-centric care.

- **Explainable AI Tools:** Explainable AI (XAI) focuses on making the decision-making process of complex AI models transparent and understandable to human users, especially clinicians. In healthcare, this means showing not just the prediction, but why and how it was made—what features or data patterns influenced the model's output. This is crucial for building trust in AI recommendations and ensuring safe clinical adoption. Tools like SHAP (SHapley Additive exPlanations) and LIME (Local Interpretable Model-agnostic Explanations) help visualize and interpret these decisions. Clinicians can use XAI to verify AI insights, refine diagnoses and communicate findings with patients. As AI grows more sophisticated, interpretability will remain a cornerstone for ethical and effective implementation in healthcare.
- **Population Health Insights:** AI-driven pattern recognition can extend beyond individual patients to identify trends and risks at the community or population level. By analyzing aggregated health data from clinics, wearables or public sources, AI can detect emerging public health threats—such as flu outbreaks, chronic disease trends or environmental health hazards. For instance, during the COVID-19 pandemic, AI models helped identify regional spikes, predict hospital demand and assess the effectiveness of containment strategies. These insights inform policy decisions, guide resource allocation and enable targeted interventions. Population-level pattern recognition enhances public health surveillance and supports proactive, data-driven responses to both local and global health challenges.

Pattern recognition is revolutionizing health data analysis by enabling early detection, improving diagnosis accuracy and personalizing treatment plans. By leveraging AI's ability to uncover hidden trends across various data types, healthcare providers can move toward more proactive, precise and preventative care. However, addressing issues like interpretability, data quality and bias remains crucial for safe and ethical implementation.

2.6 CLOUD COMPUTING AND DATA STORAGE IN DIGITAL HEALTH

Cloud computing and modern data storage solutions have fundamentally reshaped the landscape of digital health, offering unprecedented capabilities for storing, accessing and managing healthcare data. As healthcare systems generate massive volumes of information—from electronic health records (EHRs) and imaging files to genomic sequences and real-time wearable data—the need for scalable and reliable infrastructure has become essential. Cloud platforms meet this demand by providing virtually unlimited storage capacity, flexible computing resources and seamless access across locations. Unlike traditional on-premises servers that are often costly, rigid and prone to downtime, cloud environments offer dynamic scalability, allowing healthcare organizations to expand or contract their resources based on workload and patient volume. In clinical practice, cloud computing enables real-time access to patient data, empowering physicians and care teams to make informed decisions from anywhere with a secure internet connection. This is particularly crucial for telemedicine, emergency care and collaborative treatment models where time and communication are critical. Through cloud-based EHR systems, clinicians can instantly retrieve medical histories, lab results and diagnostic images, facilitating continuity of care and reducing redundant testing. For patients, cloud integration means greater control over their own health information. Patient portals allow individuals to view lab reports, schedule appointments and track treatment progress, fostering engagement and transparency in the care process. From a data analytics perspective, the cloud serves as a launchpad for advanced tools like artificial intelligence (AI), machine learning (ML) and big data analytics. These technologies thrive on large, diverse datasets—something cloud platforms can accommodate effortlessly. Healthcare researchers and data scientists use cloud services to process complex datasets for predictive modeling, drug discovery, population health studies and personalized medicine development. Cloud computing accelerates these workflows, reducing the time from discovery to deployment and enabling faster innovation in diagnostics and therapeutics. Security is another critical domain where cloud solutions excel. Major cloud service providers implement state-of-the-art cybersecurity measures, including data encryption, multi-factor authentication, access control and continuous monitoring. These tools help healthcare organizations comply with strict regulatory standards such as HIPAA in the U.S., GDPR in Europe and other national privacy laws. Moreover, cloud providers offer advanced backup and disaster recovery systems, ensuring that sensitive health data remains available and intact even in the event of hardware failure, cyberattack or natural disaster. Redundant storage across multiple data centers increases system resilience and minimizes downtime.

Interoperability is another transformative benefit. Cloud platforms often support open standards and APIs (e.g., HL7 FHIR), allowing diverse healthcare systems and third-party applications to communicate and exchange data efficiently. This integration fosters a more unified and patient-centered approach to care, breaking down data silos that traditionally hampered coordination between providers, insurers, pharmacies and labs. For example, a patient being treated by multiple specialists in different locations can have a consolidated record accessible to all involved clinicians, improving care coordination and reducing medical errors. Furthermore, cloud computing is instrumental in enabling remote patient monitoring and the Internet of Medical Things (IoMT). Wearable devices like smartwatches, glucose monitors and portable ECGs continuously collect health metrics and transmit the data to cloud servers for real-time analysis. Healthcare providers can monitor patients outside of clinical settings, detect early signs of deterioration and intervene before emergencies occur. This model of continuous care helps manage chronic diseases more effectively and reduces hospital readmission rates. In terms of cost-effectiveness, cloud solutions offer a shift from capital expenditure (CapEx) to operational expenditure (OpEx). Organizations pay only for the resources they use, eliminating the need for expensive hardware purchases and IT maintenance. This model is especially advantageous for small clinics and startups seeking to leverage cutting-edge technology without heavy financial burdens. The flexibility and scalability of the cloud democratize access to digital health tools, making innovation more inclusive. As the healthcare sector continues to evolve, cloud computing and data storage will remain foundational technologies enabling digital transformation. Future developments, such as federated learning, edge-cloud integration and serverless architecture, will further enhance cloud capabilities. These innovations promise faster data processing, stronger data privacy and more intelligent health systems that respond adaptively to patient needs. In essence, the cloud is not just a storage solution—it is the backbone of a smarter, more connected and more efficient healthcare ecosystem.

2.6.1 Scalable Data Storage

Cloud computing provides healthcare systems with virtually limitless storage capacity to manage the massive and ever-growing volume of health data. This includes structured data like EHRs and lab results, as well as unstructured data such as medical imaging, genomic sequences and continuous data from wearables. Cloud storage is elastic, meaning it automatically adjusts to meet storage demands, whether scaling up during periods of heavy usage or scaling down to reduce costs. This flexibility is crucial for large hospital networks and national health systems dealing with terabytes or petabytes of clinical data. Technologies like Amazon S3 and Microsoft Azure Blob Storage offer robust durability, ensuring long-term data integrity. Redundant data centers also provide fault tolerance and availability. Healthcare organizations no longer need to worry about running out of local storage or managing complex physical server infrastructures. Cloud storage solutions offer high availability with built-in replication and failover capabilities. These features support continuity of care even during hardware failures or network outages. The scalability and resilience of cloud platforms empower healthcare providers to innovate without being limited by legacy systems.

2.6.2 Data Interoperability and Integration

Interoperability remains one of the most pressing challenges in healthcare IT and cloud infrastructure plays a key role in addressing it. By leveraging standardized protocols and APIs—such as HL7, FHIR and DICOM—cloud systems enable different health IT systems to exchange and interpret data seamlessly. This allows integration of various data sources, including EHRs, imaging software, lab systems, mobile health apps and wearable devices. The result is a unified ecosystem where clinicians, pharmacists and administrators can access synchronized patient information in real time. Cloud-based platforms also enable third-party developers to create modular healthcare apps that can plug into existing systems, accelerating innovation. Integration improves care coordination by giving providers access to complete patient histories, reducing medical errors and unnecessary tests. It also enhances operational efficiency, as integrated systems eliminate duplicate data entry and streamline workflows. Ultimately, interoperable cloud solutions support the vision of connected, patient-centered care across providers, locations and even national borders.

2.6.3 Real-Time Data Access and Sharing

One of the greatest advantages of cloud computing in healthcare is its ability to provide real-time access to patient data from virtually any location. This feature supports mobile health applications, telemedicine and remote consultations, which are especially vital in rural and underserved communities. Clinicians can instantly retrieve lab results, imaging and patient notes using secure, cloud-based dashboards. Real-time access enhances clinical decision-making during time-sensitive scenarios like trauma care or infectious disease outbreaks. Cloud systems also enable seamless data sharing among different departments, hospitals or even countries, supporting collaborative care and medical tourism. Patients, too, benefit from real-time portals where they can view health records, receive medication reminders and communicate with providers. This transparency fosters patient engagement, adherence and satisfaction. Cloud platforms offer secure sharing tools with role-based access to ensure that only authorized users can view sensitive data. In emergencies, rapid data access can be life-saving by helping physicians understand a patient's history before initiating treatment. Cloud-facilitated real-time data sharing has thus become a pillar of modern, responsive healthcare.

2.6.4 Enhanced Data Security and Compliance

Security is a top concern in digital health and leading cloud providers offer advanced security frameworks to safeguard sensitive healthcare data. These include end-to-end encryption (at rest and in transit), multi-factor authentication, intrusion detection systems and firewall protections. Cloud platforms also support detailed access controls, allowing administrators to assign permissions based on roles and responsibilities. These measures help healthcare institutions meet rigorous legal and regulatory requirements like HIPAA in the U.S., GDPR in the EU and others worldwide. Regular compliance checks and penetration testing are conducted to identify vulnerabilities proactively. Additionally, cloud services provide audit logs that record who accessed what data and when, aiding accountability and compliance audits. Security updates and patches are automatically deployed across the infrastructure, ensuring protection against emerging cyber threats. Cloud providers also train personnel in secure operations and offer tools for security risk management. By outsourcing much of the cybersecurity burden to experienced providers, healthcare organizations can focus more on patient care while maintaining data integrity and trust.

2.6.5 Disaster Recovery and Backup

Disaster recovery is essential in healthcare, where data loss or downtime can impact lives. Cloud platforms provide built-in redundancy, automated backups and geographic data replication to ensure business continuity. In the event of hardware failure, ransomware attacks or natural disasters, cloud systems enable rapid restoration of critical applications and patient records. Snapshots and versioning features allow for precise rollback to previous states without disrupting clinical operations. Failover mechanisms automatically switch workloads to backup data centers, minimizing downtime. This level of preparedness is costly and complex to achieve with on-premise systems but is a standard feature of major cloud providers. Automated backup schedules and data integrity checks ensure that the most current and accurate data is always retrievable. By protecting data from corruption and unauthorized tampering, these solutions increase reliability and regulatory compliance. Cloud-based disaster recovery also supports legal requirements for medical record retention. Ultimately, this resilience improves trust among providers, administrators and patients by ensuring that data is always secure and accessible.

2.6.6 Cost Efficiency

One of the most compelling benefits of cloud computing in healthcare is its cost-effectiveness. Unlike traditional IT systems that require substantial capital investment in servers, infrastructure and maintenance, cloud computing follows a pay-as-you-go model. This shift to operational expenditure (OpEx) allows organizations to pay only for the storage, bandwidth and computing resources they actually use. For small clinics, startups and nonprofit hospitals, this lowers the barrier to accessing cutting-edge digital health technologies. Additionally, cloud providers handle maintenance, upgrades and security, reducing the need for large in-house IT teams. Organizations can avoid unexpected downtime and costly system overhauls. The savings extend to energy usage as well—cloud data centers are more energy-efficient than local server rooms. Cost transparency is improved with detailed billing reports and usage analytics, allowing smarter budgeting and forecasting. Cloud computing also supports faster deployment of new applications and services, which can enhance revenue generation through telehealth, diagnostics or patient engagement platforms. In a sector where financial sustainability is critical, cloud adoption offers an efficient, scalable alternative to traditional IT infrastructure.

2.6.7 Support for Big Data and AI Analytics

Modern healthcare increasingly relies on big data analytics and AI to derive insights and cloud platforms are uniquely suited to support these capabilities. Cloud infrastructure can handle the storage and processing of massive datasets, such as whole-genome sequences, longitudinal EHRs and imaging archives. High-performance computing (HPC) clusters in the cloud allow for the training and deployment of complex AI models used for tasks like disease prediction, drug discovery and clinical decision support. Tools like Google Cloud's AutoML and AWS SageMaker simplify the development of AI workflows, even for non-experts. These platforms enable real-time analytics and interactive dashboards that help clinicians monitor patient populations or track health outcomes. Cloud-based AI also supports natural language processing (NLP) for extracting insights from clinical notes or unstructured texts. Importantly, cloud resources scale elastically AI workloads can spike during training and taper off after deployment without financial penalty. The integration of cloud and AI is thus central to the future of precision medicine, operational efficiency and evidence-based care.

2.6.8 Telemedicine and Remote Monitoring Integration

Telemedicine has rapidly expanded and cloud computing plays a vital role in enabling its scalability, reliability and security. Cloud-based platforms support secure video conferencing, asynchronous messaging and remote diagnostics—all critical components of virtual care. Through cloud integrations, patient data from wearable devices, home monitoring systems or mobile apps is automatically uploaded, analyzed and visualized for care teams. These data streams feed into EHRs and decision-support systems in real time, enabling clinicians to detect early signs of deterioration or non-adherence. The cloud ensures that these services can be delivered with high uptime and compliance with health regulations, regardless of patient location. This is especially impactful in remote or underserved areas where access to specialists is limited. Patients also benefit from the continuity of care, as their virtual consultations and monitoring data are securely stored and accessible across multiple providers. As digital health expands beyond the clinic, cloud-based telehealth infrastructure ensures seamless care delivery across virtual and physical domains.

2.6.9 Collaboration in Research and Clinical Trials

Cloud computing enhances collaboration among researchers, clinicians and institutions by offering centralized access to shared data and analysis tools. Large-scale clinical trials often span multiple locations and require coordination across time zones and regulatory frameworks. Cloud-based platforms facilitate this by allowing researchers to upload, access and analyze datasets in real time. Secure, role-based access controls ensure data privacy while still enabling international collaboration. Tools like Google Colab, Microsoft Azure Notebooks and JupyterHub allow teams to develop and test AI models together in a virtual environment. Additionally, cloud platforms support data versioning, tracking and reproducibility—key pillars of modern research. Anonymized patient data stored in the cloud can be aggregated for meta-analyses or AI model training, accelerating scientific discovery. Cloud solutions also simplify compliance with ethical guidelines by logging data access and maintaining audit trails. Overall, cloud computing fosters faster, safer and more collaborative research that benefits both academia and clinical practice.

2.6.10 Future Trends and Innovation

The future of cloud computing in digital health lies in advanced innovations like serverless architecture, federated learning and edge-cloud hybrid models. Serverless computing allows developers to run healthcare applications without managing infrastructure, leading to faster deployment and cost savings. Federated learning supports privacy-preserving AI by enabling model training across decentralized datasets without moving sensitive patient data—a major advance in compliance and ethics. Meanwhile, edge-cloud hybrid models push processing power closer to data sources, like wearable devices or remote sensors. This reduces latency and bandwidth use while still syncing with centralized cloud systems. Cloud-native innovations are also driving forward concepts like digital twins—virtual replicas of patients used for simulation and treatment planning. Real-time epidemic surveillance, AI-powered diagnostics and personalized care pathways are being powered by these futuristic architectures. As cloud technologies continue to evolve, they will form the foundation for intelligent, connected and adaptive healthcare ecosystems that respond dynamically to both individual and population-level needs.

3 Chapter
HEALTH PARAMETERS MONITORED DIGITALLY

3.0 INTRODUCTION: AN OVERVIEW

In recent years, the integration of digital technologies into healthcare has revolutionized the way health parameters are monitored, assessed and managed. With the advent of wearable devices, smartphone applications, telemedicine platforms and advanced health informatics systems, individuals and healthcare professionals now have unprecedented access to real-time data that can significantly enhance preventive care, chronic disease management and emergency response. Digitally monitoring health parameters involves the continuous or periodic tracking of vital signs and physiological functions using electronic devices that transmit, store and analyze health information.

Key health parameters such as heart rate, blood pressure, blood glucose levels, body temperature, respiratory rate, oxygen saturation and physical activity levels can now be tracked using devices ranging from smartwatches to specialized medical-grade equipment. These digital tools are equipped with sensors that can detect subtle changes in the body's condition, providing insights that might otherwise go unnoticed in traditional, episodic healthcare visits. For example, continuous glucose monitors (CGMs) enable diabetic patients to receive constant feedback about their blood sugar trends, allowing for more precise insulin management. Similarly, wearable ECG monitors can detect abnormal heart rhythms and notify users and physicians before a serious event occurs. The digital monitoring of health parameters is particularly transformative in managing chronic diseases such as diabetes, hypertension, asthma and cardiovascular disorders. These conditions require ongoing monitoring and lifestyle adjustments, which digital solutions make more manageable and personalized. Patients are empowered to take charge of their own health through user-friendly apps that interpret data and offer actionable recommendations. Moreover, remote monitoring reduces the need for frequent hospital visits, thereby saving time, lowering healthcare costs and reducing strain on medical infrastructure—especially vital in underserved or rural areas. The integration of digital health technologies is depicted in Fig. 1.

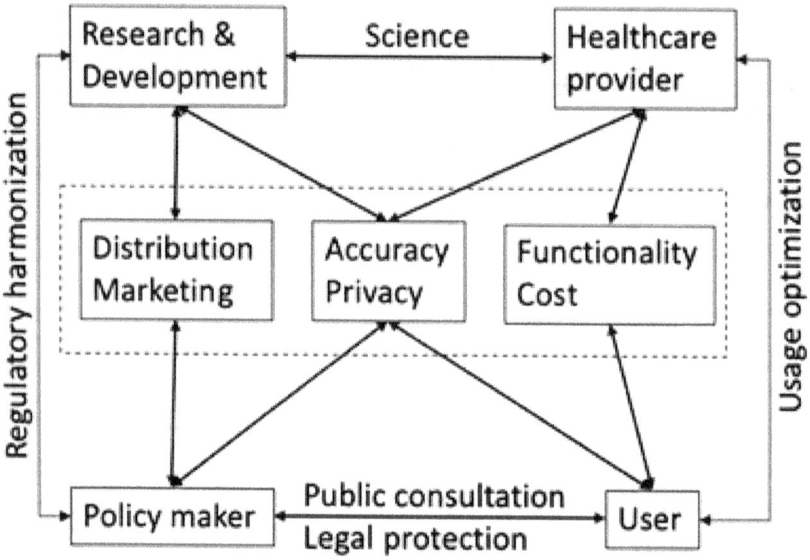

Fig. 1 The integration of digital health technologies

Telemedicine platforms (Fig. 2) have further enhanced the capabilities of digital monitoring. Through video consultations and remote diagnostics, healthcare providers can access a patient's health data in real-time, facilitating timely interventions and better continuity of care. Integration with electronic health records (EHRs) allows for seamless data sharing between devices, patients and providers, leading to more coordinated and informed decision-making. This level of connectivity supports proactive rather than reactive healthcare, allowing for the early detection of diseases, faster treatment and improved health outcomes. Furthermore, advancements in artificial intelligence and machine learning are making digital health monitoring smarter. Predictive algorithms can analyze large datasets to forecast health risks, detect patterns and personalize treatment plans. These technologies are especially promising for elderly care, mental health tracking, rehabilitation and prenatal monitoring. Smart home systems with integrated sensors can detect falls, monitor sleep quality and even assess mood changes through voice analysis or facial recognition, providing a holistic view of a person's health and well-being. Despite its numerous advantages, digital health monitoring also raises concerns about data privacy, security and the need for regulation. Ensuring that health information is protected against cyber threats and used ethically is crucial to maintaining trust in these technologies. Moreover, equitable access to digital health tools remains a challenge, particularly among older adults, low-income groups and those with limited digital literacy. To fully harness the potential of digital health monitoring, stakeholders must invest in user-friendly designs, inclusive infrastructure and robust health education.

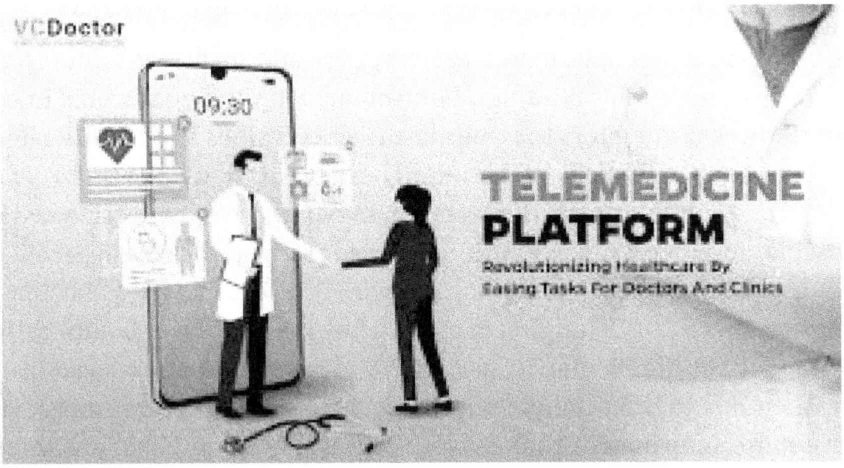

Fig. 2 Telemedicine Platform

The digital monitoring of health parameters marks a significant leap forward in modern healthcare. It bridges the gap between patient and provider, supports preventive health strategies and personalizes care in ways that were unimaginable a decade ago. As technology continues to evolve, the integration of digital tools into everyday health practices will become even more seamless, making healthcare not only more efficient but also more human-centered and proactive. By embracing these innovations thoughtfully and inclusively, we can create a future where optimal health is within reach for all.

3.1 VITAL SIGNS MONITORING

Vital signs monitoring is the continuous or periodic assessment of the body's fundamental physiological functions that are essential to life. These measurements—heart rate, blood pressure, body temperature and oxygen saturation—provide immediate and valuable insights into a person's health status. Monitoring these parameters is crucial in various healthcare settings, from routine check-ups to emergency care and intensive monitoring of critically ill patients. The data gathered from vital signs allows healthcare providers to detect early signs of deterioration, initiate timely interventions and track the progress or response to treatment. Each vital sign represents a specific aspect of bodily function: heart rate indicates cardiac activity and perfusion, blood pressure reflects circulatory dynamics and vascular health, temperature shows thermoregulatory status and potential infections and oxygen saturation reveals the efficiency of respiratory gas exchange. Together, these indicators form the foundation of clinical assessment. Advances in medical technology have led to the development of both invasive and non-invasive methods to measure these parameters accurately and continuously. For example, wearable monitors now allow for real-time tracking of heart rate and oxygen saturation in outpatient settings. Automated blood pressure monitors enhance precision and reduce manual errors. Core and surface thermometers offer quick, reliable temperature readings. Continuous monitoring systems in hospitals integrate all these parameters to issue alarms when values fall outside safe ranges, ensuring immediate medical attention. These vital signs are interdependent; changes in one often affect the others, making their collective assessment indispensable. In emergency scenarios, such as trauma, stroke or cardiac arrest, rapid evaluation of vital signs can be life-saving. In chronic disease management, like hypertension or COPD, long-term monitoring helps prevent complications and improves quality of life. Pediatric, geriatric and neonatal patients require special considerations due to their unique physiological baselines. Furthermore, vital sign trends are more informative than single readings, helping clinicians understand whether a condition is stable, improving or worsening. Medical professionals are trained to interpret both absolute values and patterns over time. In critical care, invasive techniques such as arterial lines for blood pressure or core body probes for temperature offer enhanced accuracy. In contrast, non-invasive methods are preferred for routine assessments due to their safety and ease of use. Accurate documentation and interpretation are essential, as misreadings can lead to misdiagnosis or inappropriate interventions. Patient cooperation, proper equipment calibration and standardized procedures all play a role in ensuring valid results. In modern healthcare, vital signs monitoring extends beyond hospitals, with home monitoring kits and telehealth platforms enabling remote assessments. This is especially important for elderly patients or those in rural areas who may have limited access to clinics. Additionally, during global health emergencies like pandemics, remote monitoring helps reduce the risk of cross-infection. In conclusion, vital signs monitoring is a cornerstone of clinical practice, offering rapid, non-invasive and reliable insight into the human body's internal environment. It bridges technology, clinical skill and patient care, forming the bedrock of both emergency response and long-term health management.

The core vital signs include:

1. Heart Rate (HR)

Heart rate refers to the number of times the heart beats per minute (bpm) and serves as a vital indicator of the heart's efficiency and overall cardiovascular function. It reflects how hard the heart is working to pump blood throughout the body, supplying oxygen and nutrients to tissues while removing waste products. A normal resting heart rate for adults typically ranges from 60 to 100 bpm, though well-trained athletes may exhibit lower rates due to superior cardiac conditioning. Several factors can influence heart rate, including physical activity, emotional state, medications, body temperature and overall health status. Monitoring heart rate is essential in both acute and chronic healthcare settings, as it can reveal signs of stress, fever, dehydration or underlying cardiac abnormalities. Tachycardia or an abnormally high heart rate, may indicate fever, anxiety, anemia or arrhythmias, while bradycardia or a slow heart rate, might suggest heart block, hypothyroidism or be normal in fit individuals. An irregular rhythm could be a sign of atrial fibrillation or other arrhythmic conditions requiring further investigation. Heart rate is typically measured through palpation of peripheral pulses or more precisely using devices like ECGs and pulse oximeters. Continuous monitoring allows clinicians to track trends, detect early warning signs of deterioration and assess response to interventions.

Normal Range:

- Adults: 60–100 bpm
- Athletes: May be as low as 40–60 bpm

Methods of Measurement:

- **Manual Palpation:** Manual palpation is a traditional and widely used method to measure heart rate by physically feeling the pulse with the fingertips. It is typically performed by placing the index and middle fingers over a palpable artery, such as the radial (wrist), carotid (neck) or brachial (inner arm) arteries. This method allows healthcare providers to assess not only the rate but also the rhythm and strength of the pulse. It is especially useful in emergency or low-resource settings where equipment may not be available. Manual palpation is non-invasive, quick and cost-effective. However, it requires proper technique and clinical skill to avoid inaccuracies. The pulse is usually counted for 15, 30 or 60 seconds, depending on the situation. Irregularities in rhythm, such as skipped or extra beats, can often be detected through this method. While useful, it is not as precise as electronic methods, especially in critically ill or unstable patients.
- **Electronic Monitors:** Electronic monitors are modern, reliable tools used to measure heart rate with precision and consistency across various healthcare and personal settings. Electrocardiograms (ECGs) are widely regarded as the gold standard for heart rate and rhythm assessment. They record the heart's electrical activity through electrodes placed on the chest, providing detailed information about heart rhythm, conduction abnormalities and potential cardiac conditions such as arrhythmias or ischemia. Pulse oximeters, often clipped onto a patient's finger, use light-based technology to measure both heart rate and blood oxygen saturation (SpO_2) non-invasively. They are quick, portable and especially useful in

monitoring patients with respiratory or cardiovascular issues. Wearable devices, such as smartwatches and fitness bands, use photoplethysmography (PPG) sensors to continuously monitor heart rate. These are popular for personal health tracking, fitness monitoring and even early detection of cardiac issues. In clinical settings, electronic monitors provide continuous, real-time data, essential for critically ill patients. Many of these devices include alarms to notify healthcare providers of abnormal heart rate readings. Their accuracy, ease of use and ability to integrate with electronic medical records make electronic monitors indispensable in both hospital and home care environments.

Clinical Significance:

- **Tachycardia (>100 bpm):** Tachycardia is defined as a heart rate exceeding 100 beats per minute and often reflects the body's response to stress or illness. It can be physiological, such as during exercise or emotional stress or pathological when associated with medical conditions. Common causes include fever, pain, anxiety, dehydration, anemia or overuse of stimulants like caffeine or certain medications. It may also indicate underlying cardiac issues such as supraventricular tachycardia or ventricular arrhythmias. Persistent tachycardia can strain the heart over time, reducing cardiac efficiency and oxygen delivery. In severe cases, it may result in dizziness, shortness of breath or chest pain. Clinical evaluation often includes ECG monitoring and blood tests to identify the root cause. Treatment depends on addressing the underlying issue and may involve medications, fluid replacement or lifestyle changes. Recognizing and managing tachycardia early can help prevent complications and improve patient outcomes.
- **Bradycardia (<60 bpm):** Bradycardia refers to a slower-than-normal heart rate, typically below 60 beats per minute. While often benign in well-trained athletes due to increased cardiac efficiency, it can also be a sign of medical concern. Causes of pathological bradycardia include hypothyroidism, aging, medication side effects (like beta-blockers) or conduction system disorders such as heart block. Symptoms may include fatigue, dizziness, fainting (syncope) or shortness of breath, particularly if cardiac output is compromised. In some cases, bradycardia is detected incidentally and does not require treatment. However, if it causes symptoms or indicates an underlying heart condition, further evaluation through ECG or Holter monitoring is warranted. Severe or symptomatic bradycardia may require interventions such as medication adjustment or pacemaker implantation. Early detection is essential to prevent complications such as falls, fainting or sudden cardiac arrest.

- **Irregular Rhythm:** An irregular heart rhythm or arrhythmia, is characterized by an inconsistent or abnormal pattern of heartbeats. This can range from benign occasional skipped beats to serious conditions like atrial fibrillation (AF), where the atria beat chaotically and out of sync with the ventricles. AF is particularly important to detect, as it increases the risk of stroke and heart failure. Other arrhythmias include premature ventricular contractions (PVCs), atrial flutter and ventricular tachycardia. Symptoms may include palpitations, chest discomfort, dizziness or even fainting. Diagnosis is typically confirmed through ECG, Holter monitoring or event recorders. Treatment depends on the type and severity of the arrhythmia and may involve medications like antiarrhythmics or beta-blockers, lifestyle changes or procedures like cardioversion or ablation. Regular rhythm monitoring is crucial in at-risk individuals to ensure timely management and reduce the risk of complications.

2. Blood Pressure (BP)

Blood pressure (BP) is a critical physiological parameter that measures the force exerted by circulating blood against the walls of the body's arteries. It is a key indicator of cardiovascular health and reflects how efficiently the heart is pumping and how flexible or resistant the arteries are. Blood pressure is recorded as two values: systolic pressure, which is the force during heart contraction and diastolic pressure, which is the pressure when the heart rests between beats. A normal BP ensures that organs and tissues receive adequate oxygen and nutrients. High blood pressure (hypertension) increases the risk of heart disease, stroke, kidney damage and other serious conditions. Low blood pressure (hypotension) may lead to dizziness, fainting and inadequate organ perfusion. Various factors such as age, stress, activity level, diet and medical conditions influence BP levels. Regular monitoring is essential for early detection of abnormalities. Accurate blood pressure assessment helps guide diagnosis, treatment and long-term management of many health conditions.

It is expressed as two numbers:

- **Systolic Pressure (Upper Value):** Systolic pressure is the top number in a blood pressure reading and represents the force exerted on artery walls when the heart contracts and pumps blood into the circulation. It is the highest pressure in the arteries and reflects the strength and efficiency of the heart's contraction. Normal systolic values typically range between 90 and 120 mmHg in healthy adults. Elevated systolic pressure can indicate increased cardiac workload, arterial stiffness or conditions like hypertension. Persistent high systolic pressure, especially in older adults, is a major risk factor for heart disease, stroke and kidney problems. Factors such as stress, exercise, smoking and stimulants can temporarily raise systolic pressure. Monitoring this value over time helps detect trends and potential health risks. A significantly high systolic reading, even with a normal diastolic value, may still require medical attention. Proper lifestyle changes or medications can help regulate systolic pressure effectively.

- **Diastolic Pressure (Lower Value):** Diastolic pressure is the bottom number in a blood pressure reading and measures the pressure in the arteries when the heart is at rest between beats. This resting phase is crucial, as it allows the heart to refill with blood and prepare for the next contraction. Normal diastolic pressure typically ranges from 60 to 80 mmHg. A low diastolic reading may suggest poor vascular tone or internal bleeding, while a high reading may point to stiff or narrowed arteries. Chronic elevation in diastolic pressure is associated with a higher risk of heart attack, stroke and kidney disease. Unlike systolic pressure, diastolic values are particularly important in younger adults. Factors such as high sodium intake, obesity and sedentary lifestyle can contribute to elevated diastolic pressure. Accurate measurement and regular monitoring can help detect underlying issues early. Treatment often includes diet modification, exercise, stress management and, if necessary, antihypertensive medication.

Normal Range:

- Normal: <120/80 mmHg
- Elevated: 120–129/<80 mmHg
- Hypertension Stage 1: 130–139/80–89 mmHg
- Hypertension Stage 2: ≥140/90 mmHg
- Hypotension: <90/60 mmHg

Methods of Measurement:

- **Auscultatory Method:** The auscultatory method is a traditional and widely used technique to measure blood pressure. It involves the use of a sphygmomanometer (blood pressure cuff) and a stethoscope. The cuff is wrapped around the upper arm and inflated to restrict blood flow. As the cuff deflates, the healthcare provider listens with a stethoscope over the brachial artery. The first sound heard (Korotkoff sound) indicates the systolic pressure. When the sound disappears, that marks the diastolic pressure. This method requires proper technique and positioning for accurate results. It is generally performed manually by trained personnel. While reliable, it may be affected by human error or background noise. It is often used in clinics and hospitals.

- **Oscillometric Devices:** Oscillometric devices are automatic digital blood pressure monitors commonly used for home and clinical monitoring. These devices measure blood pressure by detecting oscillations in the arterial wall as the cuff deflates. Unlike the auscultatory method, no stethoscope is needed. The machine automatically inflates and deflates the cuff and calculates systolic, diastolic and mean arterial pressure. They are easy to use and require minimal training. Oscillometric devices are useful for patients to monitor blood pressure at home. However, they may be less accurate in people with irregular heart rhythms. Readings can also be influenced by movement or improper cuff placement. These devices are widely available and convenient for routine monitoring.
- **Invasive Monitoring:** Invasive blood pressure monitoring is performed using an arterial catheter inserted directly into an artery, typically the radial artery. This method provides continuous and highly accurate blood pressure readings. It is mainly used in intensive care units and during major surgeries. The catheter is connected to a transducer that converts arterial pressure into an electrical signal displayed on a monitor. It allows real-time monitoring of systolic, diastolic and mean arterial pressure. Invasive monitoring is essential for critically ill patients who require precise cardiovascular management. The procedure carries risks such as infection, bleeding or arterial damage. It must be performed by trained medical professionals under sterile conditions. This method is not suitable for routine or outpatient blood pressure measurement.

Clinical Significance:

- **Hypertension:** Hypertension or high blood pressure, is a chronic medical condition where the force of the blood against artery walls is consistently too high. It often develops over many years without obvious symptoms, which is why it's called the "silent killer." If left untreated, it significantly increases the risk of serious health problems. Hypertension can damage blood vessels and organs, especially the heart, brain, kidneys and eyes. It is a major risk factor for stroke, heart attack, heart failure and kidney disease. Lifestyle changes such as a healthy diet, regular exercise and stress reduction can help manage it. In many cases, medication is also needed. Regular monitoring is important for early detection and control. Effective management reduces long-term health risks.
- **Hypotension:** Hypotension refers to abnormally low blood pressure, which can cause inadequate blood flow to vital organs. It may lead to symptoms such as dizziness, fainting, blurred vision, nausea and fatigue. In severe cases, it can result in shock—a life-threatening condition where organs fail

due to lack of oxygen. Hypotension can occur due to dehydration, blood loss, heart problems or certain medications. While mild hypotension may not require treatment, persistent or symptomatic cases must be investigated. It can be especially dangerous in the elderly, increasing fall risk. Managing the underlying cause is essential for treatment. Sometimes, increasing salt intake or adjusting medication is needed. Medical attention is necessary when symptoms are severe or sudden.

- **Blood Pressure Trends:** Monitoring blood pressure trends over time provides valuable insight into a patient's cardiovascular health. It helps identify patterns, fluctuations and responses to treatment. In conditions like preeclampsia, a pregnancy-related complication, tracking rising blood pressure is critical for early intervention. Similarly, in sepsis, low blood pressure indicates worsening infection and possible organ failure. In heart failure, both high and low pressures can signal deterioration. Consistent tracking can help guide medication adjustments and fluid management. Wearable devices and home monitors assist in capturing long-term data. Clinicians rely on these trends rather than single readings for diagnosis and management. Recognizing abnormal trends early can prevent complications and improve outcomes. Thus, regular and accurate monitoring is vital in chronic and acute care.

3. Body Temperature

Body temperature is a vital sign that reflects the dynamic balance between heat production and heat loss within the body. It serves as a key indicator of the body's thermoregulatory status, helping to maintain internal stability despite external environmental changes. Normal body temperature typically ranges around 36.5°C to 37.5°C (97.7°F to 99.5°F), though it can slightly vary between individuals and throughout the day. The hypothalamus in the brain plays a central role in regulating body temperature by receiving input from temperature receptors and triggering responses like sweating or shivering. Heat is generated mainly through metabolic processes, muscular activity and hormone function, while it is lost through radiation, evaporation, convection and conduction. Abnormal temperature changes can signal underlying health issues. A rise in temperature or fever, often indicates infection or inflammation, whereas a drop, known as hypothermia, may result from prolonged exposure to cold. Hyperthermia, on the other hand, can occur due to heatstroke or impaired thermoregulation. Monitoring body temperature is crucial in both routine and emergency clinical settings. It helps assess patient response to treatment, detect infection and guide medical interventions. Various methods are used to measure temperature, including oral, tympanic, axillary and rectal routes. Advances in digital thermometers have improved speed and accuracy in readings.

Overall, body temperature is a critical marker of physiological homeostasis and systemic function.

Normal Range:

- 36.1°C to 37.2°C (97°F to 99°F), depending on measurement site.

Methods of Measurement:

- Oral: Under the tongue; most common.
- Rectal: Most accurate core temperature.
- Axillary: Underarm; less accurate.
- Tympanic: Ear canal; uses infrared sensors.
- Temporal Artery: Forehead scan using infrared.

Clinical Significance:

- **Fever (>38°C / 100.4°F):** Fever is a temporary elevation of body temperature, often indicating an underlying condition such as infection or inflammation. It is a natural defense mechanism where the hypothalamus raises the body's set-point to help fight off pathogens. Common causes include viral or bacterial infections, autoimmune diseases and some cancers. Fever may also accompany symptoms like chills, sweating, headache or muscle aches. While generally not harmful on its own, a high or persistent fever warrants medical attention. In children, fever can sometimes trigger febrile seizures. Antipyretics like paracetamol or ibuprofen are used to manage symptoms. Monitoring the trend of fever helps track illness progression. Accurate temperature measurement is essential for diagnosis and treatment.
- **Hypothermia (<35°C / 95°F):** Hypothermia occurs when the body loses heat faster than it can produce it, causing a dangerous drop in core temperature. It is commonly caused by prolonged exposure to cold weather or immersion in cold water. Medical conditions like sepsis, hypothyroidism and hypoglycemia can also contribute. Symptoms include shivering, confusion, slurred speech, drowsiness and loss of coordination. As hypothermia progresses, the body's ability to shiver stops and organs begin to fail. Severe cases can lead to unconsciousness and death if not treated promptly. Management includes gentle rewarming, dry clothing and warmed IV fluids in clinical settings. Early detection and intervention are key. Elderly individuals and infants are particularly at risk.
- **Hyperthermia (>40°C / 104°F):** Hyperthermia is a dangerously high body temperature caused by the body's inability to dissipate heat effectively. Unlike fever, it is not regulated by the hypothalamus and can rapidly

escalate to life-threatening levels. Common causes include heatstroke, strenuous activity in hot environments and reactions to certain drugs (e.g., anesthetics causing malignant hyperthermia). Symptoms may include confusion, flushed skin, rapid pulse, nausea and loss of consciousness. Without prompt cooling and medical intervention, it can lead to seizures organ failure or death. Treatment involves immediate cooling methods like ice packs, cooling blankets or cold IV fluids. Hospitalization is often required for severe cases. Prevention includes hydration, rest and avoiding extreme heat exposure.

4. Oxygen Saturation (SpO_2)

Oxygen saturation (SpO_2) is a critical physiological parameter that reflects the percentage of hemoglobin in the blood that is saturated with oxygen. It is a key indicator of how effectively oxygen is being transported from the lungs to the tissues throughout the body. In healthy individuals, normal SpO_2 levels typically range from 95% to 100%. Levels below 90% are considered low (hypoxemia) and may indicate inadequate oxygen delivery, which can be life-threatening if not addressed promptly. SpO_2 is most commonly measured using a non-invasive device called a pulse oximeter, which is placed on a fingertip, toe or earlobe. The device uses light sensors to estimate oxygen levels by analyzing the color of arterial blood. Monitoring SpO_2 is especially important in patients with respiratory or cardiac conditions, such as COPD, asthma, pneumonia or heart failure. It is also routinely monitored during surgery, anesthesia and in critical care settings. Persistent low oxygen saturation can lead to symptoms such as shortness of breath, confusion, restlessness and cyanosis (bluish discoloration of skin or lips). In severe cases, it may result in organ dysfunction or cardiac arrest. Factors such as poor circulation, nail polish, cold extremities or movement can affect the accuracy of pulse oximetry readings. Supplemental oxygen therapy may be required to restore normal levels. Overall, SpO_2 is a vital sign that helps guide clinical decisions and evaluate the effectiveness of oxygenation and ventilation in patients.

Normal Range:

In healthy individuals, oxygen saturation (SpO_2) levels typically range from 95% to 100%, indicating adequate oxygen delivery to tissues and organs. This range reflects optimal lung function and efficient gas exchange in the alveoli. When SpO_2drops below 90%, it is classified as hypoxemia, a condition where the blood carries insufficient oxygen. Hypoxemia can result from respiratory disorders such as COPD, pneumonia, pulmonary embolism or acute respiratory distress. It may also occur at high altitudes or during severe asthma attacks. Symptoms of low oxygen levels include shortness of breath, rapid breathing, confusion and cyanosis (bluish skin or lips). Persistent or severe hypoxemia requires immediate medical attention and often oxygen therapy. Monitoring SpO_2 is crucial for early detection and management of respiratory compromise. Maintaining levels within the normal range supports vital organ function and overall health.

- 95–100% (healthy individuals)
- <90% indicates hypoxemia (low oxygen levels)

Methods of Measurement:

Pulse Oximetry: Pulse oximetry is a non-invasive, quick and widely used method for measuring peripheral oxygen saturation (SpO_2). The device, known as a pulse oximeter, is typically clipped onto a fingertip, earlobe or toe, where it uses light-emitting diodes (LEDs) and sensors to detect the color changes in blood caused by oxygenated and deoxygenated hemoglobin. This method estimates the percentage of hemoglobin saturated with oxygen, with readings above 95% considered normal in healthy individuals. Pulse oximetry is commonly used in clinical, emergency, surgical and home settings due to its simplicity and immediate results. It is essential for monitoring patients with respiratory or cardiac conditions, during anesthesia or in intensive care. However, it has limitations. Factors like poor circulation, cold extremities, nail polish, dark skin pigmentation or patient movement can affect accuracy. Despite these limitations, pulse oximetry remains a vital, user-friendly tool for real-time monitoring of oxygenation. It does not require blood samples, making it painless and patient-friendly. It is especially useful in continuous or repeated assessments. The device also often displays pulse rate, providing an additional vital sign at a glance. Overall, it's an essential part of modern clinical practice for early detection of hypoxemia.

Arterial Blood Gas (ABG): Arterial Blood Gas (ABG) analysis is an invasive but highly accurate method for measuring oxygen saturation (SaO_2), partial pressure of oxygen (PaO_2), carbon dioxide ($PaCO_2$), blood pH and other key parameters. The test involves drawing a blood sample from an artery, usually the radial artery at the wrist, using a needle and syringe. Unlike pulse oximetry, ABG provides a comprehensive snapshot of respiratory and metabolic function, making it invaluable in critical care, emergency medicine and respiratory therapy. SaO_2 from ABG reflects direct oxygen saturation in arterial blood, while PaO_2 indicates the pressure of oxygen dissolved in plasma. It helps clinicians assess gas exchange efficiency and acid-base balance. ABG is crucial in diagnosing conditions like respiratory failure, metabolic acidosis and oxygenation issues in mechanically ventilated patients. However, it is more complex and painful than pulse oximetry and requires trained professionals to perform and interpret. Risks include bleeding, infection or arterial injury at the puncture site. Because of its invasiveness, ABG is used when precise measurements are essential or when pulse oximetry readings are unreliable. It plays a vital role in monitoring patients in ICUs or those with severe respiratory diseases. Despite its discomfort, ABG remains the gold standard for evaluating blood gases and oxygenation status.

Clinical Significance:

Hypoxemia (<90%): Hypoxemia is a condition in which the oxygen saturation level in arterial blood falls below 90%, indicating insufficient oxygen delivery to body tissues. It is often a result of respiratory diseases such as chronic obstructive pulmonary disease (COPD), asthma, pneumonia or acute respiratory distress. Cardiovascular conditions like heart failure can also impair oxygenation due to reduced cardiac output. Environmental factors, such as exposure to high altitudes, can lead to hypoxemia because of reduced atmospheric oxygen. Symptoms include shortness of breath, rapid breathing, confusion, restlessness and cyanosis (bluish skin or lips). Left untreated, hypoxemia can lead to organ dysfunction, brain injury or death. Diagnosis is typically made using pulse oximetry or confirmed via arterial blood gas (ABG) analysis. Treatment involves addressing the underlying cause and may require supplemental oxygen, bronchodilators, steroids or mechanical ventilation in severe cases. Timely identification and intervention are critical to preventing complications. Regular monitoring in at-risk patients helps detect deteriorations early. Hypoxemia is a common and serious concern in emergency, critical and respiratory care settings.

Hyperoxia (>100%): Hyperoxia refers to abnormally high oxygen levels in the blood, typically resulting from the use of supplemental oxygen in clinical settings. While it may seem beneficial, excessive oxygen—especially SpO_2 consistently above 100% or PaO_2 >120 mmHg—can be harmful over time. Prolonged hyperoxia can lead to oxygen toxicity, which damages the lungs, eyes and central nervous system. It can cause oxidative stress, leading to inflammation and tissue injury. In premature infants, hyperoxia is associated with retinopathy of prematurity, a condition that can lead to blindness. In adults, it may impair respiratory drive in patients with chronic CO_2 retention, such as those with COPD. Hyperoxia can also increase the risk of absorption atelectasis, where high oxygen levels wash out nitrogen and cause lung collapse. It's most often seen during oxygen therapy, anesthesia and mechanical ventilation. Therefore, oxygen therapy must be carefully titrated to maintain saturation within safe limits—usually 92–96% for most patients. Healthcare providers must balance the need to correct hypoxemia while avoiding the risks of excessive oxygen. Monitoring with pulse oximetry and ABG is essential to avoid harm.

Trend Monitoring: Monitoring oxygen saturation trends over time is critical in both acute and chronic medical care. Rather than relying on a single reading, clinicians observe patterns and fluctuations in SpO_2 to assess patient stability and response to treatment. In post-operative care, monitoring ensures that patients recover from anesthesia without respiratory depression. In anesthesia, it helps detect hypoventilation or airway obstruction early. For patients with chronic lung diseases like COPD or interstitial lung disease, long-term SpO_2 trends guide oxygen therapy and medication adjustments. Trend monitoring is also essential in critical care, sleep studies (for sleep apnea) and home oxygen therapy. It allows for timely intervention if a patient begins to decompensate. Digital health tools and wearable pulse oximeters have improved the ability to track SpO_2continuously. Changes in saturation, especially when correlated with symptoms or activity levels, provide valuable diagnostic and prognostic information. Trend data also assists in evaluating rehabilitation progress or deterioration in chronic illness. Overall, continuous and trend-based SpO_2 monitoring is a cornerstone of effective respiratory and perioperative management. Summary of Heart Rate, Blood Pressure, Temperature, Oxygen Saturation are summarised in Table-1.

Table: 1 Summary of Heart Rate, Blood Pressure, Temperature, Oxygen Saturation

Vital Sign	Normal Range	Measurement Tools	Clinical Importance
Heart Rate	60–100 bpm	ECG, palpation, pulse oximeter	Detect arrhythmias, stress, fever
Blood Pressure	<120/80 mmHg	Sphygmomanometer, digital BP cuff	Monitors cardiovascular health
Temperature	36.1–37.2°C (97–99°F)	Oral, rectal, tympanic, axillary	Indicates infection or thermoregulation issues
SpO_2	95–100%	Pulse oximeter, ABG	Assesses respiratory and oxygenation status

3.2 METABOLIC AND BIOCHEMICAL MONITORING

Metabolic and biochemical monitoring is indispensable for comprehensive patient care. It supports early diagnosis, guides interventions, monitors therapy effectiveness, and helps prevent complications. Whether in critical care, outpatient clinics, or home monitoring, it provides essential data that reflect the internal workings of the human body. As healthcare continues to evolve toward precision medicine, the role of biochemical monitoring will only expand, offering deeper insights into individual health and improving personalized treatment strategies.

Metabolic and Biochemical Monitoring is a critical aspect of modern healthcare that involves the continuous or periodic assessment of physiological and biochemical processes within the human body. It is essential in both acute and chronic care settings, enabling healthcare professionals to evaluate a patient's metabolic status, detect abnormalities early and guide therapeutic decisions. This type of monitoring encompasses a broad range of parameters including blood glucose, electrolytes, renal and liver function, acid-base balance and metabolic waste products. By tracking these variables, clinicians can gain insights into the body's internal environment and homeostasis.

The body's metabolic system is a complex network of biochemical reactions that produce energy, synthesize vital compounds and regulate numerous bodily functions. When this system is disrupted—due to illness, injury or external interventions—biochemical markers in the blood and other bodily fluids can provide early warning signs of dysfunction. Metabolic and biochemical monitoring allows clinicians to assess organ performance, track disease progression and evaluate the effects of medications or treatments in real-time or at regular intervals.

In critical care and intensive care units (ICUs), biochemical monitoring plays a life-saving role. Parameters such as arterial blood gases (ABGs), serum lactate and glucose levels are frequently measured to assess respiratory and metabolic status. These values help guide fluid resuscitation, oxygen therapy, ventilation strategies and nutritional support. For example, elevated serum lactate levels may indicate tissue hypoxia or sepsis, prompting immediate intervention. Similarly, monitoring electrolyte levels such as sodium, potassium, calcium and magnesium is crucial in managing patients with cardiac, renal or endocrine disorders.

Chronic disease management also relies heavily on metabolic monitoring. Patients with diabetes, for instance, must routinely monitor blood glucose to prevent complications such as neuropathy, nephropathy or retinopathy. Kidney function tests, including serum creatinine and blood urea nitrogen (BUN), are vital for assessing renal health in patients with hypertension, diabetes or chronic kidney disease. Liver function tests (LFTs) provide insights into hepatic conditions and are important for monitoring the effects of medications that may be hepatotoxic.

Advances in technology have significantly enhanced the ability to monitor these parameters accurately and efficiently. Point-of-care testing (POCT) devices, continuous glucose monitors (CGMs) and bedside analyzers now allow rapid measurement of biochemical values with minimal patient discomfort. These innovations enable quicker clinical decision-making, reducing delays in treatment and improving patient outcomes.

Biochemical monitoring also plays a significant role in surgical care, anesthesiology, emergency medicine and sports medicine. During surgery, for example, electrolyte and blood gas monitoring ensures the patient remains metabolically stable under anesthesia. In emergency settings, quick assessment of glucose or acid-base status can help differentiate between types of shock or causes of altered mental status. In athletes, monitoring lactate or creatine kinase can provide insights into muscle fatigue and recovery needs.

Laboratory-based metabolic panels, such as the Basic Metabolic Panel (BMP) and Comprehensive Metabolic Panel (CMP), are routinely ordered during physical exams and diagnostic evaluations. These panels offer a snapshot of the body's chemical balance and metabolism and are critical for identifying conditions like dehydration, acidosis, alkalosis and electrolyte imbalances.

3.2.1 Blood Glucose

A blood glucose test, also known as a blood sugar test, can be performed in a few ways, but the most common is a finger-prick test using a glucometer. A blood sample is obtained by pricking the fingertip with a lancet and a small drop of blood is placed on a test strip inserted into the glucometer, which provides a reading. Other methods include blood draws from a vein, often for fasting or glucose tolerance tests.

Here's a more detailed breakdown of the process:

1. Finger-Prick Test (using a glucometer): Finger-Prick Test (using a glucometer) is a quick and simple method to measure blood glucose levels. It involves pricking the fingertip with a small lancet to obtain a drop of blood. This blood is placed on a test strip inserted into a glucometer, which displays the glucose reading within seconds. It is commonly used by individuals with diabetes for daily self-monitoring. The test helps manage blood sugar levels and guide insulin or dietary adjustments. Its convenience and speed make it a valuable tool in both home and clinical settings (Fig. 3).

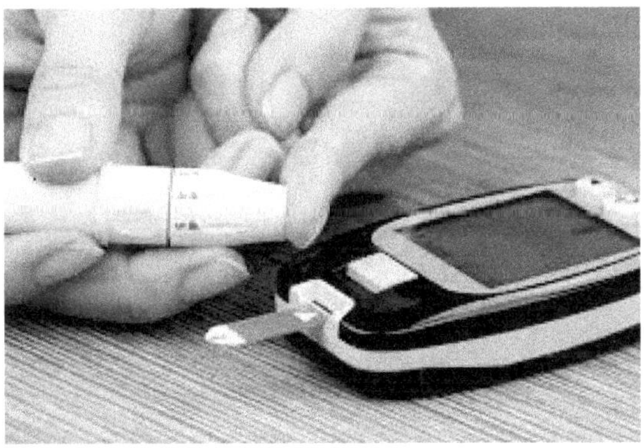

Fig.3 Finger Stick Testing

- **Preparation:** Wash and dry your hands thoroughly. Insert a test strip into the glucometer and prepare the lancet device.
- **Lancing:** Prick the side of your fingertip with the lancet.
- **Blood Sample:** Gently squeeze or massage your finger to produce a small blood drop.
- **Testing:** Apply the blood drop to the test strip and the glucometer will display your blood glucose level.

- **Post-Test:** Apply pressure to the puncture site with a cotton ball or gauze to stop the bleeding.

2. Venous Blood Draw (for fasting or glucose tolerance tests): Venous Blood Draw is a standard procedure used to collect blood from a vein, typically in the arm, for accurate laboratory analysis of glucose levels. It is commonly performed during fasting blood glucose tests or oral glucose tolerance tests (OGTT) to diagnose conditions like diabetes mellitus, prediabetes or gestational diabetes. Unlike finger-prick tests, venous samples provide more precise and comprehensive results. In a fasting test, blood is drawn after 8–12 hours without food to measure baseline glucose levels. During an OGTT, blood is drawn at intervals after consuming a glucose-rich drink to evaluate how the body processes sugar over time. This method is conducted in clinical or laboratory settings under professional supervision. It is considered a gold standard for diagnosing blood glucose disorders. The test may be repeated to confirm abnormal findings. Although slightly invasive, it yields highly reliable diagnostic data essential for long-term metabolic monitoring (Fig. 4).

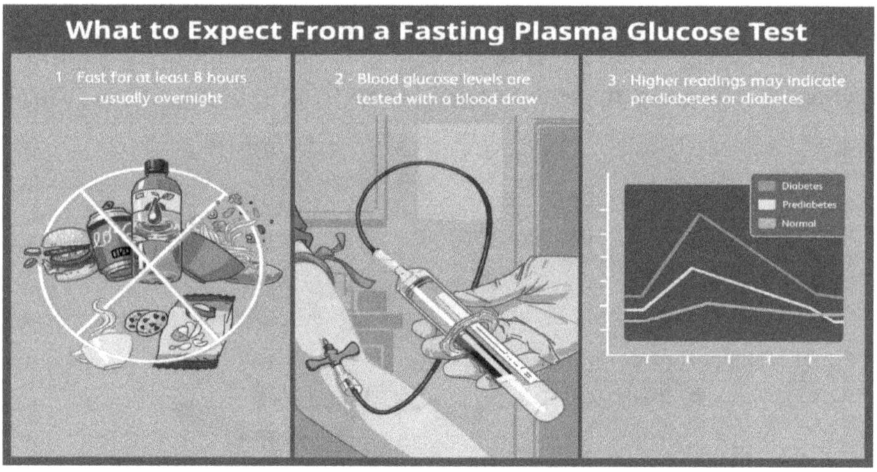

Fig. 4 What to Expect from a Fasting Glucose Test

- **Preparation:** You may need to fast (not eat or drink) for a specified period (e.g., 8-12 hours) before the test.
- **Sample Collection**: A healthcare professional will clean the puncture site (usually a vein in the arm), insert a needle and draw a blood sample.
- **Analysis:** The blood sample is sent to a lab for analysis to determine glucose levels.

Different Types of Blood Glucose Tests: Different Types of Blood Glucose Tests are essential tools used to assess how the body manages blood sugar and to diagnose or monitor conditions like diabetes and prediabetes. These tests help provide a comprehensive picture of glucose metabolism under various physiological conditions. The Fasting Blood Glucose Test is one of the most common and reliable screening methods. It measures blood sugar levels after the patient has fasted for 8–12 hours, typically overnight. This test provides a baseline reading that helps identify impaired fasting glucose or diabetes. The Postprandial Blood Glucose Test checks blood sugar levels two hours after eating, offering insights into how the body handles glucose following a meal. It is especially useful for monitoring blood sugar spikes in diabetic patients. The Glucose Tolerance Test (GTT) involves consuming a glucose-rich drink, followed by blood sampling at regular intervals—usually over two hours. This test evaluates how efficiently the body processes glucose and is often used to diagnose gestational diabetes or insulin resistance. The Random Blood Glucose Test can be conducted at any time of the day, regardless of meals. While it's convenient and fast, it is less specific than other tests and typically used for quick assessments or screening in emergency or outpatient settings.

Together, these tests help physicians tailor treatments, adjust medications and track progress in patients with glucose metabolism disorders.

- **Fasting Blood Glucose Test:** This test measures blood sugar levels after an overnight fast of 8–12 hours. It provides a baseline reading to assess how the body regulates glucose without recent food intake. It is commonly used to screen for diabetes and prediabetes. Results are typically more accurate due to the absence of dietary influence. It is a standard and reliable diagnostic tool in clinical practice.
- **Postprandial Blood Glucose Test:** This test measures blood glucose levels exactly two hours after a meal. It helps evaluate how the body responds to sugar intake and how effectively insulin is working. It is particularly useful in managing diabetes and assessing treatment response. Elevated post-meal levels may indicate poor glucose control. This test complements fasting glucose results for a fuller picture.
- **Glucose Tolerance Test (GTT):** The GTT involves drinking a glucose-rich solution, followed by timed blood samples over several hours. It assesses how efficiently the body processes sugar over time. It is commonly used to diagnose gestational diabetes and insulin resistance. The test provides detailed insight into glucose metabolism. It is more comprehensive than fasting or random tests.
- **Random Blood Glucose Test:** This test can be done at any time, regardless of when the person last ate. It is useful for rapid screening, especially in emergency situations or initial evaluations. While convenient, it is less specific and not used alone for diagnosis. Abnormally high readings may require confirmation with fasting or tolerance tests. It's often used as a preliminary check in outpatient settings.

Comparison of different types blood glucose test are summarised in Table-2.

Table.2 Comparison of different types blood glucose test

Test Type	Description	Purpose/Use	Advantages	Limitations
Fasting Blood Glucose Test	Measures blood sugar after an overnight fast of 8–12 hours.	Screens for diabetes and prediabetes.	Accurate baseline without food influence.	Requires fasting; may be inconvenient for some patients.
Postprandial Blood Glucose Test	Measures blood glucose exactly 2 hours after eating.	Evaluates glucose response post-meal; monitors diabetes control.	Complements fasting test; reflects real-life impact.	Not suitable for diagnosis on its own.
Glucose Tolerance Test (GTT)	Involves drinking a glucose-rich solution with blood samples taken at intervals.	Diagnoses gestational diabetes, insulin resistance and impaired glucose tolerance.	Detailed and comprehensive assessment.	Time-consuming; requires multiple blood draws.
Random Blood Glucose Test	Taken at any time, regardless of meals.	Used for quick screening, especially in emergency or outpatient settings.	Fast and convenient; no preparation needed.	Less specific; needs confirmation with other tests.

3.2.2 Ketones

A ketones test, whether performed using a blood sample or urine strip, is a diagnostic tool used to detect the presence and concentration of ketone bodies in the body. Ketones are chemical byproducts produced during the breakdown of fat for energy, a process that occurs when glucose is insufficient or unavailable as the body's primary fuel source. While small amounts of ketones can be normal during fasting, low-carb diets or intense exercise, elevated ketone levels can be dangerous, especially for individuals with diabetes. The test is commonly used to screen for or monitor diabetic ketoacidosis (DKA)—a potentially life-threatening complication of uncontrolled diabetes, particularly type 1 diabetes. In DKA, due to a lack of insulin, the body cannot use glucose effectively, prompting the breakdown of fat stores for energy. This results in a sharp increase in ketone production and can cause blood to become acidic, disrupting many of the body's metabolic processes.

There are three primary types of ketones detected: acetone, acetoacetate and beta-hydroxybutyrate. Blood tests are more accurate and measure beta-hydroxybutyrate, the predominant ketone in DKA. Urine tests, on the other hand, are more accessible and commonly used at home. They detect acetoacetate and provide a rough estimate of ketone levels through color changes on a dipstick. While useful for general monitoring, urine tests may lag behind real-time changes in ketone status.

Ketone testing is especially important during periods of illness, stress, missed insulin doses or persistent hyperglycemia (blood glucose > 250 mg/dL). These conditions increase the risk of ketone accumulation and progression to DKA. Early detection through regular monitoring can prompt immediate medical intervention, potentially preventing severe complications such as dehydration, electrolyte imbalance, coma or death. Besides diabetes, ketone testing is also relevant in nutritional and metabolic contexts. Individuals following ketogenic or low-carbohydrate diets may use ketone tests to verify they are in a state of nutritional ketosis, where fat is the primary energy source. However, this form of ketosis is generally mild and safe, in contrast to the harmful ketosis seen in DKA.

The test is quick, simple and can be performed at home or in clinical settings. Blood ketone meters function similarly to glucometers, requiring just a small finger-prick blood sample, while urine dipsticks require urine collection and are especially popular for children or at-home use. For accuracy, blood ketone testing is preferred in emergency or hospital settings. Regular ketone monitoring helps guide treatment decisions such as adjusting insulin doses, increasing fluid intake or seeking urgent care. In hospitalized patients or those on parenteral nutrition, ketone testing can be part of broader metabolic monitoring protocols. In summary, ketone testing provides vital information about the body's metabolic state. It is a critical tool in diabetes care, especially for preventing and managing DKA. It also plays a supportive role in nutritional science and metabolic therapy. Understanding when and how to test for ketones can help both patients and healthcare providers detect risks early, intervene appropriately and maintain better overall metabolic health.

Ketones in Urine: Ketones in Urine indicate the presence of ketone bodies being excreted by the body, typically when fat is being used as the primary energy source instead of glucose. This occurs in situations like prolonged fasting, low-carbohydrate diets, starvation or uncontrolled diabetes. The body produces ketones—mainly acetoacetate—during fat metabolism and when levels become too high, excess ketones are filtered out through the urine. A urine ketone test uses a simple dipstick that changes colour based on ketone concentration, making it a quick, non-invasive diagnostic tool. It is commonly used at home or in clinics to monitor people with type 1 diabetes, especially when they are sick or experiencing high blood sugar levels. Detecting ketones in urine can help identify early signs of diabetic ketoacidosis (DKA), a serious condition that requires immediate medical attention. Mild ketonuria may be harmless in some cases, such as during dieting or pregnancy, but persistent or high levels require evaluation. Regular monitoring helps prevent complications and guides treatment adjustments.

- **Purpose:** Urine ketone tests are used to determine whether the body is producing an abnormal number of ketones, which occurs when fat is broken down for energy instead of glucose. This process may be triggered by insufficient insulin, fasting or carbohydrate restriction. The test helps detect metabolic imbalances early, especially in individuals with diabetes. It's commonly used to monitor for diabetic ketoacidosis (DKA). Timely detection can prevent severe complications.
- **When to Test:** People with type 1 diabetes are advised to test for urine ketones when blood glucose levels are consistently above 240 mg/dL. It's also important during periods of illness, infection, stress or symptoms like nausea, vomiting or abdominal pain. These conditions may trigger a rise in ketone production. Testing helps determine if emergency care is needed. It is a vital part of sick day management plans.
- **How It's Done:** Urine ketone testing is simple and can be performed at home or in a healthcare facility. At-home kits include test strips or tablets that react with urine and change color based on ketone concentration. The user compares the strip to a color chart for interpretation. For clinical accuracy, laboratory tests can provide more detailed measurements. The process is non-invasive and fast, making it convenient for frequent monitoring.
- **Normal Range:** A trace amount of ketones in urine may be considered normal, especially after fasting, prolonged exercise or dieting. However, moderate to high levels can signal abnormal fat metabolism and potential risk for DKA. Color chart readings typically range from negative, trace, small, moderate, to large. Values outside the normal range require closer medical evaluation. Monitoring trends is more important than a single result.
- **High Levels:** High ketone levels in the urine often suggest a serious metabolic disturbance, especially in people with uncontrolled diabetes. It may indicate diabetic ketoacidosis (DKA), a life-threatening condition that requires immediate treatment. Symptoms may include rapid breathing, dehydration, fruity breath odor, confusion or even unconsciousness.

Prompt recognition and intervention can prevent complications like coma or death. Emergency care should not be delayed.

Ketones in Blood: Ketones in Blood refers to the measurement of ketone bodies circulating in the bloodstream, which provides a direct and accurate assessment of the body's metabolic state. Unlike urine tests that detect ketones excreted after some delay, blood ketone testing measures the current level of beta-hydroxybutyrate (BHB)—the primary ketone presents during ketosis and diabetic ketoacidosis (DKA). This test is especially important for people with type 1 diabetes or insulin-dependent diabetes, as it helps detect dangerous levels of ketones before severe complications arise. When insulin is insufficient or the body cannot use glucose effectively, fat metabolism increases, producing ketones as an alternative fuel source. Elevated ketones in the blood may indicate the onset of DKA, a medical emergency characterized by metabolic acidosis, dehydration and electrolyte imbalance. Blood ketone testing is performed using small portable meters, similar to glucose meters, requiring just a drop of blood from a finger prick. This method offers real-time, quantitative results that are more reliable and faster than urine tests. Monitoring blood ketone levels is crucial during illness, stress, missed insulin doses or unexplained high blood glucose levels. It aids in timely decision-making about insulin adjustments, hydration and seeking medical care. Blood ketone testing is also used by individuals following ketogenic diets to confirm nutritional ketosis. Overall, this test is a vital tool in diabetes management and emergency care, providing critical information to prevent life-threatening complications and optimize metabolic health.

- **Purpose:** Blood ketone tests measure the concentration of ketone bodies, primarily beta-hydroxybutyrate (BHB), circulating in the bloodstream. This provides a more immediate and accurate indication of ketosis compared to urine testing, which reflects ketone levels delayed by hours. The test helps identify metabolic changes when the body shifts from using glucose to fat as a primary energy source. It is crucial for early detection of dangerous conditions like diabetic ketoacidosis (DKA). By measuring blood ketones, healthcare providers and patients can better manage metabolic status and prevent complications. It's also used to monitor nutritional ketosis in specific diets. Overall, blood ketone testing is an essential tool for both medical and lifestyle purposes.
- **When to Test:** Blood ketone testing is particularly important for people with type 1 diabetes or insulin-dependent diabetes during periods of illness, pregnancy or whenever blood glucose levels are consistently elevated—usually above 240 mg/dL. These conditions increase the risk of ketone buildup and progression to DKA, which requires immediate

intervention. It is also recommended when symptoms such as nausea, vomiting, abdominal pain or rapid breathing occur. Testing can guide timely treatment adjustments such as insulin dosage or hospitalization. Additionally, individuals following ketogenic diets may test regularly to monitor their ketosis levels. In all cases, blood ketone testing provides critical real-time information for safety and management.

- **How It's Done:** Blood ketone tests can be performed in a clinical laboratory using a standard blood draw or conveniently at home using specialized portable meters similar to glucometers. The process requires a small drop of blood, usually obtained by a finger prick. The blood sample is applied to a test strip inserted into the meter, which then displays a quantitative ketone level within seconds. Home blood ketone meters allow for frequent monitoring without visiting a lab, making it easier to catch early signs of metabolic distress. Laboratory testing may provide more comprehensive panels but is less convenient for everyday use. Proper technique and meter calibration ensure accurate results.
- **Normal Range:** Normal blood ketone levels are generally less than 0.6 mmol/L, indicating that the body is not in significant ketosis. This range reflects a state where glucose is the primary energy source and fat metabolism is minimal. Slight elevations may occur during fasting, exercise or mild dietary changes but usually remain below this threshold. Maintaining ketone levels within the normal range helps prevent metabolic complications and indicates well-managed blood glucose. Values within this range usually do not require medical intervention. Regular monitoring helps detect any upward trends that may signal metabolic imbalance.
- **High Levels:** Blood ketone readings between 0.6 and 1.5 mmol/L suggest an increased risk of developing diabetic ketoacidosis (DKA) and warrant closer monitoring and corrective actions. Levels above 1.5 mmol/L are considered dangerously high and require immediate medical evaluation, as they indicate significant metabolic acidosis and potential for serious complications. Symptoms at these levels may include rapid breathing, confusion, dehydration and abdominal pain. Prompt intervention with insulin therapy and fluid replacement is critical to prevent progression to coma or death. Regular ketone testing helps identify these risks early, enabling timely treatment to reduce morbidity and mortality.

Key points:

- Ketone tests are valuable tools for managing diabetes and other conditions where ketosis is a concern.

- Elevated ketone levels, especially in the context of high blood sugar, can be a sign of DKA, a medical emergency.
- Regular monitoring of ketones, particularly for individuals with diabetes, can help prevent serious complications.
- Consult with a healthcare professional for proper interpretation of test results and appropriate management of ketone levels.

3.2.3 Cholesterol

Cholesterol tests are essential in preventive medicine and cardiovascular risk management. Accurate measurement and interpretation allow for timely interventions that can save lives by preventing heart attacks and strokes. Both patients and healthcare providers benefit from understanding cholesterol values and their implications, making cholesterol testing a cornerstone of modern clinical practice.

Cholesterol testing is a fundamental aspect of evaluating cardiovascular health and plays a pivotal role in the prevention, diagnosis and management of heart-related diseases. Cholesterol itself is a waxy, fat-like substance naturally produced by the liver and found in every cell of the body. It is vital for numerous biological functions, including the synthesis of essential hormones such as estrogen, testosterone and cortisol. Cholesterol is also necessary for producing vitamin D, which supports bone health and immune function, as well as bile acids that aid in the digestion and absorption of dietary fats. Despite its essential functions, cholesterol's reputation is often overshadowed by its association with heart disease when present in abnormal amounts. The human body transports cholesterol through the bloodstream by binding it to lipoproteins. These include low-density lipoprotein (LDL), commonly referred to as "bad cholesterol," and high-density lipoprotein (HDL), known as "good cholesterol." LDL cholesterol contributes to the buildup of fatty deposits or plaques, along the walls of arteries—a process called atherosclerosis. This narrowing and hardening of arteries reduce blood flow, which can lead to serious cardiovascular events such as heart attacks and strokes. Conversely, HDL cholesterol helps remove excess cholesterol from the bloodstream and arterial walls, transporting it back to the liver for excretion or recycling, thus offering a protective effect against heart disease.

Due to the critical role cholesterol plays in cardiovascular health, testing cholesterol levels has become a routine and essential part of medical care, especially for individuals at risk of cardiovascular disease. Cholesterol testing provides valuable insights into a person's lipid profile—the balance between LDL, HDL, total cholesterol and triglycerides—which collectively influence cardiovascular risk. Elevated LDL cholesterol and triglycerides are strongly linked to increased risk, while higher HDL levels are generally considered protective. By evaluating these components, healthcare providers can assess an individual's risk of developing conditions like coronary artery disease, peripheral artery disease and stroke. Cholesterol tests are also invaluable for guiding treatment decisions. For individuals found to have abnormal cholesterol levels, clinicians use the test results to recommend lifestyle changes such as dietary modifications, increased physical activity, weight management and smoking cessation. In many cases, cholesterol testing prompts the initiation of pharmacological therapies like statins, which effectively lower LDL cholesterol levels and reduce cardiovascular risk. The tests also help monitor the effectiveness of these interventions, allowing adjustments to therapy as needed. Moreover, cholesterol testing is not limited to adults with apparent risk factors; it has also become important in younger populations and those with a family history of lipid disorders or premature cardiovascular disease. Early detection of abnormal cholesterol levels can facilitate preventive measures that reduce long-term health complications. Inherited conditions such as familial hypercholesterolemia, which cause extremely high LDL cholesterol from a young age, require early diagnosis and aggressive management to prevent early heart disease. High cholesterol foods are depicted in Fig. 5.

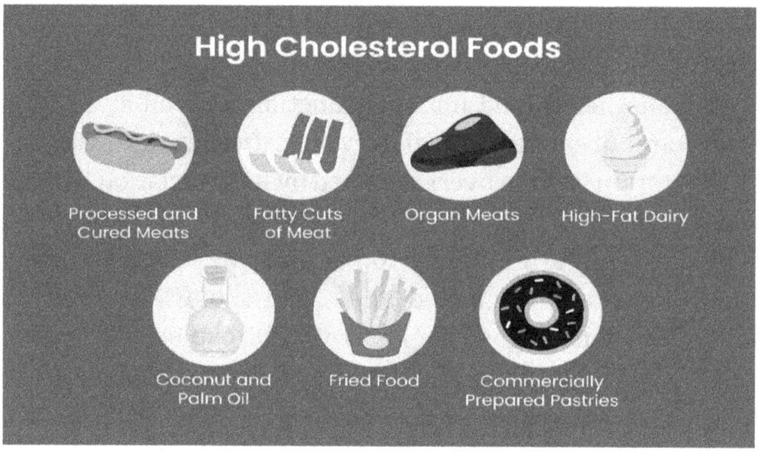
High Cholesterol Foods
Processed and Cured Meats
Fatty Cuts of Meat
Organ Meats
High-Fat Dairy
Coconut and Palm Oil
Fried Food
Commercially Prepared Pastries

Fig. 5 High Cholesterol Foods

The process of cholesterol testing is relatively simple but provides complex and clinically significant information. Typically, it involves drawing a blood sample after a period of fasting to ensure accurate measurement of LDL cholesterol and triglycerides. The results offer a comprehensive lipid profile, detailing the concentrations of total cholesterol, LDL cholesterol, HDL cholesterol and triglycerides. Emerging testing methods, including non-fasting lipid panels and advanced lipid subfraction analyses, further refine cardiovascular risk assessment by providing additional information on particle size and density. Understanding the results of cholesterol tests is crucial for both healthcare professionals and patients. Test values are interpreted within the context of overall health, existing medical conditions, lifestyle and other risk factors such as hypertension, diabetes and smoking. Guidelines from health organizations provide specific cholesterol level targets based on individual risk profiles, ensuring personalized and effective management strategies. In summary, cholesterol testing is a cornerstone of cardiovascular health assessment. It bridges the gap between basic biological processes and clinical practice, helping to identify those at risk for serious diseases early and guiding interventions that can save lives. Through regular monitoring and appropriate treatment, cholesterol tests empower patients and clinicians to work together towards better heart health and improved quality of life. This vital diagnostic tool continues to evolve with advances in medicine, reinforcing its central role in combating the global burden of cardiovascular disease.

Types of Cholesterol:

Cholesterol is a lipid or fat-like substance, essential for the body's normal functioning, but it must be present in the right balance to support good health. It circulates in the bloodstream bound to proteins, forming complexes known as lipoproteins. The main types of cholesterol include Low-Density Lipoprotein (LDL), High-Density Lipoprotein (HDL) and Very Low-Density Lipoprotein (VLDL), along with total cholesterol and triglycerides, which are measured together in a lipid panel (Fig. 6). Each type has a distinct role and impact on cardiovascular health. LDL is often called "bad" cholesterol because it can deposit in arterial walls and contribute to plaque formation. HDL or "good" cholesterol, helps clear excess cholesterol from the bloodstream. VLDL mainly carries triglycerides and also contributes to plaque buildup. Understanding these types helps clinicians assess heart disease risk and guide appropriate treatment strategies. Accurate cholesterol profiling is essential in both the prevention and management of cardiovascular conditions.

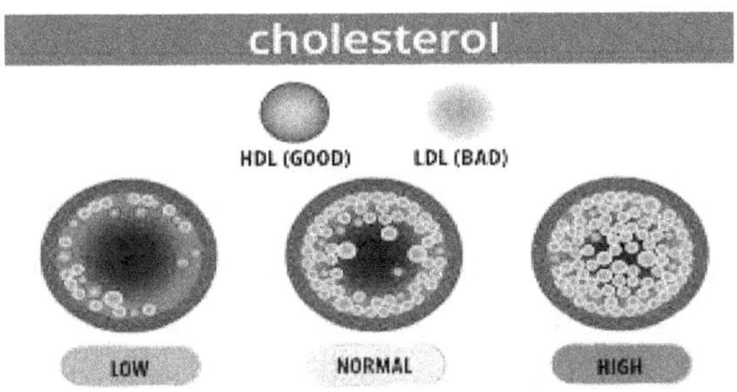

Fig.6 Cholesterol

Cholesterol in the blood is carried by lipoproteins and the main types measured are:

- **Low-Density Lipoprotein (LDL) Cholesterol:** Low-Density Lipoprotein, commonly known as LDL cholesterol or "bad" cholesterol, plays a central role in the development of cardiovascular disease. LDL carries cholesterol from the liver to the cells, but when present in excess, it deposits cholesterol onto the walls of arteries. This leads to the formation of fatty plaques that narrow and stiffen the arteries, a condition called atherosclerosis. Over time, these plaques can rupture, triggering blood clots that may cause heart attacks or strokes. High LDL levels are strongly associated with increased risk of coronary artery disease and peripheral vascular disease. Monitoring and managing LDL cholesterol is crucial for preventing these life-threatening conditions. Lifestyle changes and medications like statins effectively lower LDL cholesterol to reduce cardiovascular risk. Elevated LDL often requires long-term management strategies. Regular cholesterol testing helps track LDL levels and guide therapy. It remains a primary target in cardiovascular disease prevention.

- **High-Density Lipoprotein (HDL) Cholesterol:** High-Density Lipoprotein or HDL cholesterol, is often referred to as "good" cholesterol due to its protective effects on heart health. HDL functions by scavenging excess cholesterol from the bloodstream and artery walls and transporting it back to the liver for breakdown and excretion. This reverse cholesterol transport helps prevent the buildup of plaques that cause artery narrowing and blockages. Higher HDL levels are generally associated with a lower risk of cardiovascular disease, as HDL helps reduce inflammation and oxidative damage in blood vessels. Factors such as regular exercise, a healthy diet and not smoking can increase HDL cholesterol levels. Conversely, low HDL levels are considered a risk factor for heart disease. While HDL is protective, it's important to view it alongside other lipid measurements to get a complete picture of cardiovascular risk. Maintaining balanced cholesterol levels, including healthy HDL, supports overall cardiovascular health.
- **Total Cholesterol:** Total cholesterol is a comprehensive measure that represents the sum of all cholesterol types circulating in the blood, including LDL, HDL and other lipid fractions. It provides an overall snapshot of cholesterol status but does not distinguish between "good" and "bad" cholesterol on its own. Total cholesterol levels help identify individuals at risk for heart disease when used alongside other lipid measurements and clinical factors. High total cholesterol often indicates elevated LDL cholesterol or triglycerides, which increase cardiovascular risk. However, a high total cholesterol value might not always signify risk if HDL levels are also elevated. Physicians use total cholesterol as part of a lipid panel to evaluate heart disease risk, but further interpretation is necessary to tailor treatment. Regular testing of total cholesterol guides lifestyle and

medication decisions aimed at reducing heart disease risk. It is an accessible and widely used screening tool in clinical practice.

- **Triglycerides:** Triglycerides are a type of fat found in the blood that, while not cholesterol, are closely related to cardiovascular health. They are the main form of stored fat in the body, providing energy between meals. Elevated triglyceride levels often result from excess calorie intake, obesity, physical inactivity, excessive alcohol consumption or uncontrolled diabetes. High triglycerides can contribute to the hardening and narrowing of arteries, increasing the risk of heart disease and stroke. Elevated triglycerides are also linked to pancreatitis when levels are extremely high. They are typically measured alongside cholesterol levels in a lipid panel to provide a fuller picture of heart disease risk. Managing triglyceride levels through diet, exercise and sometimes medication is essential for comprehensive cardiovascular care. Keeping triglycerides within a healthy range helps reduce overall lipid-related risks. Regular monitoring of triglycerides complements cholesterol testing in heart disease prevention.

Purpose of Cholesterol Testing:

Cholesterol tests help screen for and monitor lipid disorders that increase cardiovascular risk. They are essential for:

- Assessing risk of coronary artery disease (CAD) and stroke.
- Guiding lifestyle and pharmacological interventions, such as diet changes, exercise and cholesterol-lowering medications like statins.
- Monitoring the effectiveness of ongoing treatment.
- Identifying inherited lipid disorders such as familial hypercholesterolemia.
- Helping evaluate secondary causes of abnormal cholesterol, such as diabetes, hypothyroidism or liver disease.

Types of Cholesterol Tests:

- **Lipid Panel (Lipid Profile):** The lipid panel, also known as a lipid profile, is the most commonly ordered blood test for assessing cardiovascular risk. It measures key components of blood lipids, including total cholesterol, LDL cholesterol, HDL cholesterol and triglycerides. To ensure accurate results, patients are usually required to fast for 9 to 12 hours before the blood draw, as eating can temporarily affect triglyceride and LDL levels. The lipid panel provides a comprehensive overview of an individual's cholesterol status and helps identify imbalances that could increase the risk of heart disease and stroke. Physicians use these results to guide preventive strategies and treatment plans. This test is essential in routine health screenings and in monitoring the effectiveness of lifestyle changes or medications. It remains a cornerstone of cardiovascular risk assessment worldwide.

- **Non-Fasting Lipid Test:** The non-fasting lipid test has gained acceptance as a convenient alternative to the traditional fasting lipid panel for routine cholesterol screening. It measures total cholesterol and HDL cholesterol without requiring the patient to fast beforehand, improving patient comfort and compliance. While non-fasting tests are generally reliable for assessing total cholesterol and HDL levels, triglyceride and LDL cholesterol measurements may be less precise due to post-meal fluctuations. Despite this limitation, non-fasting tests are especially useful in outpatient settings and large-scale screenings where fasting may be impractical. They enable timely evaluation of lipid status and help identify individuals who need further investigation or intervention. Recent guidelines support their use for initial cardiovascular risk assessment in many populations.
- **Direct LDL Measurement:** Direct LDL measurement is a specialized blood test used when traditional LDL calculation methods, such as the Friedewald equation, may be inaccurate. This is particularly important in patients with very high triglyceride levels or when fasting samples are unavailable. Instead of estimating LDL from other lipid values, direct LDL assays measure the concentration of LDL cholesterol in the blood precisely. This test provides clinicians with a more reliable LDL value, crucial for accurate risk assessment and treatment decisions in complex cases. Direct LDL measurement is valuable for patients with metabolic disorders, diabetes or those undergoing intensive lipid-lowering therapies. It enhances the clinician's ability to tailor treatment plans and monitor therapy effectiveness more accurately.
- **Advanced Lipid Testing:** Advanced lipid testing includes a range of assays that go beyond standard lipid panels to analyze the detailed characteristics of lipoproteins. These tests evaluate LDL particle size, number, density and other lipid subfractions that influence cardiovascular risk more precisely than traditional cholesterol measurements. Small, dense LDL particles, for example, are more atherogenic and linked to higher heart disease risk than larger LDL particles. Advanced lipid testing is particularly useful for patients with normal standard lipid levels but who have other risk factors or a family history of premature cardiovascular disease. These tests provide deeper insights into lipid metabolism and help in stratifying risk, guiding personalized treatment strategies. Though more costly and less widely available, advanced lipid testing represents the frontier of cardiovascular diagnostics (Table-3).

Table: 3 Summarizing the types of cholesterol tests

Type of Test	Description	Fasting Required	Primary Use
Lipid Panel (Lipid Profile)	Measures total cholesterol, LDL, HDL and triglycerides. Most commonly used test for overall lipid status.	Yes (9–12 hours)	Routine screening, diagnosis and monitoring of cholesterol levels.
Non-Fasting Lipid Test	Measures total cholesterol and HDL without fasting. Triglycerides and LDL may be less accurate.	No	Convenient initial screening, especially in outpatient or emergency settings.
Direct LDL Measurement	Directly measures LDL cholesterol without calculation. Useful when triglycerides are high or results from standard tests are unclear.	No	Accurate LDL assessment in complex or high-risk patients.
Advanced Lipid Testing	Analyzes LDL particle size, number and subfractions. Provides detailed cardiovascular risk assessment beyond standard lipids.	Varies	Used in patients with normal lipids but high cardiovascular risk or family history.
Apolipoprotein B (ApoB) Test	Measures the protein component of atherogenic lipoproteins (like LDL and VLDL). Offers a direct count of harmful particles.	No	Better risk prediction, especially in metabolic syndrome or diabetes.
Lipoprotein(a) [Lp(a)] Test	Measures a genetic variant of LDL associated with increased heart disease risk, not usually affected by lifestyle.	No	Evaluating inherited cholesterol risk or premature heart disease.

How the Test is Performed

Blood is drawn via venipuncture, usually from a vein in the arm. For fasting lipid panels, the patient avoids food and drink except water for 9-12 hours before the test. The sample is sent to a laboratory where cholesterol and triglyceride levels are quantified using enzymatic assays or other biochemical methods.

Interpretation of Results:

- **Total Cholesterol:**
    - Desirable: Less than 200 mg/dL (5.2 mmol/L)
    - Borderline High: 200–239 mg/dL (5.2–6.2 mmol/L)
    - High: 240 mg/dL (6.2 mmol/L) and above
- **LDL Cholesterol:**
    - Optimal: Less than 100 mg/dL (2.6 mmol/L)
    - Near Optimal: 100–129 mg/dL (2.6–3.3 mmol/L)
    - Borderline High: 130–159 mg/dL (3.4–4.1 mmol/L)
    - High: 160–189 mg/dL (4.1–4.9 mmol/L)

- Very High: 190 mg/dL (4.9 mmol/L) and above

◉ **HDL Cholesterol:**

- Low (risk factor): Less than 40 mg/dL (1.0 mmol/L) for men, less than 50 mg/dL (1.3 mmol/L) for women
- Acceptable: 40–59 mg/dL (1.0–1.5 mmol/L)
- High (protective): 60 mg/dL (1.5 mmol/L) and above

◉ **Triglycerides:**

- Normal: Less than 150 mg/dL (1.7 mmol/L)
- Borderline High: 150–199 mg/dL (1.7–2.2 mmol/L)
- High: 200–499 mg/dL (2.3–5.6 mmol/L)
- Very High: 500 mg/dL (5.6 mmol/L) and above

Clinical Significance: High LDL and triglyceride levels promote the formation of fatty plaques inside artery walls, leading to narrowing and hardening of arteries (atherosclerosis). This can result in reduced blood flow, causing angina, heart attacks, strokes or peripheral artery disease. Conversely, higher HDL levels help clear cholesterol from arteries and transport it back to the liver for elimination, offering a protective effect. Cholesterol testing therefore helps assess risk, motivate lifestyle changes and guide treatment to reduce cardiovascular events.

Factors Affecting Cholesterol Levels: Cholesterol levels can be influenced by genetics, diet, physical activity, age, gender, weight, smoking, alcohol use, medications and underlying medical conditions. For example, diets high in saturated fats and trans fats raise LDL cholesterol. Physical activity can increase HDL cholesterol. Some medical conditions like hypothyroidism or diabetes can also affect lipid levels. Therefore, cholesterol results must be interpreted in the context of the whole patient.

Follow-Up and Monitoring: Patients with abnormal cholesterol often require follow-up testing to monitor treatment efficacy and adherence. Lifestyle modifications such as diet and exercise are first-line interventions. If insufficient, lipid-lowering medications are prescribed. Regular testing ensures cholesterol targets are met to minimize cardiovascular risk.

3.2.4 Hormones

Hormones are chemical messengers secreted by specialized organs called endocrine glands, such as the pituitary, thyroid, adrenal glands and pancreas. These molecules play a vital role in maintaining the body's internal balance, known as homeostasis. Once produced, hormones are released directly into the bloodstream, which transports them to specific target organs or cells. These target cells have specialized receptors that recognize and bind to particular hormones, initiating a cascade of biochemical reactions. Hormones regulate a wide range of physiological processes, including growth, metabolism, reproduction, immune response and mood. There are various types of hormones classified based on their chemical structure, such as peptide hormones (e.g., insulin), steroid hormones (e.g., cortisol) and amino acid-derived hormones (e.g., adrenaline and thyroxine). Some hormones, like insulin, help control blood sugar levels, while others like growth hormone promote tissue development and regeneration. Sex hormones such as estrogen and testosterone are crucial for the development of secondary sexual characteristics and fertility. The endocrine system works in close coordination with the nervous system to ensure quick and precise regulation of bodily functions. Hormones often function through feedback mechanisms, especially negative feedback loops, which help prevent overproduction or underproduction. For example, when blood calcium levels drop, the parathyroid glands release PTH to restore balance. Similarly, thyroid hormones regulate metabolism and are tightly controlled by TSH from the pituitary gland. Hormonal imbalances can lead to various disorders, such as diabetes, hyperthyroidism or Cushing's syndrome. Because of their essential roles, even tiny deviations in hormone levels can have widespread effects on physical and mental health. Overall, hormones are integral to life, influencing nearly every function in the body continuously and precisely. Major endocrine glands and their hormones is summarised in Table-4.

Main Features of Hormones

Secreted by endocrine glands (ductless glands)

- Travel through the blood
- Affect target cells/organs that have specific receptors
- Work in small quantities
- Help maintain homeostasis

Classification of Hormones

By Chemical Structure

Type	Examples	Solubility	Receptor Location
Peptide/Protein	Insulin, ADH, GH	Water-soluble	Cell membrane
Steroid	Cortisol, Estrogen	Lipid-soluble	Intracellular
Amino acid-derived	Thyroxine, Epinephrine	Water or lipid-soluble	Membrane or intracellular
Fatty acid-derived (Eicosanoids)	Prostaglandins	Lipid-soluble	Cell membrane

By Origin

- Endocrine glands: Pituitary, thyroid, adrenal, pancreas, etc.
- Other organs: Heart (ANP), kidneys (erythropoietin), stomach (gastrin)

The major endocrine glands and their hormones are summarised in Table-4.

Table 4: Major Endocrine Glands and Their Hormones

Gland	Hormone(s)	Function(s)
Hypothalamus	TRH, CRH, GnRH	Regulate pituitary
Pituitary(Master Gland)	GH, TSH, LH, ACTH, FSH, PRL	Growth, metabolism, reproduction
Thyroid	T3, T4, Calcitonin	Metabolism, calcium regulation
Parathyroid	PTH	Increases blood calcium
Adrenal glands	Cortisol, Aldosterone, Adrenaline	Stress, metabolism, BP
Pancreas	Insulin, Glucagon	Blood sugar regulation
Ovaries	Estrogen, Progesterone	Female sex traits, cycle
Testes	Testosterone	Male sex traits
Pineal gland	Melatonin	Circadian rhythm
Kidneys	Erythropoietin	RBC production

Hormonal Mechanism of Action

The hormonal mechanism of action refers to how hormones produce their effects on target cells and organs after being secreted by endocrine glands. Hormones act as chemical messengers, traveling through the bloodstream to reach specific target cells that have receptors for those hormones. The nature of their action depends largely on their chemical structure—whether they are water-soluble or lipid-soluble. Water-soluble hormones, like insulin and adrenaline, cannot pass through the cell membrane, so they bind to receptors on the cell surface, triggering a second messenger system such as cAMP. This leads to rapid changes in cellular activity. In contrast, lipid-soluble hormones like steroid hormones (e.g., cortisol, estrogen) can easily pass through the cell membrane and bind to intracellular receptors, often within the nucleus. This binding directly affects gene transcription, leading to protein synthesis and long-term physiological changes. Some hormones act within seconds, while others take hours or days to exert their full effect. The action of hormones is highly specific and tightly regulated, ensuring that each hormone only affects its intended targets. This complex signaling network helps coordinate vital processes such as growth, metabolism, reproduction and homeostasis, maintaining the body's internal balance.

1. **Water-soluble hormones (e.g., insulin, epinephrine):**
    - Bind to receptors on the cell membrane
    - Trigger second messengers (like cAMP)
    - Cause rapid, short-term responses
2. **Lipid-soluble hormones (e.g., cortisol, thyroxine):**
    - Pass through cell membrane

- Bind to intracellular receptors
- Influence gene transcription
- Effects are slower but longer-lasting

Hormonal Regulation

Hormonal regulation is the process by which the body controls the production, release and action of hormones to maintain internal stability or homeostasis. This regulation ensures that hormones are secreted in the right amounts, at the right time and only when needed. One of the most important mechanisms involved is the feedback system, especially negative feedback loops. In this system, a hormone's effects inhibit further hormone production, preventing overactivity. For example, high levels of thyroid hormones (T3 and T4) inhibit TSH release from the pituitary gland.

On the other hand, positive feedback occurs in rare cases, where a hormone's effect stimulates further secretion, such as oxytocin during childbirth. Hormonal regulation involves communication between the hypothalamus, pituitary gland and peripheral endocrine glands, forming the hypothalamic-pituitary axis. External factors like stress, sleep, diet and environment can also influence hormone levels. Disruption in regulation can lead to disorders such as diabetes, hypothyroidism or Cushing's syndrome. Overall, hormonal regulation is a dynamic and complex process that ensures physiological balance and supports the body's ability to adapt to changing conditions.

Feedback Loops

- **Negative Feedback:** Most common. Hormone release inhibits further secretion. Example: High cortisol inhibits ACTH and CRH release.
- **Positive Feedback:** Rare. Hormone release stimulates more secretion. Example: Oxytocin during childbirth.

Functions of Hormones

Function	Hormones Involved
Growth & development	GH, Thyroxine, IGF
Metabolism	Insulin, Glucagon, T3/T4
Reproduction	FSH, LH, Estrogen, Testosterone
Stress response	Cortisol, Adrenaline
Water balance	ADH, Aldosterone
Calcium balance	PTH, Calcitonin
Sleep cycles	Melatonin

Disorders Related to Hormones

Condition	Hormone Involved	Description
Diabetes mellitus	Insulin deficiency/resistance	High blood glucose
Hypothyroidism	Low thyroxine (T3/T4)	Fatigue, weight gain
Hyperthyroidism	High thyroxine	Weight loss, anxiety
Cushing's syndrome	Excess cortisol	Moon face, obesity
Addison's disease	Low cortisol & aldosterone	Fatigue, low BP
Acromegaly	Excess GH in adults	Enlarged hands/face
Dwarfism	GH deficiency in children	Short stature

Hormone Testing

Common Blood Tests

1. TSH, T3, T4 – Thyroid Function Tests

TSH (Thyroid Stimulating Hormone) Test: The Thyroid Stimulating Hormone (TSH) test is a crucial diagnostic tool used to evaluate thyroid gland function. TSH is a hormone produced by the pituitary gland, located at the base of the brain, which plays a central role in regulating the thyroid gland's activity. The thyroid gland itself, situated in the neck, produces hormones like thyroxine (T4) and triiodothyronine (T3) that are essential for regulating the body's metabolism, energy production and overall growth and development. The TSH test measures the concentration of this hormone in the bloodstream, providing important insights into whether the thyroid is functioning normally or if there are underlying disorders. When the thyroid hormones in the blood are low, the pituitary gland responds by releasing more TSH to stimulate the thyroid to produce more hormones. Conversely, if thyroid hormone levels are high, the pituitary reduces TSH production. This feedback loop makes the TSH test an indirect but reliable indicator of thyroid health. The test is commonly used to diagnose conditions such as hypothyroidism, where the thyroid is underactive and produces insufficient hormones or hyperthyroidism, where the gland is overactive. Clinicians often order the TSH test when patients present with symptoms like fatigue, weight changes, mood swings or irregular heartbeats, all of which can be related to thyroid dysfunction. It's also a routine screening tool during pregnancy and for monitoring the effectiveness of thyroid hormone replacement therapy. The test requires a simple blood sample and results are typically available within a short timeframe. The normal reference range for TSH levels can vary slightly between laboratories but generally falls between 0.4 and 4.0 milli-international units per liter (mIU/L). Values above or below this range may indicate hypothyroidism or hyperthyroidism, respectively, though further testing is often necessary to confirm a diagnosis. Additionally, factors such as age, pregnancy, medications and overall health can influence TSH levels, highlighting the importance of professional interpretation. The TSH test is a fundamental part of assessing thyroid function, guiding diagnosis and treatment of thyroid disorders and ensuring patients maintain optimal hormonal balance for their overall well-being. Its simplicity, reliability and clinical significance make it a cornerstone in endocrine health evaluation.

- **Purpose:** Measures how much TSH the pituitary gland is producing to stimulate the thyroid.
- **Normal Range:** 0.4 – 4.0 mIU/L
- **High TSH:** May indicate hypothyroidism
- **Low TSH:** May indicate hyperthyroidism

T3 (Triiodothyronine) Test:

The T3 (Triiodothyronine) test is a laboratory blood test used to measure the level of the hormone triiodothyronine in the bloodstream. T3 is one of the primary hormones produced by the thyroid gland, along with thyroxine (T4) and plays a critical role in regulating various physiological processes, including metabolism, heart rate, body temperature and growth. Although T3 is produced directly by the thyroid, the majority of T3 in the blood is generated by conversion from T4 in other tissues, such as the liver and kidneys. The T3 test helps provide a more detailed understanding of thyroid function and complements other thyroid tests like the TSH and T4 tests. Because T3 is the active form of thyroid hormone, its levels can more accurately reflect how well the body's cells are responding to thyroid hormone stimulation. This test is particularly useful in diagnosing and monitoring hyperthyroidism, a condition where the thyroid produces excessive amounts of hormones, causing symptoms like rapid heartbeat, anxiety, weight loss and sweating. Elevated T3 levels often confirm an overactive thyroid, especially in cases where T4 levels may still be within normal ranges. Conversely, low T3 levels can indicate hypothyroidism or other health issues, such as severe illness or malnutrition. Doctors may order the T3 test when a patient exhibits signs of thyroid imbalance or when the TSH test results are abnormal but inconclusive. It is also used to monitor treatment efficacy in thyroid disorders, helping physicians adjust medication dosages to achieve optimal hormone balance. The test involves drawing a small blood sample, typically from a vein in the arm, which is then analyzed in a clinical laboratory. There are two types of T3 tests: total T3, which measures both bound and free hormone in the blood and free T3, which measures the active unbound hormone that is available to tissues. Free T3 testing is often considered more clinically relevant because it reflects the hormone that is biologically active. Reference ranges for T3 can vary by laboratory and testing method, but generally, total T3 levels range from about 80 to 200 ng/dL and free T3 levels range between 2.0 and 4.4 pg/mL. The T3 test is an important tool for assessing thyroid function and diagnosing disorders related to abnormal thyroid hormone production. When interpreted alongside TSH and T4 tests, it helps provide a comprehensive view of thyroid health, supporting accurate diagnosis and effective treatment planning. The T3 test ultimately aids in maintaining the body's metabolic balance and overall well-being by ensuring the thyroid hormones are functioning properly.

- **Purpose:** Assesses the level of active thyroid hormone.
- **Normal Range:** 80 – 200 ng/dL (total T3)
- **High T3:** Suggests hyperthyroidism
- **Low T3:** Suggests hypothyroidism or poor conversion from T4

T4 (Thyroxine) Test:

The T4 (Thyroxine) test is a blood test that measures the levels of thyroxine, a key hormone produced by the thyroid gland. Thyroxine, often referred to as T4, is one of the primary hormones responsible for regulating metabolism, growth and development in the body. It is synthesized by the thyroid gland and released into the bloodstream, where it influences how cells use energy, produce proteins and respond to other hormones. Because T4 plays a vital role in maintaining the body's overall energy balance, the T4 test is an important diagnostic tool for assessing thyroid gland function. Most of the T4 hormone in the blood is bound to proteins and inactive, while a small fraction remains unbound or "free," which is the biologically active form that can enter cells and exert its effects. There are two types of T4 tests: total T4, which measures both bound and free thyroxine and free T4, which specifically measures the hormone available to tissues. The free T4 test is generally considered more accurate in evaluating thyroid function because it reflects the hormone that is active in the body. Doctors order the T4 test when patients exhibit symptoms of thyroid disorders such as fatigue, unexplained weight changes, hair thinning, mood swings or irregular heart rhythms. The test is also used to help diagnose conditions such as hypothyroidism, where the thyroid produces too little hormone or hyperthyroidism, where excess hormone is produced. Additionally, the T4 test is used to monitor patients receiving thyroid hormone replacement therapy or medications that affect thyroid function. The thyroid gland is regulated by the pituitary hormone called Thyroid Stimulating Hormone (TSH), which signals the thyroid to produce and release T4. This relationship creates a feedback loop that keeps hormone levels balanced. When T4 levels are low, TSH levels typically increase to stimulate more production and when T4 is high, TSH decreases to reduce production. Measuring T4 alongside TSH gives a more complete picture of thyroid health. Normal reference ranges for total T4 vary but typically fall between 5.0 and 12.0 micrograms per deciliter (μg/dL), while free T4 levels usually range from 0.8 to 1.8 nanograms per deciliter (ng/dL). Variations can occur due to factors like age, pregnancy, medications and illness, which must be considered when interpreting results. The T4 test is a fundamental component in diagnosing and managing thyroid diseases, providing crucial information about hormone levels that affect metabolic processes. It helps physicians understand thyroid function, guide treatment decisions and monitor the effectiveness of therapies, thereby supporting patients' overall health and metabolic balance.

- **Purpose:** Measures the main hormone produced by the thyroid gland.
- **Normal Range:** 5 – 12 µg/dL (total T4)
- **High T4:** Hyperthyroidism
- **Low T4:** Hypothyroidism

2. FSH, LH, Estrogen, Testosterone – Fertility Hormones

FSH (Follicle Stimulating Hormone) Test:

The Follicle Stimulating Hormone (FSH) test is a blood test used to measure the level of FSH, a vital hormone produced by the pituitary gland located at the base of the brain. FSH plays a key role in regulating the reproductive processes in both males and females. In women, FSH is responsible for stimulating the growth and maturation of ovarian follicles, which contain the eggs and it also helps regulate the menstrual cycle and ovulation. In men, FSH supports the production of sperm by acting on the testes. Because of its central role in reproductive health, measuring FSH levels provides important insights into fertility, hormonal balance and the function of the ovaries or testes. The FSH test is commonly ordered when a patient is experiencing issues related to fertility, irregular menstrual cycles or symptoms of menopause. It helps doctors diagnose conditions such as primary ovarian insufficiency, menopause, polycystic ovary syndrome (PCOS) and certain pituitary disorders. For men, it assists in evaluating causes of infertility and testicular function. Additionally, the FSH test can be used to assess the functioning of the hypothalamic-pituitary-gonadal axis, the hormonal system that controls reproduction. FSH levels fluctuate naturally during the menstrual cycle, with peaks occurring just before ovulation, so timing of the test is important for accurate interpretation. For women, the test is often done on specific cycle days to get meaningful results. Elevated FSH levels in women can indicate diminished ovarian reserve or menopause, while low levels may suggest pituitary gland problems or hypothalamic dysfunction. In men, abnormal FSH levels can point to issues with sperm production or testicular failure. The test involves a simple blood draw and results are usually available within a short period. FSH values are measured in international units per liter (IU/L) and normal ranges vary depending on age, sex and reproductive status. For example, women of reproductive age typically have FSH levels between 4.7 and 21.5 IU/L, which vary throughout their cycle, while postmenopausal women usually have higher levels due to reduced ovarian function. The FSH test is a critical tool in assessing reproductive health and diagnosing disorders related to fertility and hormonal imbalances. It guides physicians in developing appropriate treatment plans for individuals facing reproductive challenges, providing valuable information about the complex interplay between the brain and reproductive organs. The FSH test ultimately supports patients in understanding their reproductive status and managing their reproductive health effectively.

- **Purpose:** Evaluates reproductive function and ovarian/testicular reserve.
- **Normal Range:**
    - Women (follicular phase): 4.7 – 21.5 mIU/mL
    - Men: 1.5 – 12.4 mIU/mL
- **High FSH:** Ovarian failure or menopause
- **Low FSH:** Pituitary dysfunction

LH (Luteinizing Hormone) Test:

The Luteinizing Hormone (LH) test is a blood test that measures the levels of LH, a hormone produced by the pituitary gland, which plays a crucial role in regulating the reproductive system in both men and women. LH works closely with Follicle Stimulating Hormone (FSH) to control the function of the ovaries in women and testes in men. In women, LH triggers ovulation—the release of a mature egg from the ovary—and stimulates the production of progesterone, which supports the early stages of pregnancy. In men, LH stimulates the production of testosterone by acting on the Leydig cells in the testes, which is essential for sperm production and the development of male secondary sexual characteristics.

The LH test is commonly used to evaluate fertility issues, menstrual irregularities and pituitary gland function. It is also useful in diagnosing conditions such as polycystic ovary syndrome (PCOS), primary ovarian insufficiency and hypothalamic or pituitary disorders. In men, the test helps assess causes of infertility and testicular function. Because LH levels vary throughout the menstrual cycle, the timing of the test is important for accurate interpretation, often being performed on specific days to coincide with the mid-cycle LH surge that triggers ovulation. In women, abnormally high or low levels of LH can indicate various reproductive disorders. Elevated LH levels are commonly seen in PCOS and menopause, while low levels may suggest hypothalamic or pituitary dysfunction. In men, low LH levels may point to problems with the pituitary gland or hypothalamus, whereas high levels can indicate testicular failure or damage. Monitoring LH levels can also help doctors evaluate the effectiveness of treatments related to fertility or hormone replacement therapy. The LH test is typically performed by drawing a blood sample, which is then analyzed in a laboratory. Results are measured in international units per liter (IU/L), with reference ranges varying based on age, sex and reproductive status. For example, LH levels in women fluctuate widely during the menstrual cycle, ranging from 2 to 15 IU/L during the follicular phase and peaking between 20 to 100 IU/L during ovulation. Men generally have steady LH levels ranging from about 1.8 to 8.6 IU/L. The LH test is a vital diagnostic tool for understanding reproductive health and hormone function. By measuring LH levels, healthcare providers gain insight into ovulatory function, fertility status and underlying endocrine disorders. The information derived from this test aids in diagnosis, treatment planning and monitoring of reproductive and hormonal health, helping patients manage conditions related to fertility and hormonal imbalances effectively.

- **Purpose:** Assesses ovulation in women and testosterone production in men.
- **Normal Range:**
  - Women (mid-cycle peak): 25 – 105 mIU/mL
  - Men: 1.8 – 8.6 mIU/mL
- **High LH:** PCOS or menopause
- **Low LH:** Hypopituitarism

Estrogen (Estradiol, E2) Test:

The Estrogen test, specifically measuring estradiol (E2), is a blood test used to evaluate the levels of estradiol, the most potent and prevalent form of estrogen in the body. Estrogen is a primary female sex hormone responsible for the development and regulation of the female reproductive system and secondary sexual characteristics. Estradiol is produced mainly by the ovaries, but also in smaller amounts by the adrenal glands and fat tissue. This hormone plays a vital role in regulating the menstrual cycle, supporting pregnancy and maintaining bone density, cardiovascular health and overall well-being. Measuring estradiol levels through the E2 test provides valuable insights into reproductive health, hormonal balance and certain medical conditions. The estradiol test is commonly ordered for women experiencing menstrual irregularities, infertility or symptoms of menopause. It is also used to monitor ovarian function during fertility treatments, assess the health of the ovaries and evaluate suspected hormonal imbalances. In men, estradiol testing may be conducted when symptoms of hormonal imbalance, such as gynecomastia or infertility, are present. Additionally, the test can help diagnose conditions such as polycystic ovary syndrome (PCOS), ovarian cysts or estrogen-producing tumors. Estradiol levels fluctuate throughout the menstrual cycle, peaking just before ovulation, which makes timing of the test critical for accurate interpretation. Normal estradiol values vary by age, sex and phase of the menstrual cycle. For premenopausal women, estradiol levels typically range from 15 to 350 picograms per milliliter (pg/mL), while postmenopausal women generally have lower levels, often below 30 pg/mL. Men usually have estradiol levels between 10 and 40 pg/mL. The test involves a simple blood draw and results are analyzed to help healthcare providers understand a patient's hormonal status. Abnormally high or low estradiol levels can indicate various health issues. Elevated estradiol may suggest ovarian hyperactivity, hormone replacement therapy effects or certain tumors, while low levels can be seen in menopause, ovarian failure or hypothalamic disorders. The estradiol (E2) test is an essential tool for assessing estrogen-related health and reproductive function. It aids in diagnosing hormonal imbalances, guiding fertility treatments and monitoring therapeutic interventions. By providing detailed information about estradiol levels, this test helps clinicians optimize care and support overall hormonal health and reproductive wellness.

- **Purpose:** Measures female sex hormone levels.
- **Normal Range:**
  - Women (reproductive age): 15 – 350 pg/mL
- **High Estrogen:** Tumors, liver disease
- **Low Estrogen:** Menopause, ovarian failure

Testosterone Test:

The Testosterone test is a blood test that measures the level of testosterone, the primary male sex hormone, in the bloodstream. Testosterone is essential for the development of male reproductive tissues such as the testes and prostate, as well as for promoting secondary sexual characteristics like increased muscle and bone mass and the growth of body hair. While testosterone is predominantly produced in the testes in men, it is also produced in smaller amounts by the adrenal glands. In women, testosterone is produced in the ovaries and adrenal glands but at much lower levels. This hormone plays a vital role not only in sexual development and function but also in overall health, mood regulation and energy levels in both sexes. The testosterone test is commonly ordered when there are symptoms of hormonal imbalance, such as decreased libido, erectile dysfunction, infertility, fatigue or unexplained changes in muscle mass or mood. It is also used to evaluate delayed or early puberty, monitor hormone replacement therapy and investigate potential causes of gynecomastia (enlargement of male breast tissue) in men. For women, abnormal testosterone levels may indicate conditions such as polycystic ovary syndrome (PCOS), adrenal gland disorders or hormone-secreting tumors. Testosterone exists in the blood in two forms: bound and free. Most testosterone is bound to proteins such as sex hormone-binding globulin (SHBG), which makes it biologically inactive. The free testosterone fraction, which is unbound, is the active form that can enter cells and exert physiological effects. Because of this, doctors may order tests measuring total testosterone, free testosterone or both, depending on the clinical context. Normal testosterone levels vary by age, sex and time of day, often peaking in the morning. In adult men, typical total testosterone levels range from about 300 to 1,000 nanograms per deciliter (ng/dL), whereas in women, normal levels are significantly lower, usually between 15 and 70 ng/dL. Levels outside these ranges can indicate a range of health issues, from hypogonadism and infertility to hormone-secreting tumors or metabolic disorders. The test requires a blood sample, usually taken in the morning to capture peak hormone levels and results help guide diagnosis and treatment plans. In summary, the testosterone test is a vital diagnostic tool for assessing reproductive health, hormonal balance and overall well-being in both men and women. It provides key insights into conditions affecting sexual development, fertility and endocrine function.

- **Purpose:** Measures male sex hormone level.
- **Normal Range:**
  - Men: 300 – 1,000 ng/dL
  - Women: 15 – 70 ng/dL
- **Low Testosterone:** Hypogonadism, pituitary disorders
- **High Testosterone:** PCOS (in women), tumors

3. Cortisol, ACTH – Adrenal Function Tests

Cortisol Test:

The Cortisol test is a blood, urine or saliva test that measures the level of cortisol, a steroid hormone produced by the adrenal glands located on top of the kidneys. Cortisol is often referred to as the "stress hormone" because it plays a critical role in the body's response to stress. It helps regulate various vital functions such as metabolism, immune response, blood sugar levels and blood pressure. Cortisol follows a daily rhythm, typically peaking in the early morning and gradually decreasing throughout the day. Measuring cortisol levels provides valuable information about adrenal gland function and the body's ability to manage stress and maintain homeostasis. The cortisol test is commonly used to diagnose disorders related to abnormal cortisol production, such as Cushing's syndrome, which results from excessive cortisol and Addison's disease, which occurs due to insufficient cortisol levels. It is also helpful in evaluating symptoms like unexplained weight changes, fatigue, muscle weakness, high blood pressure and mood disturbances, all of which can be linked to cortisol imbalance. In addition, cortisol testing assists in monitoring treatment for adrenal or pituitary gland disorders. Because cortisol levels fluctuate throughout the day, the timing of sample collection is critical for accurate results. Blood cortisol is typically measured in the morning when levels are highest, while late-night cortisol levels may be tested to identify abnormal patterns. Urine cortisol tests often involve a 24-hour collection to assess total cortisol production and saliva tests offer a non-invasive way to monitor cortisol's daily cycle. Normal cortisol levels vary depending on the testing method and time of day but generally range from 6 to 23 micrograms per deciliter (μg/dL) in the morning. Abnormally high cortisol can indicate conditions like Cushing's syndrome, stress or tumors of the adrenal or pituitary glands. Low cortisol levels may suggest Addison's disease, adrenal insufficiency or damage to the pituitary gland. The cortisol test is an essential diagnostic tool for assessing adrenal gland function and hormone regulation related to stress and metabolism. It helps healthcare providers diagnose hormonal disorders, guide treatment plans and monitor the effectiveness of therapies aimed at restoring hormonal balance. Understanding cortisol levels is key to managing a range of health conditions and ensuring overall well-being.

- **Purpose:** Checks adrenal gland function; used to diagnose Cushing's or Addison's disease.
- **Normal Range (morning):** 6 – 23 μg/dL
- **High Cortisol:** Cushing's syndrome, chronic stress
- **Low Cortisol:** Addison's disease

ACTH (Adrenocorticotropic Hormone) Test:

The ACTH (Adrenocorticotropic Hormone) test is a blood test that measures the level of ACTH, a hormone produced by the pituitary gland located at the base of the brain. ACTH plays a critical role in regulating the adrenal glands, which sit atop the kidneys and produce important hormones such as cortisol. Specifically, ACTH stimulates the adrenal cortex to release cortisol, a hormone essential for managing stress, metabolism, immune response and blood pressure. Because of its central role in the hypothalamic-pituitary-adrenal (HPA) axis, measuring ACTH levels provides valuable insight into adrenal and pituitary gland function and helps diagnose disorders related to hormone imbalances. The ACTH test is commonly ordered when there is suspicion of conditions like Addison's disease, where the adrenal glands produce insufficient cortisol or Cushing's syndrome, characterized by excessive cortisol production. It also helps differentiate between causes of abnormal cortisol levels, such as whether they originate from the pituitary gland or the adrenal glands themselves. Symptoms that might prompt an ACTH test include unexplained fatigue, weakness, weight changes, blood pressure abnormalities and changes in skin pigmentation. Since ACTH and cortisol have a closely linked regulatory relationship, these tests are often ordered together to better understand the feedback loop within the HPA axis. ACTH levels naturally fluctuate throughout the day, typically peaking in the early morning and dropping at night, so timing of the blood draw is important for accurate assessment. In some cases, stimulation or suppression tests may be performed alongside to evaluate how the adrenal glands respond to ACTH or to other regulatory hormones. Normal ACTH levels vary by laboratory but generally range from about 10 to 60 picograms per milliliter (pg/mL) in the morning when levels peak. High ACTH levels can indicate primary adrenal insufficiency (Addison's disease), where the pituitary produces excess ACTH to compensate for failing adrenal glands. Conversely, low ACTH levels may suggest secondary adrenal insufficiency due to pituitary or hypothalamic dysfunction. The ACTH test is an essential tool for diagnosing and managing disorders of the adrenal and pituitary glands. By measuring ACTH levels, healthcare providers gain critical insights into hormone regulation, aiding in the diagnosis of complex endocrine disorders and guiding appropriate treatment strategies. This test supports the maintenance of hormonal balance crucial for overall health and stress adaptation.

- **Purpose:** Assesses pituitary function and adrenal responsc.
- **Normal Range:** 10 – 60 pg/mL (morning)
- **High ACTH:** Addison's disease
- **Low ACTH:** Cushing's syndrome (from adrenal tumor or steroid use)

4. Insulin, Glucose – Diabetes Screening

Glucose Test (Fasting Blood Sugar):

The Glucose Test, commonly known as the Fasting Blood Sugar (FBS) test, is a fundamental blood test used to measure the amount of glucose—commonly referred to as blood sugar—in the bloodstream after a period of fasting, typically 8 to 12 hours. Glucose is the primary source of energy for the body's cells and is derived from the foods we eat, particularly carbohydrates. Maintaining balanced blood glucose levels is essential for normal body function, as both excessively high and low glucose levels can lead to serious health complications. The fasting glucose test is an important tool for assessing how well the body regulates blood sugar and is widely used in diagnosing and monitoring diabetes mellitus and other metabolic disorders. The Fasting Blood Sugar test is usually ordered when a person shows symptoms suggestive of diabetes, such as increased thirst, frequent urination, unexplained weight loss, fatigue or slow healing of wounds. It is also used as a routine screening test for individuals at risk of developing diabetes, including those with obesity, a family history of diabetes or certain ethnic backgrounds. The test helps differentiate between normal glucose metabolism, prediabetes—a condition where blood sugar levels are elevated but not high enough to be classified as diabetes—and diabetes itself. To perform the test, the patient must fast overnight, refraining from eating or drinking anything except water. This fasting period ensures that the blood glucose measurement is not influenced by recent food intake, providing a clear picture of the body's baseline glucose level. Blood is drawn from a vein, usually in the arm and sent to a laboratory for analysis. Normal fasting blood glucose levels typically range from about 70 to 100 milligrams per deciliter (mg/dL). Levels between 100 and 125 mg/dL suggest prediabetes, while levels of 126 mg/dL or higher on two separate tests indicate diabetes. The fasting glucose test is often used alongside other tests such as the oral glucose tolerance test (OGTT) and hemoglobin A1c to provide a comprehensive assessment of blood sugar control over time. These tests help doctors diagnose diabetes, monitor the effectiveness of treatment plans and guide lifestyle or medication adjustments. The Glucose Test (Fasting Blood Sugar) is a vital diagnostic and monitoring tool for blood sugar regulation and metabolic health. It enables early detection of diabetes and prediabetes, helping prevent complications by facilitating timely intervention. Maintaining healthy glucose levels through diet, exercise and medication when necessary is crucial for long-term health and quality of life.

- **Purpose:** Screens for diabetes and insulin resistance.
- **Normal Range:** 70 – 99 mg/dL (fasting)
- **100–125 mg/dL:** Prediabetes
- **126 mg/dL or higher:** Diabetes

Insulin Test:

The Insulin test is a blood test that measures the level of insulin, a vital hormone produced by the pancreas, in the bloodstream. Insulin plays a crucial role in regulating blood sugar (glucose) by facilitating its uptake into the body's cells for energy production or storage. It helps maintain blood glucose levels within a narrow range, preventing hyperglycemia (high blood sugar) and hypoglycemia (low blood sugar). The insulin test is an important tool for assessing how well the body produces and uses insulin, which is critical in diagnosing and managing various metabolic disorders, including diabetes and insulin resistance. This test is commonly ordered when there is suspicion of abnormal insulin levels due to symptoms such as unexplained weight changes, excessive thirst, frequent urination, fatigue or signs of hypoglycemia like dizziness and confusion. It is also used to evaluate conditions such as type 1 and type 2 diabetes, metabolic syndrome and polycystic ovary syndrome (PCOS), where insulin resistance often plays a key role. Additionally, the insulin test can help diagnose rare disorders like insulinomas, tumors of the pancreas that produce excessive insulin.

The insulin test typically requires a fasting blood sample to provide accurate baseline insulin levels without the influence of recent food intake. It may also be performed in conjunction with a glucose tolerance test to assess how insulin levels change in response to glucose consumption. Normal fasting insulin levels generally range from 2 to 25 micro-units per milliliter (μU/mL), although reference ranges can vary depending on the laboratory and testing methods. Abnormally high insulin levels may indicate insulin resistance, a condition where the body's cells do not respond effectively to insulin, often leading to type 2 diabetes. Low insulin levels, on the other hand, may suggest type 1 diabetes or pancreatic dysfunction where insulin production is impaired. Monitoring insulin levels helps healthcare providers tailor treatment plans, including lifestyle modifications, medications or insulin therapy, to better manage blood sugar and metabolic health. The insulin test is a valuable diagnostic and monitoring tool for understanding the body's insulin production and function. It plays a pivotal role in the detection and management of diabetes, metabolic disorders and related conditions. By providing insight into insulin dynamics, this test supports effective interventions aimed at maintaining optimal blood sugar control and overall health.

- **Purpose:** Measures insulin levels to evaluate insulin resistance.
- **Normal Range (fasting):** 2 – 25 μIU/mL
- **High Insulin:** Insulin resistance, PCOS
- **Low Insulin:** Type 1 diabetes

5. PTH, Calcium – Calcium Balance and Parathyroid Function

PTH (Parathyroid Hormone) Test:

The PTH (Parathyroid Hormone) test is a blood test that measures the level of parathyroid hormone in the bloodstream. PTH is produced by the parathyroid glands—four small glands located in the neck near the thyroid gland—and plays a crucial role in regulating calcium, phosphorus and vitamin D levels in the body. This hormone helps maintain stable calcium concentrations in the blood, which is essential for normal functioning of nerves, muscles and bones. By controlling calcium absorption from the intestines, calcium release from bones and calcium excretion through the kidneys, PTH ensures proper mineral balance critical for metabolic and skeletal health. The PTH test is typically ordered when there is suspicion of calcium imbalance or related disorders, such as hypercalcemia (high calcium levels) or hypocalcemia (low calcium levels). It is commonly used to diagnose conditions such as hyperparathyroidism, where excessive PTH is produced, leading to elevated calcium levels or hypoparathyroidism, characterized by insufficient PTH and low calcium levels. The test also aids in evaluating bone diseases, kidney problems and vitamin D disorders that affect calcium metabolism.

In clinical practice, the PTH test is often performed alongside blood calcium and phosphorus tests to provide a comprehensive picture of mineral balance and parathyroid function. Normal PTH levels typically range from about 10 to 65 picograms per milliliter (pg/mL), although reference ranges can vary depending on the laboratory. Abnormally high PTH levels may indicate primary or secondary hyperparathyroidism, vitamin D deficiency or chronic kidney disease, while low levels can be seen in hypoparathyroidism or after parathyroid gland removal. The test involves a simple blood draw, usually from a vein in the arm and is often performed in the morning since PTH levels can fluctuate throughout the day. Interpreting PTH results requires careful consideration of calcium and vitamin D levels, as well as the patient's overall health and symptoms. The PTH test is a vital diagnostic tool for assessing parathyroid gland function and calcium metabolism. It helps healthcare providers diagnose and manage disorders that impact bone health, mineral balance and kidney function. By providing critical information about hormone levels that regulate calcium, the PTH test supports effective treatment strategies aimed at maintaining bone strength and metabolic stability.

- **Purpose:** Evaluates parathyroid gland function and calcium regulation.
- **Normal Range:** 10 – 65 pg/mL
- **High PTH:** Hyperparathyroidism, low calcium
- **Low PTH:** Hypoparathyroidism

Calcium Test:

The Calcium test is a blood test that measures the level of calcium in the bloodstream, an essential mineral critical for numerous physiological functions. Calcium plays a vital role in building and maintaining strong bones and teeth, facilitating muscle contraction, transmitting nerve signals and enabling blood clotting. Because calcium is so important for overall health, maintaining its levels within a precise range is necessary to support the body's normal functioning. The calcium test helps evaluate calcium balance and can provide important insights into bone health, parathyroid gland function, kidney function and certain metabolic conditions. This test is often ordered when patients exhibit symptoms such as muscle spasms, numbness or tingling in the fingers, bone pain, fatigue or irregular heart rhythms—signs that may indicate calcium imbalances. It is also routinely performed to monitor chronic conditions like osteoporosis, kidney disease and parathyroid disorders, as well as to assess patients taking medications or supplements that could affect calcium levels. The calcium test is a key component of metabolic panels that evaluate overall mineral and electrolyte status.

Calcium in the blood exists in two main forms: bound to proteins such as albumin and in a free, ionized form which is biologically active. Because protein levels can influence total calcium measurements, doctors sometimes order an ionized calcium test or adjust calcium results based on albumin levels to obtain a more accurate assessment of physiologically active calcium. Normal total calcium levels generally range from about 8.5 to 10.5 milligrams per deciliter (mg/dL), although reference ranges may vary slightly between laboratories. Abnormal calcium levels can indicate a variety of health issues. High calcium levels, known as hypercalcemia, may suggest hyperparathyroidism, certain cancers, excessive vitamin D intake or kidney disease. Low calcium levels or hypocalcemia, can be caused by hypoparathyroidism, vitamin D deficiency, kidney failure or conditions that affect calcium absorption.

Because calcium balance is tightly linked to parathyroid hormone and vitamin D levels, these tests are often conducted together to diagnose underlying causes. The calcium test is a crucial diagnostic tool for assessing mineral balance, bone health and metabolic function. It aids healthcare providers in detecting disorders related to calcium metabolism and guides appropriate treatment plans to restore balance and support overall health. Monitoring calcium levels is especially important for preventing complications related to bones, muscles, nerves and cardiovascular function.

- **Purpose:** Measures total calcium in the blood.
- **Normal Range:** 8.5 – 10.5 mg/dL
- **High Calcium:** Hyperparathyroidism, cancer
- **Low Calcium:** Hypoparathyroidism, vitamin D deficiency

3.3 SLEEP AND CIRCADIAN RHYTHM MONITORING

Sleep and circadian rhythm monitoring are essential components in understanding human health, behavior and overall well-being. Sleep, a naturally recurring state of rest, is vital for physical restoration, cognitive function, emotional regulation and metabolic balance. It is during sleep that the body repairs tissues, consolidates memories and regulates hormones critical for maintaining homeostasis. The circadian rhythm, often referred to as the body's internal clock, is a roughly 24-hour cycle that governs physiological processes, including the sleep-wake cycle, hormone secretion, body temperature and metabolism. These rhythms are synchronized primarily by environmental cues such as light and darkness, ensuring that bodily functions occur at optimal times throughout the day and night. Monitoring sleep and circadian rhythms provides crucial insights into both normal biological patterns and disruptions that may contribute to various health problems. Sleep disorders such as insomnia, sleep apnea, restless leg syndrome and narcolepsy can significantly impair quality of life, leading to fatigue, impaired concentration, mood disturbances and increased risk of chronic diseases like diabetes, cardiovascular disease and obesity. Likewise, circadian rhythm disorders, including delayed sleep phase syndrome and shift work disorder, arise from misalignment between the internal clock and external environment, causing difficulties in sleeping at conventional times and negatively affecting daytime functioning. Technological advances have greatly improved the ability to monitor sleep and circadian rhythms accurately and non-invasively. Polysomnography, the gold standard for sleep studies, records brain waves, eye movements, heart rate, respiratory effort and muscle activity during sleep, providing detailed information about sleep architecture and identifying disorders. Actigraphy, involving wearable devices like wristbands, tracks movement patterns to estimate sleep duration and quality over extended periods in natural settings. Additionally, monitoring circadian rhythms can include measuring core body temperature, melatonin levels and other biomarkers to assess the timing and robustness of the internal clock. Understanding the interplay between sleep quality and circadian rhythms is fundamental in designing effective treatments for sleep-related disorders. For example, chronotherapy and light therapy are used to realign circadian rhythms in individuals with delayed or advanced sleep phase syndromes. Lifestyle interventions promoting good sleep hygiene—such as regular sleep schedules, limiting screen time before bed and creating a comfortable sleep environment—are critical components in maintaining healthy sleep patterns. Furthermore, identifying circadian misalignment in shift workers and travellers crossing time zones can guide strategies to minimize adverse effects like fatigue and impaired cognitive performance. Sleep and circadian rhythm monitoring also have implications beyond clinical settings. They are valuable in occupational health to improve productivity and safety, in athletic performance to optimize recovery and training and in mental health to manage mood disorders like depression and bipolar disorder, which are often linked to disrupted sleep and circadian cycles. The growing interest in personalized medicine highlights the need for individualized assessment of sleep and circadian rhythms, enabling tailored interventions based on each person's unique biological profile. Sleep and circadian rhythm monitoring are indispensable tools for advancing our understanding of human biology, diagnosing disorders and promoting health and well-being. By capturing detailed data on sleep patterns and internal biological clocks, these monitoring techniques help unravel the complex relationship between rest, physiology and disease. Continued research and technological innovation in this field hold promise for enhancing diagnostic accuracy, improving therapeutic outcomes and supporting healthier lifestyles across diverse populations.

3.3.1 Sleep Staging

Sleep staging refers to the classification of sleep into distinct phases or "stages," which reflect the brain's activity and physiological processes during rest. Sleep is not a uniform state but rather a dynamic cycle composed of multiple stages that repeat throughout the night. These stages are categorized into two main types: Non-Rapid Eye Movement (NREM) sleep and Rapid Eye Movement (REM) sleep. Understanding these stages is essential for evaluating sleep quality, diagnosing sleep disorders and guiding therapeutic interventions.

NREM sleep is further divided into three stages: N1, N2 and N3.

- Stage N1 is the lightest stage of sleep, where a person transitions from wakefulness to sleep.

- Stage N2 is a deeper form of light sleep, characterized by slower brain waves and features like sleep spindles and K-complexes.
- Stage N3, also known as deep sleep or slow-wave sleep (SWS), is the most restorative stage, essential for physical recovery and immune function.

REM sleep, on the other hand, is associated with vivid dreaming, muscle atonia (temporary paralysis of voluntary muscles) and heightened brain activity similar to wakefulness. REM sleep plays a key role in memory consolidation, emotional processing and brain development. A typical night's sleep cycles through these stages in 90–120-minute intervals, repeating 4 to 6 times. Sleep staging is commonly performed using polysomnography (PSG), a comprehensive sleep study that records brain waves (EEG), eye movements (EOG), muscle tone (EMG), heart rate and breathing patterns. These physiological signals allow for precise identification of each sleep stage and how long the individual spends in each. In recent years, wearable sleep trackers and home-based EEG devices have also emerged, providing more accessible but less detailed staging information. Monitoring sleep stages is crucial for detecting abnormalities such as reduced deep sleep or disrupted REM cycles, which may indicate conditions like insomnia, sleep apnea, narcolepsy or REM behavior disorder. Changes in sleep architecture can also be influenced by age, medications, stress and lifestyle. Normal sleep architecture involves more deep NREM sleep early in the night and longer REM periods closer to morning. Deviations from this pattern can impact cognitive function, mood, physical health and overall quality of life. Therefore, analyzing the balance and progression of sleep stages provides valuable insight into sleep health. Sleep staging is a foundational aspect of sleep science that reveals how the brain and body function during rest. It helps clinicians diagnose sleep disorders, researchers study the impact of sleep on health and individuals understand their own sleep patterns. As technology evolves, sleep staging continues to play a pivotal role in advancing personalized sleep medicine and improving global sleep health.

3.3.2 Sleep Quality Analysis

Sleep quality analysis is the process of evaluating how well a person sleeps—not just how long they sleep, but how restful, uninterrupted and restorative that sleep is. While sleep duration is often the most discussed metric, sleep quality provides a deeper understanding of whether sleep supports optimal physical, mental and emotional health. High-quality sleep is characterized by ease of falling asleep, staying asleep throughout the night, minimal awakenings, spending adequate time in deeper sleep stages and waking up feeling refreshed and alert. Unlike simple sleep duration tracking, sleep quality analysis looks at a wide range of parameters. These include sleep latency (how long it takes to fall asleep), sleep efficiency (the percentage of time in bed actually spent asleep), number of awakenings, time spent in each sleep stage (NREM and REM) and variability in sleep patterns across nights. Together, these indicators provide a comprehensive picture of sleep health. Poor sleep quality can occur even if a person gets the recommended 7–9 hours of sleep per night. Factors such as stress, anxiety, sleep apnea, restless legs syndrome, chronic pain, inconsistent sleep schedules and environmental disturbances (like light or noise) can fragment sleep and reduce its restorative value. Over time, inadequate sleep quality is associated with cognitive decline, mood disorders, weakened immunity, metabolic dysfunction and cardiovascular problems. Sleep quality is typically assessed using both subjective and objective methods. Subjective tools include self-reported sleep diaries and questionnaires like the Pittsburgh Sleep Quality Index (PSQI), which help identify perceived sleep issues. Objective tools, such as polysomnography, actigraphy and wearable trackers, measure real-time physiological data to evaluate sleep patterns, movements, breathing and brain activity. Advanced technologies now allow sleep quality to be monitored at home using smart devices that record sleep stages, heart rate variability, breathing patterns and ambient noise or light levels. These technologies make it easier to identify factors disrupting sleep and track progress during treatment or behavioral changes. Clinicians use this data to diagnose conditions like insomnia, obstructive sleep apnea and circadian rhythm disorders and to tailor interventions such as cognitive-behavioral therapy for insomnia (CBT-I), lifestyle modifications or medical treatments. In research settings, analyzing sleep quality helps scientists explore how sleep impacts learning, memory, immune response and disease progression. In occupational health, it plays a role in assessing risks for shift workers and improving productivity and safety. Sleep quality analysis is an essential aspect of modern health assessment. It helps distinguish between merely "sleeping" and truly "restorative sleep." By combining subjective experiences with objective data, sleep quality analysis supports personalized care, promotes better sleep habits and contributes to long-term physical and mental well-being.

3.4 PHYSICAL ACTIVITY AND MOBILITY

Physical activity and mobility are fundamental aspects of human health, closely tied to overall well-being, independence and quality of life. Physical activity refers to any movement of the body that requires energy expenditure, ranging from structured exercises like walking, running or weight training to everyday tasks such as climbing stairs, gardening or cleaning. Mobility, on the other hand, refers to a person's ability to move freely and easily in their environment. It encompasses balance, coordination, strength and flexibility—key components that enable individuals to perform daily activities and engage in social and occupational roles. Together, physical activity and mobility are strong indicators of functional health. Regular movement promotes cardiovascular fitness, muscle and bone strength, weight management, metabolic efficiency and mental resilience. In contrast, reduced mobility or sedentary behavior is associated with increased risks of chronic diseases like type 2 diabetes, hypertension, cardiovascular disease, osteoporosis, depression and certain cancers. Moreover, poor mobility can contribute to a loss of independence, social isolation and a higher risk of falls, especially among the elderly. Assessment of physical activity and mobility has become an important component in preventive medicine, rehabilitation, geriatrics, sports science and chronic disease management. It can be evaluated through both subjective methods, like questionnaires and activity logs and objective tools such as pedometers, accelerometers, wearable fitness trackers and gait analysis systems. These technologies allow for continuous monitoring of activity levels, step counts, movement patterns and energy expenditure in real-world settings, offering valuable insights into a person's physical capabilities and lifestyle habits. Mobility assessments often include tests like the Timed Up and Go (TUG) test, 6-Minute Walk Test (6MWT) and gait speed analysis, which help clinicians measure endurance, stability and risk of falling. These tools are especially important for aging populations and individuals recovering from injury or surgery. Advanced motion-sensing systems and wearable sensors can now provide detailed feedback on joint movement, posture and muscle activation during movement, allowing for early detection of mobility impairments and optimization of rehabilitation strategies. Maintaining good physical activity levels and mobility across the lifespan is crucial not only for disease prevention but also for preserving autonomy and enhancing mental health. Interventions such as strength training, flexibility exercises, balance training and aerobic activity are often recommended to improve mobility and prevent decline, particularly in older adults or those with chronic illnesses. Physical activity and mobility are critical determinants of health and functional independence. Monitoring and enhancing these areas through modern technology, clinical assessment and lifestyle interventions can greatly improve an individual's physical performance, reduce health risks and support long-term well-being.

3.4.1 Step Counting

Step counting is a simple yet powerful method for measuring physical activity by tracking the number of steps a person takes throughout the day. It has gained widespread popularity due to its ease of use, accessibility and effectiveness in promoting movement and healthier lifestyles. With the rise of smartphones, smartwatches and fitness bands, millions of people now monitor their daily steps to stay active and motivated. Step counting not only encourages regular movement but also serves as a key indicator of overall mobility, endurance and cardiovascular health.

Traditionally, step counting was done using mechanical pedometers, which detected motion from the hips. Today, modern accelerometer-based devices and wearable sensors provide far more accurate, real-time step tracking, often integrated with apps that display activity trends, calories burned, heart rate and sleep. These tools are used in both personal fitness goals and clinical settings, such as rehabilitation, geriatric care and chronic disease management, where step counts can reflect recovery progress or daily function. The commonly recommended target of 10,000 steps per day originated as a marketing slogan in Japan but has since been supported by research suggesting that it promotes cardiovascular fitness, weight control and reduced risk of chronic diseases. However, recent studies show that even as few as 6,000 to 8,000 steps per day can offer significant health benefits, especially in older adults or sedentary individuals. What matters most is consistency and gradual increase based on personal health status. Step counting is especially useful for tracking incidental activity—small movements like walking to the kitchen, taking the stairs or walking during phone calls—that may not be captured by traditional workout tracking. For individuals with limited mobility, step goals can be tailored to realistic targets, helping maintain engagement and motivation. In medical and research settings, step count data is used to monitor mobility decline, evaluate treatment outcomes and detect early signs of health deterioration. For instance, a sudden drop in daily steps might indicate illness, depression or injury. Step counts also correlate with fall risk, especially in older adults, making them a valuable metric in preventative care. Step counting is a practical, cost-effective and evidence-based way to measure and encourage physical activity. It empowers individuals to take control of their movement habits and provides valuable data to healthcare providers and researchers alike. As wearable technology advances, step counting remains a cornerstone in the pursuit of a more active, healthy lifestyle.

3.4.2 Fall Detection

Fall detection is a safety and health-monitoring technology designed to automatically identify when a person has experienced a fall and, in many systems, alert caregivers, emergency contacts or medical personnel. Falls are a leading cause of injury, hospitalization and even death among older adults, making fall detection a critical component in elder care, rehabilitation and chronic condition management. Prompt detection and response can significantly reduce the severity of injuries and improve outcomes for individuals living alone or at high risk of falling. Modern fall detection systems use a combination of sensors, such as accelerometers, gyroscopes and barometers, often embedded in wearable devices, smartphones or in-home monitoring systems. These sensors detect sudden changes in motion orientation or impact consistent with a fall. Some systems incorporate artificial intelligence (AI) or machine learning algorithms to distinguish between actual falls and non-fall activities like sitting down quickly or dropping the device.

There are two main types of fall detection systems:

- Wearable-based systems, such as smartwatches or pendants, that continuously monitor movement.
- Environmental or vision-based systems, including cameras or radar sensors installed in homes to detect falls without requiring the user to wear a device.

Many modern fall detection devices include automatic emergency alert features, which notify caregivers or emergency services within seconds of a detected fall. Some allow manual confirmation by the user, preventing false alarms if the device misinterprets motion. Fall detection is often paired with GPS tracking in mobile devices, enabling help to be dispatched quickly to the correct location.

In clinical and home settings, fall detection enhances independent living, especially for older adults or individuals with neurological conditions like Parkinson's disease, multiple sclerosis or post-stroke disabilities. These systems provide peace of mind to both users and family members, ensuring rapid response in potentially life-threatening situations. Despite their benefits, fall detection systems face challenges such as false positives, battery life limitations and privacy concerns with in-home monitoring. Ongoing advancements aim to improve accuracy, comfort and user compliance. Fall detection is a life-saving innovation that blends technology with healthcare. It empowers vulnerable individuals to live more safely and independently while enabling caregivers to respond swiftly in emergencies. As populations age globally, fall detection will continue to play a vital role in modern health monitoring and elderly care.

3.4.3 Gait Analysis

Gait analysis is the systematic study of human walking patterns, often used to assess mobility, balance and movement efficiency. It involves measuring and evaluating the way a person walks (their "gait") to detect abnormalities or asymmetries that may indicate underlying health issues. Gait is a complex motor function that relies on the coordination of the nervous system, musculoskeletal system and sensory input. Subtle changes in gait can provide early signs of conditions such as Parkinson's disease, stroke, multiple sclerosis, arthritis or musculoskeletal injuries. Traditionally, gait analysis was conducted visually by trained clinicians observing a patient walk. However, modern gait analysis systems use advanced technologies including motion capture cameras, force plates, pressure sensors and wearable inertial sensors (IMUs) to measure precise biomechanical parameters. These systems can assess step length, stride length, cadence, gait speed, symmetry and ground reaction forces, among many other variables.

Gait analysis is widely used in multiple fields:

- In clinical settings, to diagnose and monitor neurological and orthopedic disorders.
- In rehabilitation, to evaluate progress after surgeries, injuries or strokes.
- In sports science, to optimize athletic performance and prevent injury.
- In geriatric care, to assess fall risk and mobility decline in older adults.

Wearable technology has revolutionized gait analysis, enabling continuous and real-world monitoring outside of laboratories or clinics. Small, lightweight sensors placed on the legs, waist or shoes can record movement data over days or weeks, providing insights into how a person walks in daily life, not just under clinical observation. Gait abnormalities, such as limping, shuffling, unsteady walking or asymmetrical stride, can point to specific issues with joints, muscles, balance or neurological function. Identifying and quantifying these patterns helps healthcare providers personalize treatment plans, choose appropriate mobility aids and guide physical therapy. Early detection of gait changes is especially valuable for aging populations or individuals with progressive neurological conditions. Regular gait analysis can help prevent falls, maintain independence and improve quality of life. Fait analysis is a powerful, non-invasive tool for understanding human movement. By combining clinical insight with modern technology, it plays a critical role in diagnosis, rehabilitation, fall prevention and performance enhancement across a wide range of populations.

3.5 MENTAL AND COGNITIVE HEALTH MONITORING

Mental and cognitive health monitoring is an essential part of modern healthcare and wellness, focusing on understanding and managing emotional well-being, stress levels and brain function. As mental health issues such as depression, anxiety and cognitive decline become increasingly prevalent, especially in aging populations and high-stress lifestyles, continuous monitoring offers the opportunity for early detection, prevention and timely intervention. By leveraging technology, psychology and neuroscience, mental and cognitive health monitoring helps individuals and clinicians track changes, assess risks and personalize care.

3.5.1 Mood tracking

Mood tracking is a widely used method that involves regularly recording emotional states—such as happiness, sadness, irritability or anxiety—over time. This can be done through self-reported digital diaries, smartphone apps or wearable devices that infer mood through behavioral data like speech tone, typing patterns, facial expressions, sleep and physical activity. Regular mood monitoring can reveal patterns linked to daily routines, life events or medication changes, helping individuals better understand their emotional triggers and regulate mental well-being. In clinical contexts, mood tracking supports diagnosis and management of mood disorders like depression, bipolar disorder and seasonal affective disorder (SAD).

3.5.2 Stress detection

Stress detection uses both subjective feedback and physiological markers to identify signs of acute or chronic stress. Wearable sensors and smart devices now measure stress indicators such as heart rate variability (HRV), skin conductance (electrodermal activity), respiration rate and cortisol levels. Elevated stress can impact sleep, immune function, cognitive clarity and emotional stability. Stress monitoring enables early intervention through relaxation techniques, therapy or lifestyle changes, making it valuable in both personal wellness and workplace mental health programs.

3.5.3 Cognitive assessments

Cognitive assessments evaluate brain functions such as memory, attention, problem-solving and executive function. These assessments may be conducted via standardized tests in clinical environments or through mobile-based cognitive games and questionnaires. Continuous digital cognitive testing helps detect early signs of mild cognitive impairment (MCI), dementia, Alzheimer's disease or neurological changes following injuries like concussions or strokes. Repeated monitoring allows for trend analysis over time, making it easier to assess treatment effectiveness or disease progression.

Together, mood, stress and cognitive data provide a 360-degree view of mental and cognitive health. When integrated, these tools can highlight early red flags and inform individualized treatment plans involving medication, psychotherapy, cognitive training or lifestyle interventions. Mental and cognitive health monitoring is also crucial for populations at high risk—such as the elderly, caregivers, frontline workers and individuals with chronic illnesses—where early signs of mental strain may otherwise go unnoticed. Modern mental health platforms increasingly use AI and machine learning to analyze large volumes of user data, identify behavioral patterns and predict potential crises such as depressive episodes or burnout. This makes mental health support more proactive, accessible and personalized. However, privacy, data security and ethical concerns remain important challenges that need careful consideration when deploying these technologies at scale.

3.6 REPRODUCTIVE AND WOMEN'S HEALTH MONITORING

Reproductive and women's health monitoring is a vital aspect of healthcare that focuses on tracking biological, hormonal and physical processes related to the female reproductive system. It encompasses a wide range of areas, including menstrual health, fertility, pregnancy, menopause and hormonal balance. With advancements in digital health technologies, women today have access to powerful tools that allow them to monitor and manage their reproductive health with greater precision, convenience and autonomy. One of the most common applications is menstrual cycle tracking, which helps women monitor period patterns, ovulation timing and symptoms like cramps, mood changes or acne. This is especially useful for identifying irregularities, managing premenstrual syndrome (PMS) and planning or preventing pregnancy. Fertility tracking goes a step further by monitoring ovulation windows using basal body temperature, hormone levels (like LH) and cervical mucus data to aid in conception efforts or natural contraception. During pregnancy, health monitoring includes tracking fetal growth, maternal vitals, sleep, nutrition and signs of complications like gestational diabetes or preeclampsia. Wearables, smart scales and mobile apps can support expectant mothers in maintaining a healthy pregnancy and staying connected to healthcare providers.

For women going through perimenopause or menopause, monitoring hormonal changes, sleep disruptions, mood swings and hot flashes helps manage symptoms and guides hormone therapy or lifestyle interventions. Reproductive health tracking also plays a critical role in identifying early signs of disorders like polycystic ovary syndrome (PCOS), endometriosis and thyroid dysfunction, which often affect fertility and menstrual health. Reproductive and women's health monitoring empowers women to better understand their bodies, make informed health decisions and detect issues early. It supports a more personalized approach to care and contributes to long-term health, well-being and reproductive autonomy.

3.6.1 Fertility

Fertility monitoring involves tracking biological signs and hormonal changes to understand and optimize the chances of conception. It is widely used by individuals or couples trying to conceive, as well as those practicing natural family planning methods. The most fertile days typically occur around ovulation, the time when an egg is released from the ovary. By identifying this fertile window, individuals can increase the likelihood of pregnancy or avoid it naturally. Modern fertility tracking combines multiple physiological indicators, such as basal body temperature (BBT), luteinizing hormone (LH) surges, cervical mucus changes and ovarian cycle patterns. Devices like ovulation predictor kits, fertility monitors and smartphone apps help track these changes with daily input or sensor data. Some wearable devices even detect subtle temperature shifts or nighttime heart rate variations to signal ovulation more accurately. Fertility tracking can also help diagnose reproductive health issues, such as anovulation (lack of ovulation), luteal phase defects or hormonal imbalances. It's especially useful in managing conditions like PCOS, thyroid disorders or irregular cycles that affect fertility. With increasing interest in personalized reproductive care, fertility monitoring empowers individuals with insights into their unique cycle patterns and reproductive readiness.

3.6.2 Menstrual Cycle

Menstrual cycle monitoring is a key aspect of women's health, providing valuable insight into hormonal health, reproductive status and overall well-being. The menstrual cycle typically spans around 28 days and includes four main phases: menstrual, follicular, ovulation and luteal. Monitoring this cycle helps identify patterns in symptoms, track regularity and detect changes that may signal health issues. Using mobile apps or wearable devices, women can log daily symptoms such as cramping, bloating, mood swings and flow intensity. This data supports better understanding of premenstrual syndrome (PMS), cycle length variability and hormonal fluctuations. Some apps now use AI algorithms to predict future periods, ovulation days and symptom cycles, enhancing accuracy over time. Cycle tracking is especially helpful for women managing hormonal disorders like endometriosis, PCOS or those transitioning through perimenopause. It also aids in planning for events or activities by anticipating discomfort or fatigue. Clinically, menstrual data supports gynecological consultations, fertility planning and hormonal therapy decisions. Regular cycle tracking not only promotes body awareness but also fosters proactive reproductive and hormonal health management.

3.6.3 Pregnancy Tracking

Pregnancy tracking is the continuous monitoring of maternal and fetal health throughout gestation, offering both reassurance and vital information during a transformative life stage. From the moment of conception to delivery, expectant mothers can track symptoms, growth milestones and health metrics to stay informed and connected to their healthcare providers. Most pregnancy tracking tools include features such as fetal development updates, kick counts, weight gain tracking, appointment reminders and symptom logs. More advancSed wearables may track maternal heart rate, sleep quality, activity levels and even detect signs of complications like gestational diabetes or preeclampsia through vital signs. Pregnancy tracking helps identify warning signs early, allowing for timely medical intervention. It also supports emotional health by guiding mindfulness, stress reduction and self-care practices. Educational content delivered via apps can inform expecting mothers about each trimester, dietary needs, safe exercises and labour preparation. Pregnancy tracking bridges the gap between clinical visits, enhances maternal awareness and contributes to healthier pregnancy outcomes for both mother and baby.

Chapter 4 INTEGRATION WITH CLINICAL CARE

4.0 INTRODUCTION: AN OVERVIEW

Integration with clinical care refers to the process of connecting personal health monitoring technologies—such as wearables, mobile health apps, and remote sensing devices—with formal healthcare systems and providers. This integration creates a unified, real-time picture of an individual's health, bridging the gap between daily life and clinical decision-making. It represents a shift from episodic, in-clinic care to continuous, data-driven, personalized health management. The rise of digital health tools has empowered individuals to monitor vital signs, physical activity, sleep, menstrual cycles, mental health, and chronic conditions outside of clinical environments. However, the true value of these tools is realized when their data is meaningfully shared and interpreted by healthcare professionals. Integrated health systems allow real-time or periodic syncing of patient-generated data with electronic health records (EHRs), enabling clinicians to make more informed decisions, monitor trends over time, and intervene early when necessary (Fig. 1).

For example, a cardiologist may track a patient's blood pressure and heart rate remotely using connected devices, reducing the need for frequent office visits while improving hypertension management. Diabetics can log blood glucose readings via smartphone apps, which automatically alert care teams if readings fall outside safe ranges. Mental health professionals can monitor mood or stress levels through validated digital assessments, providing timely support between therapy sessions. In maternal care, data from pregnancy tracking apps can be reviewed to detect early signs of gestational complications, improving outcomes for both mother and baby.

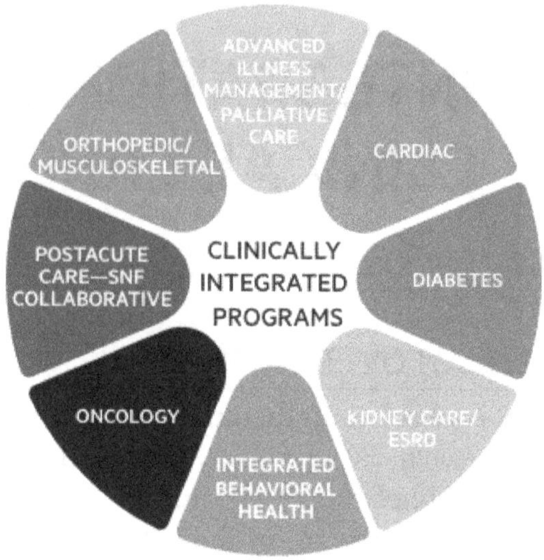

Fig. 1 Clinically Integrated Programs

Integration also enhances chronic disease management, where ongoing monitoring is essential. Patients with asthma, COPD, or heart failure can use wearable sensors or connected inhalers and scales that share information with clinical teams. This enables proactive care models, helping to prevent hospitalizations and reduce emergency visits. For elderly or mobility-impaired individuals, fall detection and activity tracking devices alert caregivers or physicians to sudden changes, allowing rapid intervention. One of the most promising aspects of integration is in telemedicine and remote patient monitoring (RPM). These technologies allow patients to consult doctors virtually, while real-time biometric data (such as oxygen saturation, ECG, glucose levels, etc.) provides objective insights. This model was especially valuable during the COVID-19 pandemic and continues to transform care delivery for rural or underserved populations. Successful integration requires interoperability, where devices and software platforms can communicate seamlessly across healthcare systems. This often involves standards like HL7, FHIR (Fast Healthcare Interoperability Resources), and secure APIs. Privacy and security are also critical, as sensitive health data must be encrypted, anonymized, and protected under laws like HIPAA and GDPR. Clinicians benefit from dashboards and analytics tools that visualize incoming data in actionable formats—highlighting trends, flagging anomalies, and supporting clinical decision-making. Some platforms use AI algorithms to assist in early diagnosis or to predict disease progression based on continuous data input. Patients, in turn, feel more engaged in their health journeys, knowing their data contributes meaningfully to their care plans.

Healthcare providers are also increasingly using integrated systems for population health management, where aggregated patient data helps identify at-risk groups, improve resource allocation, and track public health trends. Insurance companies and health systems may incentivize the use of connected devices to lower long-term healthcare costs through prevention and early detection. Despite its promise, integration faces challenges such as data overload, clinician burnout from excessive alerts, inconsistent device accuracy, and limited reimbursement models. However, ongoing collaboration between technology developers, healthcare institutions, policymakers, and patients is steadily overcoming these barriers. Integration with clinical care transforms isolated health monitoring into collaborative, continuous care. It empowers individuals, supports healthcare professionals, and leads to better health outcomes through earlier intervention, personalized treatment, and more efficient care delivery. As technology continues to evolve, integrated care will become the foundation of a smarter, more responsive healthcare system.

4.1 TELEMEDICINE AND VIRTUAL HEALTH CONSULTATIONS:

Telemedicine and virtual health consultations represent a paradigm shift in how healthcare is delivered. They offer efficient, patient-centered care options that transcend geographical and logistical barriers. When integrated with traditional care pathways and enhanced by digital tools, telemedicine is not only a convenience—it's a cornerstone of modern, accessible, and resilient healthcare systems.

Telemedicine refers to the use of telecommunications technology to deliver healthcare services remotely. It allows patients to consult with healthcare professionals without the need for in-person visits, using video calls, phone calls, secure messaging, or dedicated telehealth platforms. Virtual health consultations are a key application of telemedicine, enabling real-time interaction between patients and providers from the comfort of home or other non-clinical settings. Telemedicine has seen significant growth in recent years, driven by advances in digital health technology, increased internet connectivity, and growing demand for accessible, efficient healthcare. The COVID-19 pandemic further accelerated adoption, as providers and patients turned to virtual care to maintain continuity while minimizing exposure risk.

Components of Virtual Health Consultations

- **Technology Platform:** Virtual consultations typically occur via secure web-based portals, mobile apps, or video conferencing tools that comply with privacy regulations (e.g., HIPAA in the U.S.). These platforms often include features like appointment scheduling, patient intake forms, electronic prescriptions, and integration with electronic health records (EHRs).
- Types of Services Offered: Telemedicine supports a wide range of services-
  - General primary care (fever, cold, infections, etc.)
  - Chronic disease management (diabetes, hypertension, asthma)

- Mental health counseling (therapy, medication management)
- Follow-up visits post-surgery or hospitalization
- Second opinions and specialist consultations
- Remote dermatology, cardiology, and pediatrics, among others.

- **Remote Monitoring Integration:** Devices like blood pressure monitors, glucometers, pulse oximeters, and wearable ECGs can sync with virtual care platforms, allowing providers to view real-time physiological data during or before the consultation.

- **E-Prescriptions and Referrals:** After assessing the patient, the provider can issue prescriptions electronically or refer the patient to in-person services, diagnostic tests, or specialist care.

Benefits of Telemedicine and Virtual Consultations

Telemedicine and virtual health consultations offer numerous benefits that enhance both patient experience and healthcare delivery. One of the most significant advantages is convenience—patients can consult with doctors from home, avoiding travel time, waiting rooms, and time off work. This makes healthcare more accessible, especially for individuals in rural or underserved areas where clinics and specialists may be far away. Telemedicine also supports continuity of care, allowing regular check-ins for chronic disease management, mental health, and post-operative follow-ups.

Another major benefit is cost-effectiveness. It reduces the burden on emergency rooms and urgent care facilities by providing quick access for non-emergency issues. Infection control is also improved, as virtual visits limit exposure to contagious diseases—a key advantage during pandemics. For healthcare systems, telemedicine helps optimize resource use and can reduce hospital readmission rates through better outpatient monitoring. Additionally, integration with remote monitoring tools (like wearable devices and health apps) gives doctors access to real-time patient data, enabling more informed decision-making. Patients feel more engaged and empowered, as virtual care often encourages active participation in their health. Overall, telemedicine brings flexibility, efficiency, and personalized care into the healthcare experience.

- **Accessibility:** Telemedicine significantly improves healthcare accessibility, particularly for individuals living in rural, remote, or underserved areas. These populations often face barriers such as long travel distances, lack of transportation, and a shortage of local medical professionals or specialists. With virtual consultations, patients can connect with providers from their own homes, removing the geographic limitations that once prevented timely care. This is especially beneficial for elderly individuals, disabled patients, and those with mobility challenges. Telemedicine can also bridge access for marginalized communities that may face socioeconomic, linguistic, or cultural barriers in traditional healthcare settings. By reducing dependency on physical infrastructure, it enables broader and more equitable access to essential services, including mental health, chronic disease management, and preventive care. Additionally, school-based telehealth programs can support children's health in remote districts. In emergency scenarios, rural clinics can collaborate with urban specialists to manage critical cases effectively. Ultimately, telemedicine helps ensure that location no longer dictates the quality of care received.

- **Convenience:** Convenience is one of the most appreciated benefits of telemedicine, offering patients a faster, simpler way to access healthcare. Traditional in-person visits often require commuting, taking time off work, arranging childcare, or waiting for hours at the clinic. Virtual consultations eliminate these burdens, allowing people to see a doctor from home, at work, or even while traveling. This is especially valuable for follow-up appointments, prescription refills, and managing minor illnesses, which don't always require a physical exam. In busy households or for caregivers juggling multiple responsibilities, telemedicine provides much-needed flexibility. For healthcare providers, it helps maintain better appointment adherence and reduces no-show rates. The scheduling is often more adaptable, with options for early morning, evening, or even weekend consults. Ultimately, by minimizing disruptions to daily life, telemedicine empowers individuals to prioritize their health without sacrificing convenience or comfort.
- **Continuity of Care:** Telemedicine strengthens continuity of care, which is crucial for managing long-term health conditions like diabetes, hypertension, asthma, and mental health disorders. Through regular virtual check-ins, providers can monitor symptoms, adjust medications, and guide lifestyle modifications in real-time. This consistent engagement prevents gaps in care that might lead to complications, hospitalizations, or poor health outcomes. It also fosters a stronger patient-provider relationship, as communication becomes more frequent and accessible. Telehealth enables shared decision-making and personalized care planning, especially for patients with complex needs. Mental health continuity is particularly enhanced, as virtual therapy sessions remove logistical and emotional barriers to seeking help. Remote monitoring tools can be integrated to track vitals, mood, or physical activity, further enhancing clinical oversight. In short, telemedicine makes care more proactive rather than reactive, leading

to better disease control, greater patient satisfaction, and improved long-term outcomes.

- **Reduced Healthcare Burden:** By offering efficient and timely care, telemedicine helps reduce the burden on hospitals, urgent care centers, and emergency rooms. Many non-emergency medical issues—such as infections, minor injuries, medication questions, or cold and flu symptoms—can be safely managed through virtual visits. This frees up in-person healthcare resources for more critical and complex cases. During health crises like flu season or pandemics, telehealth acts as a pressure release valve, ensuring that overwhelmed healthcare systems can continue operating effectively. It also reduces unnecessary hospital admissions through remote monitoring and early intervention. For patients, avoiding an ER visit can mean significant cost savings, less time lost, and reduced exposure to infections. Healthcare providers benefit too, as streamlined workflows reduce burnout and improve patient flow. Ultimately, telemedicine contributes to a more sustainable, efficient healthcare ecosystem, ensuring the right level of care is delivered at the right time and place.
- **Infection Control:** Telemedicine plays a vital role in infection prevention and control, particularly during infectious disease outbreaks such as COVID-19. By minimizing in-person visits, it reduces the risk of exposure for both patients and healthcare workers. This is especially important for high-risk groups like the elderly, immunocompromised individuals, pregnant women, or those with chronic illnesses. Virtual care helps prevent waiting room crowding, where airborne infections can easily spread. It also limits cross-contamination within clinical environments, enhancing the safety of essential in-person visits. Telehealth supports contactless triage and ongoing symptom monitoring for those in quarantine or isolation. Moreover, providers can evaluate patients remotely before advising on the need for testing or hospitalization, reducing unnecessary physical interaction. In nursing homes, prisons, or shelters—where outbreaks can be devastating—telemedicine adds an extra layer of defense. In short, telemedicine serves as a critical public health tool, helping protect communities while maintaining access to care during health emergencies.

Challenges and Limitations

- **Digital Divide:** One of the most significant challenges in telemedicine is the digital divide—the gap between those with access to digital technology and those without. Many individuals, especially in rural areas, low-income communities, or elderly populations, may not have reliable access to high-speed internet, smartphones, computers, or even basic digital literacy.

This limits their ability to participate in virtual consultations or use health monitoring apps. Language barriers and visual or hearing impairments further complicate access. Even when devices are available, poor internet quality can cause dropped calls or miscommunication, reducing the effectiveness of virtual care. This inequality raises serious concerns about healthcare accessibility and fairness, as those who need care the most are often the least able to use telemedicine services. Bridging this gap requires investment in digital infrastructure, subsidized devices, community education, and inclusive technology design to ensure no one is left behind in the shift to digital health.

- **Clinical Limitations:** While telemedicine is suitable for many conditions, it does have clinical limitations that prevent it from replacing all in-person care. Some diagnoses and treatments require hands-on physical examinations, laboratory tests, imaging (like X-rays or MRIs), or procedures that simply can't be conducted virtually. For example, detecting a heart murmur, palpating a mass, or suturing a wound all require a clinician's physical presence. Certain acute or complex medical issues may also present subtly, making in-person evaluation safer and more accurate. Additionally, telehealth often relies on self-reported symptoms or home-measured vitals, which may not always be accurate. Providers must carefully judge when virtual care is appropriate and when to escalate to in-person evaluation. These limitations highlight the importance of hybrid models, where telemedicine complements but does not replace in-person services.
- **Privacy and Security:** With telemedicine's rise, data privacy and cybersecurity have become pressing concerns. Virtual consultations involve the transmission of sensitive health information over digital networks, which can be vulnerable to hacking, data breaches, or unauthorized access. Ensuring the confidentiality and integrity of patient data is critical—not just for compliance with laws like HIPAA (USA) or GDPR (EU), but for maintaining patient trust. Risks include insecure platforms, weak passwords, unencrypted communications, and usage of public or shared devices. Furthermore, storing patient data on third-party servers increases complexity in managing data ownership and control. Healthcare providers must use secure, encrypted, and compliant platforms and educate patients on best practices for protecting their health data. As virtual care expands, robust cybersecurity policies, frequent audits, and regulatory oversight will be essential to safeguarding digital healthcare environments.
- **Licensing and Regulation:** Telemedicine must navigate complex and often inconsistent licensing and regulatory frameworks, which vary

widely between regions, states, and countries. In many cases, healthcare providers must hold a valid license in the jurisdiction where the patient is located, creating legal barriers to cross-border virtual care. These rules limit the ability of providers to scale their services and reduce patient access to specialized care. Additionally, differing scope-of-practice laws, prescription regulations, and telehealth reimbursement policies add administrative burdens and legal risks. While some regions introduced temporary relaxations during the COVID-19 pandemic, many of these waivers have since expired, creating uncertainty for providers. Achieving long-term success in telehealth requires harmonized regulatory standards, streamlined licensing processes (such as interstate compacts), and clear guidelines for cross-jurisdictional care that protect patients while supporting innovation and growth.

- **Reimbursement Barriers:** Reimbursement models for telemedicine remain inconsistent and are a significant barrier to its wider adoption. While many insurers expanded telehealth coverage during the pandemic, permanent policies have yet to be standardized. Payment rates for virtual consultations may be lower than in-person visits, discouraging providers from offering these services. In some cases, only specific services or provider types are eligible for reimbursement, while others are excluded entirely. Differences across public (e.g., Medicare, Medicaid) and private insurance plans further complicate the landscape. Moreover, billing codes, documentation requirements, and approval processes can be complex and time-consuming. For sustainable adoption, there needs to be a clear, consistent, and fair reimbursement structure that reflects the value and cost-efficiency of virtual care. Governments and insurers must work together to design models that incentivize quality telehealth services while ensuring equitable access for all patients.

Future of Telemedicine

The future of telemedicine lies in the development and widespread adoption of hybrid care models, where virtual and in-person healthcare services are seamlessly blended to deliver comprehensive, patient-centered care. These models leverage the strengths of both formats—combining the convenience, efficiency, and accessibility of telehealth with the hands-on, diagnostic precision of traditional face-to-face visits. Hybrid systems are adaptable, scalable, and designed to match the complexity of a patient's needs, offering flexibility without compromising quality (Fig. 2).

Technological advancements are playing a central role in shaping this future. AI-powered triage bots are now capable of analyzing patient-reported symptoms and directing them to the appropriate level of care—saving time and streamlining provider workflows. Remote diagnostic tools and connected medical devices can monitor everything from blood pressure and glucose levels to oxygen saturation and ECG patterns, sending data directly to providers for real-time review. This makes virtual chronic disease management far more proactive and effective.

Wearable health sensors—from fitness trackers to medical-grade biosensors—are increasingly used to monitor daily activity, sleep, stress levels, and vital signs. These tools provide continuous, contextual data that can inform clinical decisions, predict complications, and alert providers to early signs of deterioration. Meanwhile, virtual reality (VR) therapy is revolutionizing fields like physical rehabilitation, pain management, and mental health, offering immersive treatments that patients can access from home.

Fig. 2 Future of Telemedicine

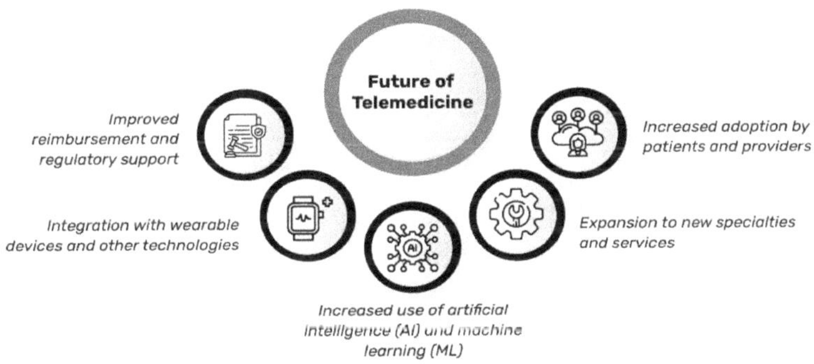

To fully realize this hybrid future, however, key systems must evolve. Regulations must be modernized to ensure that licensing, privacy, and quality standards are consistent across borders. Medical education must train future providers in digital care delivery, remote communication, and data interpretation. Digital infrastructure—including broadband access, EHR interoperability, and cybersecurity—must be robust and inclusive to close the digital divide.

As telemedicine becomes mainstream, the focus will shift from basic access to personalization, precision, and continuity. The hybrid model isn't just a backup for in-person care—it's becoming an essential pillar of modern healthcare. With thoughtful implementation and investment, it promises to deliver smarter, safer, and more equitable care for diverse populations, in both urban and remote settings.

4.2 EHR INTEGRATION AND INTEROPERABILITY

Electronic Health Record (EHR) integration and interoperability lie at the heart of healthcare's digital transformation, serving as the foundation for a more connected, intelligent, and patient-centered care ecosystem. As healthcare becomes increasingly reliant on digital tools—ranging from telemedicine platforms and mobile health apps to remote monitoring devices and AI diagnostic systems—the ability to seamlessly access, share, and update patient data across diverse platforms has become not just a goal, but a necessity. EHR integration ensures that a patient's complete health information—such as lab results, imaging, medication history, allergies, vital signs, chronic disease data, and progress notes—is consolidated into a single, longitudinal digital record. This enables physicians, nurses, specialists, pharmacists, and other care providers to access a real-time, unified view of the patient's health, regardless of where the care was provided. For patients, it means they no longer need to retell their medical history at every appointment or worry about missed information during care transitions.

Interoperability, on the other hand, refers to the ability of different health information systems to exchange, interpret, and use data accurately and meaningfully. It allows a hospital's EHR system to "talk" to a lab's reporting system, a pharmacy's prescription software, or even a patient's personal health device. This exchange is made possible through standardized data formats, structured coding systems, and APIs that support secure communication between otherwise incompatible technologies.

The interoperability landscape is defined by several key standards:

- HL7 (Health Level Seven): A widely used messaging protocol that supports data exchange across clinical systems.
- FHIR (Fast Healthcare Interoperability Resources): A modern web-based standard using APIs, making integration with mobile apps, patient portals, and remote devices easier and faster.
- LOINC and SNOMED CT: Coding systems that standardize lab results and clinical terminology to ensure semantic consistency.
- DICOM: Used in radiology for sharing imaging data across facilities.

These standards are vital for achieving not just technical connectivity, but also semantic interoperability, where systems understand and interpret data the same way. Without them, health information remains fragmented across silos—hindering care coordination, duplicating tests, and increasing costs.

The benefits of robust EHR integration and interoperability are profound. For clinicians, it reduces documentation burdens, speeds up decision-making, and provides full context for diagnoses and treatment plans. For patients, it ensures safety through medication reconciliation, avoids redundant testing, and supports continuity of care—especially when seeing multiple providers or transitioning between facilities. For health systems, it promotes efficiency, supports population health management, and enables advanced analytics for quality improvement.

In modern healthcare, interoperability also extends to patient-facing tools. Personal health apps, wearable fitness trackers, and remote monitoring devices now feed data back into EHRs, enabling a more holistic view of patient health outside the clinic. This empowers individuals to be active participants in their care while providing clinicians with richer data for preventive and personalized medicine.

However, despite progress, significant challenges remain. Legacy systems, proprietary software, vendor resistance to open data exchange, and varying national policies can all act as barriers to seamless interoperability. Data privacy and security concerns also come into play—particularly when sharing sensitive health information across platforms or borders. Healthcare organizations must ensure that patient data is shared responsibly, encrypted securely, and compliant with regulations such as HIPAA, GDPR, and local data protection laws.

Governments and regulatory bodies worldwide are increasingly mandating interoperability. In the United States, the 21st Century Cures Act and the ONC's information blocking rule compel providers and vendors to give patients easier access to their data and eliminate unnecessary restrictions on data sharing. In the European Union, the European Health Data Space (EHDS) initiative aims to create a cross-border health information infrastructure, promoting both care delivery and medical research.

Looking ahead, true interoperability will not only connect systems but also drive innovation. AI-based clinical decision support, predictive analytics, and virtual care tools all depend on rich, structured, and interoperable data. With proper implementation, EHR integration becomes the central nervous system of a smart healthcare network—enabling personalized treatment plans, improved outcomes, and real-time collaboration between care teams.

Ultimately, EHR integration and interoperability are not simply IT challenges—they are clinical, operational, and ethical imperatives. They redefine how healthcare is delivered, shifting the focus from fragmented episodes to a continuous, patient-centered journey. As digital health continues to evolve, investing in interoperable infrastructure is essential to realizing the vision of efficient, connected, and equitable care for all.

EHR Integration:

EHR integration refers to the process of connecting various digital health systems and tools—such as telemedicine platforms, remote monitoring devices, pharmacy systems, lab information systems, and patient portals—into a single, unified EHR system. This ensures that all relevant data (e.g., lab results, imaging, prescriptions, vitals, visit notes, and more) is available in one place for healthcare professionals.

Examples of integrated tools include:

- Wearable health devices syncing heart rate or glucose data to patient records
- Telehealth platforms logging virtual consultation notes directly into EHRs
- Mobile apps sharing self-reported symptoms or medication adherence
- Hospital and clinic systems exchanging discharge summaries, referrals, and medication orders

Effective integration streamlines workflows, reduces documentation burdens, prevents redundant testing, and helps clinicians make data-informed decisions quickly.

Interoperability: Types and Importance

Interoperability is the ability of different healthcare systems and software applications to exchange, interpret, and use health data consistently. It allows multiple organizations—clinics, hospitals, pharmacies, labs, and even insurers—to work together through shared digital communication standards.

There are four levels of interoperability: Foundational Interoperability: Foundational interoperability represents the most basic level of data exchange between healthcare systems. At this stage, systems are capable of sending and receiving data electronically, but without the ability to interpret the data's meaning. It's like passing along a document or image from one system to another without knowing what it contains. For example, a hospital may send a PDF lab report to a clinic, but the receiving system cannot extract or analyze the data within it. There is no standardized format or automatic integration. Foundational interoperability is often manual and limited in functionality, but it lays the groundwork for more advanced levels by establishing connectivity. It's typically used in simple referrals or file transfers via email or web portals. While useful for communication, it does not yet improve clinical decision-making or automation.

- **Structural Interoperability:** Structural interoperability builds on foundational capabilities by ensuring that data is exchanged in standardized and organized formats. This level focuses on the syntax and structure of health data, such as using HL7 or CDA (Clinical Document Architecture) formats to organize information into defined fields and layouts. With structural interoperability, data like vital signs, lab results, or medication lists are no longer shared as just text or attachments—they are shared as structured records that can be parsed and displayed consistently. This allows the receiving system to store the data in the right place within its own records. However, it still may not fully understand the meaning of the data (e.g., a diagnosis code). Structural interoperability is key for automation, data management, and basic integration between health information systems.

- **Semantic Interoperability:** Semantic interoperability enables healthcare systems not just to share structured data, but to interpret and use the data consistently and accurately. It ensures that the meaning behind clinical information—such as diagnosis codes, medications, lab values, or allergies—is understood in the same way by all systems. This is made possible through the use of standardized medical terminologies like SNOMED CT, LOINC, and ICD-10. For instance, when one system records "Type 2 diabetes," another system can recognize it precisely and trigger relevant clinical decision support tools or alerts. Semantic interoperability is essential for clinical quality reporting, population health analytics, machine learning models, and patient safety. It enables intelligent automation and meaningful use of data, ensuring the right information is interpreted correctly, no matter where it comes from.
- **Organizational Interoperability:** Organizational interoperability addresses the non-technical elements that are critical for full, secure, and ethical health data exchange. This includes policies, legal agreements, governance models, and privacy frameworks that guide how and when data is shared between institutions, providers, and even across national borders. It ensures that organizations follow common standards for data access, consent management, security protocols, and compliance (such as HIPAA or GDPR). Without organizational interoperability, even the best technical systems can't work together effectively, as there may be legal or policy barriers to data sharing. It also defines how trust is established between parties, how data responsibilities are assigned, and how audits or disputes are handled. This level is crucial for enabling cross-institutional and cross-border health collaboration, especially in public health, research, and global health networks.

Without interoperability, health data remains siloed, duplicative, and error-prone. True interoperability ensures coordinated care, especially for patients who see multiple providers across different settings or transition from inpatient to outpatient care.

Standards Enabling EHR Interoperability

Achieving interoperability depends on the adoption of industry-wide data standards, including:

- **HL7 (Health Level Seven):** Messaging standards for sharing clinical and administrative data.

- **FHIR (Fast Healthcare Interoperability Resources):** A newer, API-based standard that allows real-time access to health data across systems and apps.
- **LOINC:** Standard codes for lab tests and measurements.
- **SNOMED CT & ICD-10:** Standardized medical terminology and diagnostic codes.
- **DICOM:** Used for storing and transmitting medical imaging.

These standards ensure that when data moves from one system to another, it retains its structure, meaning, and context, enabling reliable use across platforms.

Benefits of EHR Integration and Interoperability

- **Improved Patient Safety:** Improved patient safety is one of the most significant benefits of EHR integration and interoperability. By having a complete and accurate digital record, healthcare providers can avoid common errors such as medication mistakes, allergies being overlooked, or contraindicated treatments being prescribed. Interoperability reduces redundant testing and procedures, minimizing patient exposure to unnecessary interventions. Real-time access to up-to-date patient information helps clinicians quickly identify potential risks and take preventive measures. This leads to fewer adverse events, hospital readmissions, and medical complications. In emergencies, access to comprehensive data can be life-saving, ensuring providers have the critical information they need to deliver appropriate care promptly.
- **Enhanced Care Coordination:** Enhanced care coordination is achieved when all members of a patient's healthcare team—specialists, primary care providers, pharmacists, and others—can access a single, unified source of truth for the patient's health information. This seamless sharing facilitates smoother transitions between care settings, such as hospital discharge to outpatient follow-up, preventing gaps or duplications in care. Providers can collaborate more effectively, communicating through shared notes and alerts embedded in the EHR. Patients benefit from a holistic care approach, with fewer conflicting treatments and more consistent management plans. This integrated coordination is especially vital for individuals with complex or chronic conditions requiring multi-disciplinary care.
- **Faster Clinical Decisions:** Faster clinical decisions result from the availability of real-time, comprehensive patient data at the point of care. With interoperable systems, clinicians can quickly review recent lab results, imaging, medication histories, and clinical notes without delay. This reduces the time spent searching for information or waiting for paper

records to arrive. It enables providers to make evidence-based decisions promptly, improving treatment effectiveness and patient outcomes. Rapid access to alerts about allergies, drug interactions, or abnormal test results further supports timely interventions. Faster decision-making not only enhances care quality but also increases patient satisfaction by reducing wait times and unnecessary appointments.

- **Operational Efficiency:** Operational efficiency improves significantly when healthcare organizations adopt integrated and interoperable EHR systems. Streamlined documentation processes reduce duplicate data entry, freeing clinicians to focus more on patient care than paperwork. Automated data sharing between departments, labs, and pharmacies cuts down administrative burdens and accelerates workflows. Communication is clearer and more direct, with fewer errors caused by manual transcription or lost information. Improved scheduling, billing, and resource management become possible as all relevant data is consolidated. This efficiency translates into cost savings, reduced staff burnout, and better allocation of healthcare resources, ultimately supporting a more sustainable care delivery model.
- **Empowered Patients:** Empowered patients are those who actively participate in their own healthcare journey, and interoperability facilitates this through patient portals and health apps linked to integrated EHR systems. Patients gain secure, easy access to their medical records, test results, medication lists, and appointment schedules. They can monitor their health status, track progress, and communicate directly with providers, fostering transparency and trust. This access encourages better self-management of chronic diseases, adherence to treatment plans, and informed decision-making. Additionally, patients can share their records with different providers, enabling continuity of care wherever they seek treatment. Empowerment through data access ultimately improves engagement, satisfaction, and health outcomes.
- **Population Health Insights:** Population health insights arise from aggregating interoperable health data across multiple providers, care settings, and geographic areas. This comprehensive data enables public health officials and researchers to identify trends, monitor outbreaks, and track the effectiveness of interventions at scale. It supports targeted outreach and preventive programs for at-risk populations, such as vaccination drives or chronic disease management initiatives. Analytics derived from integrated data can inform policy-making, resource allocation, and quality improvement efforts. Interoperability also facilitates clinical research

and real-world evidence generation, accelerating medical advancements. By leveraging broad, high-quality data, healthcare systems can shift from reactive to proactive and predictive models of care.

Challenges in Achieving Integration and Interoperability

- Despite the benefits, full interoperability remains a major challenge due to:
- Fragmented legacy systems with proprietary software that resists integration
- Lack of data standardization across regions or providers
- Security and privacy concerns, especially when exchanging sensitive data
- Resistance from vendors who prefer closed ecosystems for business reasons
- High implementation costs and need for workforce training
- To address these, many governments and organizations are enforcing data-sharing mandates, offering financial incentives, and promoting open standards.

Global and Policy Perspective

In the U.S., initiatives like the 21st Century Cures Act and ONC's interoperability rule mandate that patients have full access to their digital health data and that providers eliminate "information blocking." The EU's European Health Data Space (EHDS) aims to unify health data sharing across member states. These frameworks reflect a growing commitment to a patient-centric, data-driven healthcare system that crosses institutional and national boundaries.

EHR integration and interoperability are not just technical goals—they are essential enablers of high-quality, connected, and patient-centered care. They allow healthcare systems to function as cohesive networks rather than isolated silos. By adopting open standards, ensuring data security, and investing in infrastructure and education, healthcare institutions can unlock the full potential of digital transformation and deliver more efficient, equitable, and responsive care for all.

4.3 CLINICAL DECISION SUPPORT SYSTEMS (CDSS):

Clinical Decision Support Systems (CDSS) represent a pivotal advancement in healthcare technology, designed to aid clinicians by providing intelligent, data-driven guidance throughout the patient care process. These sophisticated computer-based systems integrate vast amounts of patient-specific data—including medical histories, lab results, imaging, vital signs, and medication records—with comprehensive, evidence-based medical knowledge. By doing so, CDSS can generate timely, relevant, and actionable recommendations tailored to each individual patient's unique clinical context. This integration enables healthcare providers to make more informed, precise, and effective decisions, significantly enhancing diagnostic accuracy, treatment planning, and overall patient outcomes. The importance of CDSS arises from the growing complexity of modern medicine. With rapid expansions in medical knowledge, clinical guidelines, and treatment options, it has become increasingly difficult for providers to keep up with all relevant information while managing a high volume of patients. CDSS serve as a valuable assistant by synthesizing this vast body of knowledge and applying it directly to clinical cases. They help reduce cognitive overload on clinicians by filtering, organizing, and prioritizing critical information that might otherwise be missed or overlooked during routine practice. One of the core strengths of CDSS lies in their ability to support evidence-based medicine. These systems are programmed with up-to-date clinical guidelines, research findings, and best practice protocols, ensuring that recommendations align with the latest standards of care. As new research emerges, CDSS can be updated to reflect evolving knowledge, making them dynamic tools that evolve alongside the medical field. This capability helps promote uniformity and standardization in care delivery, reducing variability between providers and improving overall quality. Beyond guiding diagnosis and treatment, CDSS can perform vital safety functions. For example, they can detect potential drug interactions, allergies, or contraindications before a medication is prescribed, preventing adverse drug events that could harm patients (Fig. 3). Additionally, they offer reminders for preventive care measures, such as vaccinations and screening tests, encouraging proactive health management. These features collectively contribute to a safer clinical environment and a reduction in medical errors. The benefits of CDSS extend to operational efficiency as well. By automating routine checks and data analysis, these systems save valuable time for healthcare providers, allowing them to focus more on patient interaction and care. Automated alerts, decision pathways, and standardized order sets reduce administrative burdens and improve workflow continuity. This enhanced efficiency can lead to faster clinical decisions, shorter patient wait times, and better resource utilization.

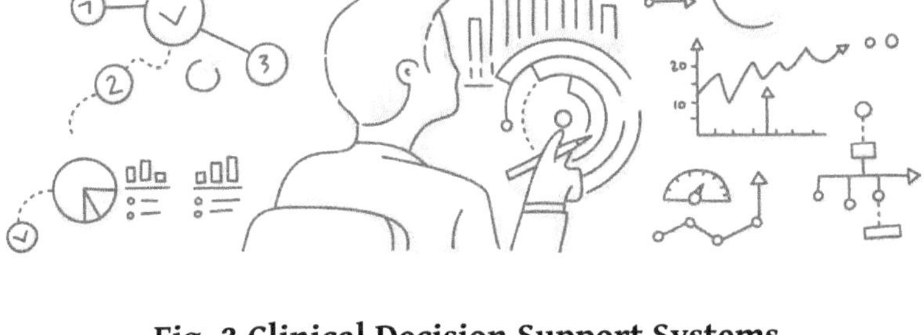

Fig. 3 Clinical Decision Support Systems

CDSS also facilitate personalized medicine by tailoring recommendations based on individual patient data, including demographics, genetics, and comorbidities. This personalization improves the relevance and effectiveness of clinical interventions. Moreover, the integration of CDSS with electronic health records (EHRs) allows seamless incorporation of decision support directly into existing clinical workflows. This real-time, contextual guidance helps ensure that recommendations are not only accurate but also timely, delivered exactly when they are needed in the decision-making process.

Despite these strengths, CDSS face certain challenges, such as alert fatigue, where excessive or irrelevant notifications may overwhelm providers and reduce the system's effectiveness. Ensuring high-quality, complete data input is critical to maintaining accurate and reliable recommendations. Additionally, clinicians' acceptance of CDSS can vary, as some may perceive these tools as intrusive or fear that reliance on automated suggestions could undermine clinical autonomy. Looking to the future, advancements in artificial intelligence and machine learning promise to greatly expand the capabilities of CDSS. These technologies can enable predictive analytics, early warning systems, and continuous learning from large datasets to refine recommendations further. Integration with wearable devices and remote patient monitoring will allow CDSS to operate beyond traditional clinical settings, supporting more proactive and preventive care models. Clinical Decision Support Systems are transforming healthcare by enhancing clinical decision-making through intelligent, data-driven support. They play a crucial role in improving patient safety, care quality, and operational efficiency while adapting to the ever-evolving landscape of medical knowledge. As technology advances and integration deepens, CDSS will continue to empower clinicians to deliver more precise, effective, and personalized care to their patients. CDSS are software applications that analyze patient-specific information and present healthcare providers with evidence-based guidance, alerts, reminders, or diagnostic suggestions. The primary purpose of CDSS is to improve clinical outcomes by reducing errors, enhancing decision-making speed, and supporting adherence to clinical guidelines and protocols.

4.3.1 Types of CDSS

CDSS can be categorized based on their mode of interaction and functionality:

- **Passive CDSS:** Provide information or knowledge resources that clinicians can consult as needed, such as drug databases or clinical guidelines.
- **Active CDSS:** Deliver proactive alerts, reminders, or diagnostic suggestions during the clinical workflow without requiring user initiation.

- **Knowledge-Based Systems:** Rely on a predefined set of clinical rules, algorithms, or decision trees derived from medical literature.
- **Non-Knowledge-Based Systems:** Use machine learning and artificial intelligence to analyze data patterns and predict outcomes without explicit rule-based logic.

Types of clinical decision support systems (CDSS) are summarised in Table-1.

Table 1 : Types of Clinical Decision Support Systems (CDSS)

Type of CDSS	Description	Characteristics
Passive CDSS	Provide reference information or resources that clinicians can consult manually, such as drug databases or clinical practice guidelines.	User-initiated, non-intrusive, used for reference and education.
Active CDSS	Offer real-time alerts, reminders, or suggestions within the clinical workflow without user initiation.	Automated, interruptive, supports timely decision-making during care delivery.
Knowledge-Based Systems	Utilize a predefined set of rules, algorithms, or decision trees derived from clinical expertise and medical literature.	Transparent logic, rule-driven, easy to audit and update.
Non-Knowledge-Based Systems	Use AI/ML techniques to analyze large datasets and identify patterns or predictions without relying on explicit clinical rules.	Data-driven, adaptive, potentially opaque (black-box models), requires large data sets.

4.3.2 Core Components of CDSS

A typical CDSS includes the following components:

- **Knowledge Base:** A curated repository of clinical guidelines, protocols, drug information, and evidence-based literature.
- **Inference Engine:** The processing unit that applies logical rules or AI algorithms to the knowledge base using patient-specific data.
- **Communication Mechanism:** Interfaces that deliver recommendations or alerts to clinicians within electronic health record (EHR) systems or standalone applications.
- **User Interface:** The platform where healthcare providers interact with the CDSS, such as through dashboards, pop-ups, or mobile apps.

Components of a typical Clinical Decision Support System (CDSS) is depicted in Table-2.

Table 2: Components of a typical Clinical Decision Support System (CDSS)

Component	Description	Function
Knowledge Base	A curated repository containing clinical guidelines, protocols, drug interactions, and evidence-based resources.	Provides the foundational medical content used for decision-making.
Inference Engine	The processing logic that applies decision rules, algorithms, or AI models to patient-specific data.	Analyzes data and generates context-specific recommendations or alerts.
Communication Mechanism	The system used to deliver alerts, recommendations, or reminders to the clinician, often integrated within EHRs or other platforms.	Ensures timely and relevant delivery of decision support during clinical workflows.
User Interface (UI)	The visual and interactive platform through which clinicians view and interact with CDSS outputs (e.g., dashboards, pop-ups, apps).	Facilitates user interaction, interpretation of suggestions, and clinical decision-making.

4.3.3 Functions and Features

CDSS offers multiple functions that support diverse clinical needs:

- **Diagnostic Support:** Suggests possible diagnoses based on symptoms, lab results, and medical history.
- **Therapeutic Guidance:** Recommends treatment options, drug dosages, and contraindications.
- **Medication Management:** Alerts providers about drug interactions, allergies, duplicate therapies, and dosing errors.
- **Preventive Care Reminders:** Notifies clinicians and patients about vaccinations, screenings, or routine check-ups.
- **Order Sets and Clinical Pathways:** Provides standardized treatment protocols to promote best practices and reduce variability.
- **Documentation Assistance:** Facilitates accurate and complete clinical documentation for quality and billing.

4.3.4 Integration with Healthcare Systems

For maximum effectiveness, CDSS is integrated tightly with EHRs and other digital health tools. This integration enables real-time access to patient data and workflow embedding, ensuring that recommendations are timely and contextually relevant. Interoperability standards like HL7 FHIR facilitate data exchange between CDSS and other clinical systems.

4.3.5 Benefits of CDSS

The adoption of CDSS offers numerous benefits:

- **Improved Patient Safety:** Reduces medication errors, adverse drug events, and diagnostic mistakes.
- **Enhanced Clinical Efficiency:** Speeds up decision-making and reduces cognitive load on providers.
- **Consistency and Standardization:** Promotes adherence to evidence-based guidelines and reduces practice variability.
- **Personalized Care:** Tailors recommendations based on individual patient data and risk factors.
- **Cost Savings:** Decreases unnecessary tests and treatments through optimized care pathways.

4.3.6 Challenges and Limitations

Despite their advantages, CDSS face several challenges:

- **Alert Fatigue:** Alert fatigue is a significant challenge in the use of Clinical Decision Support Systems, occurring when clinicians receive too many alerts, many of which may be irrelevant or low priority. This overload can lead providers to become desensitized, causing them to ignore or override important warnings that could affect patient safety. Frequent interruptions during clinical workflows disrupt concentration and increase cognitive burden. To combat alert fatigue, CDSS must be carefully calibrated to prioritize critical alerts and minimize false positives. Customizable alert settings, user feedback loops, and intelligent filtering algorithms are essential to ensure that notifications are meaningful and actionable. Addressing alert fatigue improves provider engagement, reduces burnout, and enhances the overall effectiveness of decision support.
- **Data Quality:** The accuracy and reliability of CDSS recommendations heavily depend on the quality of input data. Incomplete, outdated, or erroneous patient records can lead to incorrect suggestions, undermining clinician trust and potentially compromising patient safety. Data quality issues may arise from manual entry errors, missing lab results, or inconsistent coding practices. Ensuring high-quality data requires standardized data collection protocols, real-time updates, and integration across multiple sources. Automated data validation and cleansing techniques can help identify and correct inaccuracies before they impact decision support. Robust data governance and staff training are also critical to maintaining data integrity, which is the foundation for effective CDSS performance.

- **User Resistance:** User resistance to CDSS is a common barrier to successful implementation and utilization. Clinicians may perceive these systems as intrusive or disruptive to their established workflows, fearing that reliance on automated recommendations diminishes their professional judgment and autonomy. Some providers might distrust the technology, questioning the accuracy of algorithm-generated advice or feeling uncomfortable with computer-mediated decision-making. Overcoming resistance involves involving clinicians early in system design, offering comprehensive training, and demonstrating the clinical value of CDSS through evidence and positive outcomes. Creating flexible systems that allow clinicians to override or customize recommendations can also increase acceptance and trust.
- **Complexity of Integration:** Integrating CDSS with diverse electronic health record (EHR) platforms and healthcare IT infrastructure is technically complex. Different EHR vendors use varying data standards, architectures, and interfaces, making seamless interoperability challenging. Integration issues can result in delayed data exchange, incomplete information sharing, or system incompatibilities, reducing CDSS effectiveness. Additionally, healthcare organizations may face significant costs and resource demands during implementation. To address these challenges, adherence to industry standards like HL7 and FHIR, collaboration between vendors, and use of middleware solutions are critical. Ongoing technical support and updates ensure that CDSS remain compatible and perform optimally within evolving healthcare ecosystems.
- **Legal and Ethical Concerns:** Legal and ethical considerations surrounding CDSS revolve around accountability for clinical decisions influenced by automated recommendations. When a CDSS suggests a course of action, questions arise about who bears responsibility if an error occurs—the clinician, the software developer, or the healthcare institution. Transparency in how CDSS algorithms generate advice is vital for ethical use, allowing clinicians to understand and trust the system's reasoning. Patient consent and data privacy must also be rigorously protected, adhering to regulations like HIPAA or GDPR. Developing clear legal frameworks and professional guidelines will help define liability, protect patient rights, and foster ethical deployment of CDSS in clinical practice.

4.3.7 Future Directions

The future of Clinical Decision Support Systems (CDSS) is poised to be profoundly shaped by rapid advancements in artificial intelligence (AI), big data analytics, and the evolving field of precision medicine. As healthcare generates ever-increasing volumes of data—from electronic health records (EHRs), genomics, imaging, wearable devices, and patient-reported outcomes—CDSS will harness these vast datasets through sophisticated machine learning algorithms. These AI-driven systems will move beyond traditional rule-based logic to deliver predictive analytics, enabling clinicians to anticipate health events such as disease exacerbations, hospital readmissions, or adverse drug reactions well before they occur. This proactive approach will support early intervention and personalized treatment, improving patient outcomes while reducing costs.

Machine learning models trained on diverse patient populations will allow CDSS to identify subtle patterns and risk factors that may not be evident to human providers. By continuously learning from new data, these systems will evolve dynamically, enhancing their accuracy and clinical relevance over time. The integration of precision medicine into CDSS will tailor recommendations based on a patient's unique genetic makeup, lifestyle, and environmental factors, fostering individualized care plans that optimize efficacy and minimize side effects.Moreover, the proliferation of wearable health sensors and remote monitoring technologies will transform CDSS into real-time, continuous decision support platforms. These devices will provide uninterrupted streams of vital signs, activity levels, glucose monitoring, and other physiologic data, feeding directly into CDSS algorithms.

This continuous data flow enables early detection of deviations from baseline health and timely alerts, even when patients are outside traditional clinical settings. Such remote decision support capabilities will be particularly valuable for managing chronic diseases, post-operative care, and aging populations, allowing providers to intervene promptly and avoid complications.

Improving the user interface design of CDSS will be another crucial factor for future success. Systems that are intuitive, seamlessly integrated into clinical workflows, and customizable to provider preferences will encourage adoption and sustained use. Incorporating direct clinician feedback into system updates will ensure that CDSS remain relevant, actionable, and reduce the risk of alert fatigue. Enhancements like natural language processing (NLP) will facilitate easier interaction, allowing providers to communicate with CDSS using conversational language rather than complex commands. Ethical considerations and data privacy will also be central to the evolution of CDSS. Future systems will incorporate robust security measures to protect sensitive patient data, maintain confidentiality, and comply with regulatory standards. Transparent algorithms that provide explanations for their recommendations will build trust among clinicians and patients, addressing concerns about "black box" decision-making. Finally, the future CDSS landscape will increasingly involve interdisciplinary collaboration, combining expertise from clinicians, data scientists, informaticians, and engineers. This teamwork will drive innovations that not only improve clinical decision-making but also enhance health system efficiency and patient empowerment.

The future of CDSS is bright and transformative. Powered by AI, enriched with big data, and personalized through precision medicine, next-generation systems will offer predictive, continuous, and patient-centered decision support. These advancements will help shift healthcare from reactive to proactive, ultimately improving outcomes, reducing costs, and empowering both providers and patients in the delivery of high-quality care.

4.4 ALERT SYSTEMS AND PHYSICIAN DASHBOARDS:

Alert systems and physician dashboards are vital components of modern healthcare information systems, playing a crucial role in enhancing patient care, improving clinical outcomes, and streamlining provider workflows. These tools are deeply integrated within Electronic Health Records (EHRs) and Clinical Decision Support Systems (CDSS) to serve as dynamic, real-time interfaces that support clinicians in making timely and informed decisions. With the exponential growth of clinical data, healthcare professionals rely heavily on intelligent systems to distill vast amounts of information into actionable insights. Alert systems achieve this by providing timely notifications regarding critical or abnormal clinical events, such as drug interactions, lab abnormalities, or acute changes in a patient's condition. These alerts are designed to reduce errors, prevent adverse events, and prompt necessary interventions, thereby ensuring patient safety.

There are various types of alerts, including medication alerts, diagnostic alerts, clinical deterioration alerts, and preventive care reminders. Medication-related alerts, for instance, notify physicians of potential drug-drug interactions, allergies, or incorrect dosages, particularly in vulnerable populations like pediatrics or the elderly. Diagnostic alerts flag abnormal lab or imaging results that require immediate attention, while condition-specific alerts, such as sepsis or cardiac arrest warnings, enable rapid clinical response. Preventive alerts also play a key role by reminding providers of routine screenings, immunizations, or follow-up care, contributing to long-term population health management. However, the effectiveness of alert systems depends heavily on their design and relevance. Overuse or poorly configured alerts can lead to alert fatigue, a phenomenon where clinicians become desensitized to notifications and may ignore or override them—even those that are clinically significant. To combat this, modern systems incorporate context-aware logic, machine learning algorithms, and user feedback loops to improve the specificity and relevance of alerts. Ideally, alert systems should support—not interrupt—the clinician's workflow.

Complementing alert systems are physician dashboards, which act as centralized control panels that consolidate critical patient data, trends, and alerts into an intuitive, visual format. These dashboards provide clinicians with a comprehensive, real-time overview of patient status, including vital signs, lab trends, medication lists, allergies, imaging reports, and more. They are customizable based on specialty, role, or patient population, and can include performance metrics, quality indicators, and decision-support tools. For example, a cardiologist might use a dashboard that emphasizes ECG data, lipid panels, and heart failure risk scores, while a primary care physician may prefer population health analytics and chronic disease management tools. When alerts are seamlessly integrated into dashboards, clinicians are able to prioritize tasks, triage patients, and take immediate action—all from a single interface. This integration promotes efficiency, reduces cognitive overload, and minimizes the risk of missed information. Furthermore, modern dashboards often support interactive features, such as one-click ordering, real-time messaging, and patient tracking across shifts or departments, enhancing continuity of care.

Alert systems and physician dashboards are not merely tools for data display—they are strategic enablers of high-quality, evidence-based care. They empower healthcare professionals to navigate complex clinical environments with greater confidence and precision. As healthcare continues to embrace digital transformation, the refinement and intelligent integration of these systems will remain central to improving patient outcomes, reducing clinical errors, and supporting the evolving demands of modern medicine.

4.4.1. Alert Systems

Alert systems are designed to automatically notify physicians and healthcare staff of time-sensitive or critical clinical events. They serve as proactive tools to prevent medical errors, optimize treatment, and ensure compliance with guidelines.

Types of Alerts

- **Medication Alerts:** Medication alerts are automated notifications that warn clinicians about potential issues related to prescriptions, such as drug-drug interactions, allergies, incorrect dosages, or contraindications. These alerts are critical for ensuring medication safety, particularly in complex cases involving multiple drugs or vulnerable populations like children and the elderly. They help prevent adverse drug events (ADEs), a leading cause of harm in healthcare. Often integrated into e-prescribing workflows, they provide real-time guidance during order entry. To remain effective, alerts must be clinically relevant and intelligently filtered to avoid alert fatigue.
    - Drug-allergy interactions

- Drug-drug interactions
- Drug-dosage alerts (age/weight-based)
- Duplicate therapies

◉ **Diagnostic Alerts:** Diagnostic alerts notify clinicians about critical or abnormal test results—such as lab values, imaging findings, or pathology reports—that require prompt attention. These alerts help ensure that serious conditions like infections, organ dysfunction, or malignancies are not overlooked or delayed in diagnosis. Often triggered automatically by thresholds or predefined criteria, they support early intervention and timely follow-up. They also help bridge communication gaps between departments, such as labs and clinical teams. Well-designed diagnostic alerts reduce diagnostic errors and improve patient outcomes.

- Abnormal lab results (e.g., critical potassium levels)
- Imaging results requiring urgent follow-up

◉ **Clinical Condition Alerts:** Clinical condition alerts are triggered by specific patterns in patient data that indicate the onset or worsening of serious health conditions, such as sepsis, acute kidney injury, or cardiac arrest. These alerts analyze combinations of vital signs, lab results, and clinical notes to detect early signs of deterioration. By flagging high-risk scenarios in real time, they enable rapid response teams to intervene before a patient's condition becomes critical. These alerts are especially valuable in intensive care, emergency, and post-surgical units. Their predictive capabilities make them essential for improving survival rates and preventing complications.

- Sepsis alerts based on vitals and labs
- Deteriorating patient condition (e.g., vital sign trends)

◉ **Preventive Care Reminders:** Preventive care reminders prompt healthcare providers to perform routine screenings, immunizations, and wellness checks based on patient age, gender, and risk factors. These alerts support early detection and management of chronic diseases, helping to reduce long-term complications and healthcare costs. By ensuring adherence to evidence-based guidelines, they promote consistent, proactive care rather than reactive treatment. They also enhance patient engagement by facilitating timely follow-ups and health maintenance. Ultimately, preventive reminders contribute to improved population health and better quality of life.

- Immunizations due
- Routine screenings (e.g., mammograms, colonoscopies)

◉ **Compliance Alerts:** Compliance alerts notify clinicians and healthcare staff when documentation, protocols, or regulatory requirements are incomplete or overdue. These alerts help ensure adherence to hospital policies, clinical guidelines, and legal mandates, such as timely charting or infection control measures. By promoting consistent compliance, they reduce the risk of legal liabilities, audit failures, and penalties. They also support quality improvement initiatives by highlighting areas needing attention. Ultimately, compliance alerts help maintain high standards of care and institutional accountability.

- Missing documentation
- Protocol deviations

Delivery Methods

- **Pop-up Notifications within EHR Interfaces:** Pop-up alerts within the Electronic Health Record (EHR) interface are the most immediate form of in-system communication. These alerts appear in real-time during clinical documentation or order entry, often requiring acknowledgment before proceeding. They're useful for catching issues such as drug interactions or allergy conflicts at the point of care. While effective, overuse can lead to alert fatigue. Therefore, careful design and prioritization are essential for impact.
- **Text/Email/Pager Alerts for High-Priority Situations:** For urgent or life-threatening events, high-priority alerts are sent via text messages, emails, or traditional pagers. These are especially critical in settings like the ICU, emergency department, or surgical wards where rapid response can be lifesaving. They allow for off-site or mobile notification, ensuring timely communication regardless of location. These alerts are usually reserved for severe abnormalities or escalations. Their reliability makes them essential in emergency protocols.
- **Mobile App Push Notifications:** Push notifications through mobile health apps provide clinicians with a modern, portable method to stay informed. These alerts can include patient updates, task reminders, and urgent clinical warnings, accessible even when not logged into the EHR. They support on-the-go decision-making and are valuable for multidisciplinary teams working across departments. With growing adoption of mobile health solutions, push alerts are becoming an integral part of care coordination. Security and user control are key considerations.
- **Dashboard Integration:** Integrating alerts directly into physician dashboards allows clinicians to view and respond to notifications in a consolidated, non-disruptive format. This method supports contextual awareness, displaying alerts alongside relevant patient data such as labs, vitals, and history. It helps reduce cognitive overload and improves alert

relevance. Clinicians can take action from within the dashboard itself, enhancing workflow efficiency. It's a strategic solution to balance visibility with usability.

Challenges

- **Alert Fatigue:** Alert fatigue occurs when clinicians are bombarded with excessive, often non-critical alerts, leading to desensitization. As a result, providers may begin to ignore or override even important, potentially life-saving notifications. This undermines the purpose of the alert system and increases the risk of missed or delayed interventions. It's a common issue in poorly optimized EHRs. Reducing alert volume and improving specificity are essential to combat this problem.
- **Workflow Disruption:** Ill-timed or irrelevant alerts can interrupt clinical workflows, causing frustration and reducing efficiency. Alerts that appear during critical tasks or patient interactions can break concentration and delay care delivery. When alerts feel intrusive, clinicians may begin to view them as obstacles rather than helpful tools. This can reduce adoption and trust in the system. Designing alerts that integrate seamlessly into the workflow is key to minimizing disruption.
- **Customization Needs:** To be truly effective, alerts must be context-sensitive and tailored to both the patient's clinical profile and the provider's specialty or role. A one-size-fits-all alert system leads to irrelevant notifications that dilute the value of the system. Customization allows alerts to be filtered based on urgency, relevance, and care setting. Personalized alert thresholds and preferences improve clinician engagement. This makes the system more efficient, accurate, and trusted.

4.4.2 Physician Dashboards

A physician dashboard is a digital interface that consolidates and displays key patient data, metrics, and alerts in a single, user-friendly view. Dashboards are integrated into EHRs and help physicians monitor patient populations, track individual patient progress, and make informed decisions.

Key Features

- **Patient Summary Views:** Physician dashboards provide comprehensive patient summary views, consolidating critical data such as vitals, lab results, current medications, allergies, and medical history. This unified view eliminates the need to navigate through multiple EHR tabs. Clinicians can assess the patient's overall condition at a glance, supporting quick decision-making. It improves continuity of care by offering context-rich insights. This feature is especially valuable during time-sensitive or high-stress clinical scenarios.

- **Real-Time Alerts and Notifications:** Dashboards deliver real-time alerts that are often color-coded based on severity to draw immediate attention to urgent issues. These alerts may include abnormal labs, critical changes in vital signs, or medication errors. In addition, task lists and care reminders are integrated to support daily workflow. This helps clinicians prioritize actions and ensure nothing critical is missed. Together, they create a proactive and responsive care environment.
- **Clinical Metrics and KPIs:** Dashboards include clinical performance indicators like time to antibiotic administration, length of stay, and readmission rates. These key performance indicators (KPIs) offer valuable insight into care efficiency and effectiveness. They also track compliance with standardized quality measures such as HEDIS and MACRA. Clinicians and administrators can use this data for quality improvement initiatives. Overall, it helps align clinical practice with institutional and regulatory goals.
- **Customizable Panels:** NDashboards offer customizable panels that can be tailored based on clinical specialty or individual preferences. For example, cardiologists might view ECG data and heart failure metrics, while oncologists focus on tumor markers and treatment timelines. Personalized widgets and filters allow users to highlight the most relevant patient data. This customization enhances usability and clinical relevance. It ensures the dashboard supports diverse workflows across departments and specialties.

Benefits

- **Efficiency:** Physician dashboards provide clinicians with immediate access to the most relevant and up-to-date patient information. By organizing critical data—such as vitals, lab results, and medications—in one intuitive interface, they reduce time spent navigating complex EHR systems. This streamlined access minimizes delays in care and enhances overall workflow. Clinicians can quickly assess patient status, prioritize tasks, and respond effectively. The result is improved time management and greater clinical productivity.
- **Improved Decision-Making:** Dashboards support data-driven clinical decision-making by presenting evidence-based insights at the point of care. By integrating real-time patient data with clinical guidelines and predictive analytics, they enable more accurate assessments and timely interventions. Physicians can make better-informed choices, tailored to individual patient contexts. This enhances diagnostic precision and therapeutic

appropriateness. Ultimately, it contributes to safer, more consistent, and higher-quality care delivery.

- **Enhanced Patient Safety:** Consolidated alerts within dashboards play a key role in preventing medical errors and adverse events. These alerts notify clinicians of critical issues such as abnormal labs, medication interactions, or vital sign deterioration. By highlighting high-priority risks in a clear and actionable format, dashboards help ensure that no crucial detail is overlooked. This proactive approach to safety empowers clinicians to intervene early and appropriately. The result is better patient outcomes and reduced harm.
- **Population Health Management:** Physician dashboards allow for efficient monitoring of patient groups with shared conditions, such as diabetes, hypertension, or heart failure. Clinicians can track trends, outcomes, and compliance across entire populations, identifying gaps in care and opportunities for early intervention. These insights support targeted outreach and coordinated management plans. Over time, this approach helps reduce hospitalizations, improve chronic disease control, and lower healthcare costs. It's a powerful tool for advancing preventive and value-based care.

4.4.3 Integration of Alert Systems and Dashboards

The most effective clinical interfaces integrate alert systems directly into physician dashboards, creating a central hub for notifications, tasks, and patient data. This integration ensures that:

- Alerts are presented in context, reducing unnecessary interruptions.
- Physicians can act on alerts directly from the dashboard (e.g., ordering a lab or medication).
- Dashboards serve as control panels for patient monitoring and intervention tracking.

4.4.4 Best Practices for Implementation

- **Prioritize Critical Alerts to Reduce Fatigue:** Focusing on the most urgent and clinically significant alerts helps minimize overload and prevents desensitization among providers. By filtering out low-priority notifications, the system ensures that important warnings receive proper attention. This targeted approach improves patient safety and maintains clinician trust. It also streamlines workflow by reducing unnecessary interruptions. Effective prioritization is key to sustainable alert management.

- **Use Intelligent Filtering and Context-Aware Algorithms:** Incorporating smart algorithms that consider patient-specific data and clinical context enhances alert relevance. These systems can suppress redundant or irrelevant alerts and adjust thresholds based on the clinical scenario. Context-awareness helps tailor alerts to individual cases, reducing false positives. This intelligent filtering improves accuracy and clinician satisfaction. It also supports personalized care and decision-making.
- **Ensure User-Centric Design with Input from Clinicians:** Designing alert systems with direct feedback from end-users ensures they meet real-world needs and workflows. Clinician involvement during development helps identify pain points and practical requirements. User-centric design fosters usability, acceptance, and effective communication. It also helps balance alert frequency and content quality. Ultimately, this collaboration creates more meaningful and actionable alerts.
- **Provide Training and Feedback Loops to Improve System Relevance:** Ongoing education empowers clinicians to understand alert rationale and appropriate responses, enhancing compliance. Feedback loops allow users to report false alarms or suggest improvements, facilitating continuous refinement. Training builds confidence and helps integrate alert systems into daily practice. Iterative feedback ensures the system evolves alongside clinical needs. This dynamic process maintains system effectiveness and user engagement.
- **Monitor Alert Response Data to Optimize System Performance:** Analyzing how clinicians interact with alerts—such as overrides, dismissals, or acknowledgments—provides valuable insights for system tuning. Monitoring response patterns helps identify problematic alerts and areas for adjustment. Data-driven optimization improves alert accuracy, reduces fatigue, and enhances patient safety. It also supports quality improvement and regulatory reporting. Regular performance reviews are essential for maintaining an effective alert ecosystem.

4.5 REDUCING HOSPITAL READMISSIONS THROUGH MONITORING:

Hospital readmissions, particularly within 30 days of discharge, are a major concern for healthcare systems worldwide. They often indicate poor care transitions, inadequate follow-up, or unaddressed patient needs. Readmissions not only impact patient well-being but also burden healthcare providers with increased costs, resource strain, and potential financial penalties under value-based reimbursement models. Monitoring—especially through technology-enabled tools—is a powerful strategy to reduce unnecessary readmissions by enabling early intervention, improving care continuity, and enhancing patient self-management. Hospital readmissions are frequently preventable. Common causes include medication errors, missed follow-up appointments, poorly managed chronic conditions, patient non-adherence, and lack of education about discharge instructions. Certain patient populations, such as those with heart failure, chronic obstructive pulmonary disease (COPD), diabetes, and elderly patients, are at higher risk. Monitoring programs aim to identify early signs of deterioration or noncompliance before they lead to a medical crisis requiring hospitalization.

4.5.1 Types of Monitoring to Prevent Readmissions

- **Remote Patient Monitoring (RPM):** Remote Patient Monitoring (RPM) utilizes digital health technologies to collect and transmit patient data—such as blood pressure, glucose levels, oxygen saturation, and weight—from the comfort of their homes to healthcare providers. This continuous stream of real-time data allows clinicians to monitor patients closely, detect early signs of deterioration, and respond quickly before conditions become critical. RPM is especially effective for managing chronic diseases like heart failure, diabetes, and COPD, where small fluctuations in health indicators can lead to serious complications. By reducing the need for in-person visits, RPM improves convenience for patients while lowering healthcare costs. It also fosters patient engagement by encouraging daily self-monitoring and awareness of their health status. Alerts can be programmed to notify clinicians of dangerous trends, prompting proactive interventions. RPM is integrated with EHR systems to ensure seamless communication between patients and providers. This approach bridges the gap between hospital discharge and outpatient care. As a result, it has become a cornerstone strategy in efforts to reduce readmission rates and support long-term recovery.
- **Post-Discharge Follow-Up Monitoring:** Post-discharge follow-up monitoring involves actively checking in with patients during the crucial days and weeks after hospital discharge to ensure recovery is on track. This can be done through structured phone calls, video consultations, home health visits, or automated check-in tools. These follow-ups are essential for identifying early complications such as infections, medication side effects, or worsening symptoms. They also allow healthcare providers to assess whether patients are adhering to their care plans, understanding their medications, and following discharge instructions correctly. When issues are caught early, they can often be resolved in outpatient settings, preventing unnecessary hospital returns. Care coordinators, nurses, or case managers often lead these efforts, acting as bridges between the hospital and community care providers. Documentation from follow-up interactions is usually fed back into the patient's EHR to inform ongoing care. This

continuous communication enhances care continuity and builds trust with patients. Overall, follow-up monitoring supports safer transitions of care and plays a vital role in readmission prevention strategies.

- **Wearable Devices and Smart Tools:** Wearable devices and smart tools offer an innovative, continuous way to monitor patients' health by capturing real-time physiological and behavioral data. Devices such as smartwatches, fitness trackers, ECG patches, and Bluetooth-enabled medical equipment measure metrics like heart rate, step count, blood oxygen levels, sleep quality, and arrhythmias. These tools provide insights into patient recovery trends that might not be apparent in clinical visits alone. By detecting abnormal patterns—such as irregular heart rhythms or significant drops in activity—clinicians can intervene before an issue escalates. Wearables also empower patients by providing immediate feedback, promoting lifestyle changes, and reinforcing adherence to care plans. Many devices are designed with mobile apps that allow both the patient and provider to visualize health trends over time. Integration with healthcare platforms and telehealth systems enables real-time data sharing. These technologies are particularly valuable for patients with chronic illnesses or those recovering from surgery. In turn, they reduce emergency visits and prevent avoidable hospital readmissions. Their convenience and non-invasive nature support widespread adoption across various age groups.
- **Medication Monitoring:** Medication monitoring is a critical strategy to prevent readmissions caused by missed doses, incorrect usage, or adverse drug reactions. This approach utilizes tools such as smart pillboxes, electronic medication dispensers, mobile apps, and SMS reminders to ensure patients take their medications as prescribed. Monitoring systems can track when doses are taken, send alerts for missed doses, and notify caregivers or clinicians if problems arise. This is particularly important for patients with complex regimens, such as those managing heart disease, diabetes, or mental health conditions. Poor medication adherence is one of the leading causes of readmissions, especially within the first 30 days post-discharge. By identifying non-compliance early, healthcare providers can intervene with counseling, dose adjustments, or simplification of treatment plans. Many digital tools also include educational features, helping patients understand the importance and timing of their medications. Integration with electronic health records ensures that providers have visibility into medication adherence trends. This enables personalized support and timely adjustments. Ultimately, effective medication monitoring enhances treatment effectiveness and reduces the likelihood of costly complications and readmissions.

4.5.2 Components of an Effective Monitoring Program

- **Risk Stratification:** Risk stratification involves identifying patients who are most likely to experience complications or hospital readmissions based on clinical, behavioral, and social risk factors. Using EHR data, predictive analytics, and clinical judgment, healthcare teams can pinpoint individuals who would benefit most from close post-discharge monitoring. Algorithms may evaluate variables such as recent hospitalizations, chronic disease burden, comorbidities, medication complexity, and social determinants of health. This targeted approach ensures that monitoring resources are efficiently allocated to high-need populations. Stratification also allows for the customization of care intensity, with high-risk patients receiving more frequent or advanced interventions. Clinicians can proactively manage at-risk individuals rather than reacting to crises. Tools like readmission risk scores can be embedded into discharge workflows. Ultimately, effective risk stratification improves outcomes, reduces avoidable readmissions, and supports more equitable care delivery.
- **Personalized Care Plans:** Personalized care plans are customized roadmaps for patient recovery, tailored to individual clinical conditions, preferences, and life circumstances. These plans take into account factors such as diagnosis, functional status, cognitive ability, health literacy, caregiver support, and socioeconomic challenges. Instead of applying a one-size-fits-all protocol, clinicians design specific monitoring regimens, medication schedules, diet recommendations, and educational resources that reflect the patient's unique needs. This personalized approach increases the relevance and impact of remote monitoring and follow-up care. Patients are more likely to adhere to plans that are realistic, understandable, and aligned with their daily routines. Technology platforms can help automate plan customization using smart templates and dynamic data. Additionally, involving patients and caregivers in care plan development enhances shared decision-making and empowerment. Personalized care plans are key to optimizing health outcomes and preventing unnecessary hospital returns.
- **Care Coordination:** Effective care coordination ensures that every member of a patient's healthcare team—nurses, case managers, pharmacists, primary care providers, specialists, and home care staff—is aligned around a unified care plan. This collaborative model improves communication, closes care gaps, and enables timely action in response to monitoring alerts or clinical changes. Coordinators often serve as the central point of contact, facilitating information flow across different care settings and

ensuring patients understand their treatment instructions. Technologies like shared dashboards, secure messaging, and care management platforms enhance real-time coordination. Pharmacists can help manage medication reconciliation, while social workers address barriers like transportation or housing. Strong coordination reduces fragmentation, a common cause of readmissions. It also ensures that no aspect of patient care—medical, behavioral, or logistical—is overlooked. Ultimately, coordinated care supports safer, smoother transitions between hospital, home, and outpatient services.

- **Patient Engagement Tools:** Patient engagement tools are digital or educational resources designed to empower individuals to take an active role in their health management, especially after hospital discharge. These tools include mobile apps, patient portals, remote monitoring devices with user feedback, instructional videos, and interactive care guides. They help patients understand their conditions, follow care instructions, and recognize warning signs that require clinical attention. By teaching patients how to use monitoring devices and interpret their own health data, these tools foster a sense of ownership and accountability. Engagement tools also improve communication between patients and providers, offering platforms for questions, appointment scheduling, and real-time alerts. When patients feel informed and supported, they are more likely to adhere to treatment plans and seek help early—reducing the risk of complications or readmissions. Tailoring tools to individual preferences, language, and literacy levels enhances usability and effectiveness. In short, empowered patients are healthier patients.
- **Technology Integration in Monitoring:** Modern healthcare increasingly relies on technology integration to create seamless, real-time, and data-driven monitoring systems. These systems are connected to Electronic Health Records (EHRs) and care management platforms, enabling clinicians to access and interpret patient data without switching between tools. Automated alert systems analyze incoming data streams for abnormalities or warning signs—such as irregular vitals or medication non-adherence—and notify the care team immediately. Customizable dashboards present vital information in intuitive formats, allowing clinicians to track patient trends, risk scores, and intervention outcomes at a glance. This integration enables fast, informed decisions and promotes coordinated care across providers. Additionally, telehealth platforms work alongside monitoring tools to offer immediate virtual consultations when alerts are triggered. This hybrid model enhances response time and convenience, especially for patients in remote or underserved areas. Technology integration ensures

continuous care, reduces fragmentation, and supports a proactive approach to health management. It also enables documentation and analytics that support quality improvement and reporting.

- **Outcomes and Evidence:** A growing body of research supports the effectiveness of monitoring programs—particularly Remote Patient Monitoring (RPM)—in reducing hospital readmissions. Studies have shown that patients with chronic conditions like heart failure, COPD, diabetes, and those recovering from surgery benefit significantly from structured monitoring. RPM enables early detection of clinical deterioration, allowing timely intervention that prevents costly and potentially dangerous hospital returns. Additionally, these programs improve patient satisfaction by offering a sense of safety and continuity after discharge. Patients often report greater confidence in managing their health with ongoing support and feedback. Monitoring also boosts adherence to care plans, as regular check-ins and alerts reinforce compliance. Health systems that implement such programs often see reduced financial penalties under value-based models like the U.S. Medicare Hospital Readmissions Reduction Program (HRRP). Moreover, improved outcomes translate to lower operational costs, better quality metrics, and increased patient retention. The evidence strongly supports monitoring as a cost-effective, outcome-driven solution in modern healthcare.

4.5.3 Challenges and Considerations

Technology Access and Literacy: One of the primary barriers to the success of remote monitoring programs is unequal access to technology and digital literacy. Elderly patients, those with low socioeconomic status, or individuals in rural or underserved areas may lack smartphones, computers, or reliable internet connectivity. Even when devices are available, patients may struggle with navigating apps, interpreting health data, or responding to alerts. This digital divide can limit the effectiveness of monitoring tools and contribute to healthcare disparities. To address this, healthcare systems must provide training, simplified user interfaces, and technical support. Programs should also consider offering loaner devices or partnering with community organizations to improve access. By ensuring inclusivity and usability, healthcare providers can extend the benefits of digital monitoring to all patients—not just the tech-savvy.

Data Overload: With continuous data streaming from multiple sources—wearables, remote sensors, and apps—clinicians can quickly become overwhelmed without proper data management systems in place. This phenomenon, known as data overload, can result in important alerts being buried among less relevant information. Without intelligent filtering or prioritization, clinicians may experience "alert fatigue," where they start ignoring notifications altogether. This poses serious risks, as critical health issues could be missed or delayed. Advanced analytics, AI-driven alert triage, and customizable dashboards are essential to ensure only the most relevant and actionable data reaches providers. Efficient visualization tools can also help teams make sense of trends at a glance. Managing data volume effectively is crucial to maintaining clinician efficiency and patient safety.

Privacy and Compliance: Remote monitoring programs handle sensitive personal health data, making privacy and regulatory compliance paramount. Unauthorized access, data breaches, or improper data sharing can violate patient trust and lead to severe legal consequences. Compliance with frameworks such as HIPAA (Health Insurance Portability and Accountability Act) in the U.S. is essential to protect patient rights. Ensuring encrypted data transmission, secure storage, and controlled access protocols is a technical necessity. Additionally, providers must obtain informed consent and educate patients about how their data will be used and protected. As monitoring expands into mobile apps and cloud platforms, maintaining regulatory alignment becomes increasingly complex. Regular audits, cybersecurity measures, and updated privacy policies are critical to safeguarding data integrity and institutional credibility.

Sustainability: For monitoring programs to be successful in the long term, they must be operationally and financially sustainable. Initial implementation often requires significant investment in technology infrastructure, device procurement, software licensing, and training for clinical staff. Beyond setup, ongoing maintenance, user support, data management, and workflow integration demand continuous resources. Without dedicated funding, staff turnover or system fatigue can undermine program continuity. Reimbursement structures must also evolve to support remote care services. Sustainability also hinges on aligning the program with clinical goals and institutional priorities, ensuring it adds measurable value. Building scalability and flexibility into the design will help programs evolve with changing needs. A sustainable monitoring model ultimately balances cost-efficiency with quality care delivery.

4.5.5 Home-to-Hospital Continuum of Care

Hospital readmissions are a significant challenge for healthcare systems worldwide, often reflecting gaps in patient care transitions and resulting in increased costs, patient morbidity, and strain on healthcare resources. The home-to-hospital continuum of care is an integrated approach designed to ensure seamless coordination of healthcare services as patients move between their homes and hospital settings. This continuum emphasizes proactive monitoring and communication to reduce avoidable readmissions and improve overall patient outcomes.

- **Understanding the Continuum of Care:** The continuum of care encompasses all stages of a patient's healthcare journey—from discharge planning and post-acute care at home to potential rehospitalization. Effective management of this continuum requires collaboration among multidisciplinary teams including primary care providers, specialists, home health agencies, care coordinators, and patients themselves. The goal is to maintain continuity in treatment plans, medication management, symptom monitoring, and follow-up care, regardless of the care setting.
- **Role of Remote Monitoring in the Continuum:** One of the most powerful tools in reducing hospital readmissions is remote patient monitoring (RPM). RPM leverages technology such as wearable devices, mobile health apps, and telehealth platforms to collect and transmit real-time clinical data from patients in their homes to healthcare providers. Vital signs, medication adherence, symptom tracking, and biometric data are continuously monitored, enabling early detection of deterioration or complications. Remote monitoring helps identify warning signs—such as elevated blood pressure, irregular heart rhythms, or worsening respiratory status—before they escalate into emergencies requiring hospitalization. Alerts generated by monitoring systems can trigger timely interventions, such as medication adjustments or outpatient visits, thus preventing unnecessary readmissions.
- **Comprehensive Discharge Planning:** A critical component of the home-to-hospital continuum is effective discharge planning. Prior to discharge, healthcare teams must ensure that patients and caregivers receive clear instructions on medications, follow-up appointments, lifestyle modifications, and symptom management. Coordination with home health services, social support, and community resources is essential to address potential barriers to care, such as mobility issues or social determinants of health. Discharge plans integrated with remote monitoring tools provide continuous oversight, bridging the gap between inpatient care and home management. These plans empower patients to participate actively in their own care, improving adherence and satisfaction.
- **Enhanced Communication and Care Coordination:** Successful continuum of care depends on robust communication channels between hospital teams and outpatient providers. Electronic Health Records (EHRs) and health information exchanges facilitate real-time sharing of patient data, test results, and care plans. Care coordinators play a pivotal role in

orchestrating this communication, ensuring that all providers are updated and that the patient's needs are consistently met. Technology-enabled care coordination also includes virtual visits, telephonic check-ins, and patient portals that foster ongoing engagement and education. This continuous connection helps reduce gaps in care that often lead to readmissions.

- **Patient Engagement and Education:** Engaging patients as active participants in their care is vital for reducing readmissions. Education about their condition, medication management, symptom recognition, and when to seek help improves self-management capabilities. Home monitoring devices that provide feedback directly to patients can enhance awareness and motivation. Furthermore, involving caregivers in education and monitoring helps extend support beyond clinical settings, providing an additional safety net during the vulnerable post-discharge period.
- **Outcomes and Benefits:** Implementing a home-to-hospital continuum of care supported by remote monitoring has been shown to reduce hospital readmission rates, lower healthcare costs, and improve patient quality of life. Early intervention reduces emergency visits and the burden on acute care facilities. Patients benefit from receiving care in the comfort of their homes, with improved satisfaction and clinical outcomes. This model also supports value-based care initiatives by aligning financial incentives with quality metrics and patient-centered outcomes.

5
Chapter

APPLICATIONS ACROSS MEDICAL SPECIALTIES

5.0 INTRODUCTION: AN OVERVIEW

Clinical Decision Support Systems (CDSS) have rapidly evolved into integral tools within modern healthcare, offering advanced functionalities that support clinicians in delivering accurate, timely, and evidence-based care. These systems function by integrating patient-specific data with a robust knowledge base, thereby generating intelligent insights, recommendations, and alerts that can assist in diagnosis, treatment planning, preventive care, and risk management. Initially developed as adjuncts to help manage complex clinical information, CDSS tools are now embedded within electronic health records (EHRs), telemedicine platforms, and mobile health applications, transforming them into dynamic, workflow-enhancing technologies. What distinguishes CDSS from simple reference tools is their capacity to deliver context-aware, real-time guidance tailored to individual patients. By analyzing variables such as lab results, imaging data, medication history, and comorbidities, these systems can flag potential issues—ranging from drug interactions to missed diagnoses—before they manifest into clinical problems. This has proven particularly valuable in specialties where diagnostic uncertainty or treatment complexity is high, such as oncology, cardiology, and critical care. As medicine moves toward a data-intensive, precision-based model, CDSS plays a foundational role in translating massive volumes of clinical data into meaningful, actionable insights. Medical speciality is summarised in Fig. 1.

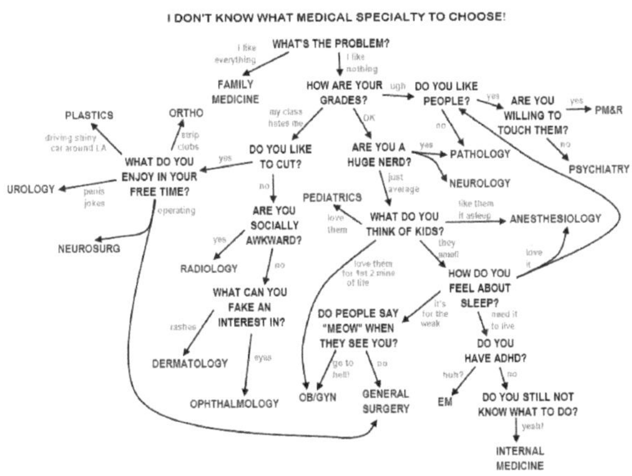

Fig. 1 Medical Speciality

One of the greatest strengths of CDSS lies in its adaptability across diverse medical specialties. In internal medicine, it supports differential diagnosis generation and chronic disease management by recommending best practices based on updated guidelines. In cardiology, CDSS can assist with interpretation of ECGs, risk stratification for heart failure, and optimization of therapy according to American Heart Association (AHA) guidelines. Similarly, in oncology, CDSS helps personalize cancer treatment plans by integrating genomic data, treatment response models, and toxicity profiles, thus supporting oncologists in selecting the most appropriate chemotherapeutic or immunotherapy regimen for each patient. In surgical specialties, CDSS enhances perioperative decision-making by identifying surgical risks, optimizing preoperative planning, and minimizing postoperative complications. Anesthesiology benefits from intraoperative decision support systems that monitor vital signs and adjust sedation in real time. In emergency medicine, where seconds can mean the difference between life and death, CDSS aids rapid triage, sepsis identification, and stroke detection using predictive scoring systems and symptom clusters. Pediatric applications of CDSS are also growing, enabling safe dosing, growth chart monitoring, and early detection of developmental delays based on age-specific parameters. Beyond diagnostics and treatment, CDSS contributes significantly to preventive medicine and population health. Systems designed for primary care often include alerts for vaccination schedules, cancer screening, and lifestyle counseling interventions based on family history and individual risk factors. In public health, CDSS platforms have been used to track disease outbreaks, assess community health metrics, and implement targeted interventions during pandemics. Behavioral health, another historically under-digitized domain, has begun leveraging CDSS for early identification of mental health disorders, suicide risk prediction, and therapeutic guidance based on psychological screening tools. Moreover, CDSS applications extend into the realm of medication safety, a critical focus area in all specialties. These systems alert clinicians to potential drug-drug interactions, dosing errors, and contraindications, significantly reducing the risk of adverse drug events. Pharmacogenomics-based CDSS further enable personalized medication prescriptions by analyzing patients' genetic profiles to determine optimal drug efficacy and minimize side effects. This is especially beneficial in specialties like psychiatry, oncology, and infectious diseases, where treatment response can vary widely.

As artificial intelligence (AI) and machine learning (ML) continue to be integrated into CDSS platforms, their predictive and adaptive capabilities are becoming more sophisticated. AI-powered CDSS can detect subtle patterns in patient data that may not be apparent to human clinicians, such as early signs of clinical deterioration or rare disease presentations. These innovations are particularly useful in radiology and pathology, where image-based data can be analyzed rapidly and with high accuracy. Despite their vast potential, CDSS must be thoughtfully integrated into clinical workflows to realize their full benefit. Poorly designed interfaces, irrelevant alerts, or lack of interoperability can hinder rather than help, causing alert fatigue or clinician resistance. Therefore, a user-centered design, ongoing training, and feedback loops are essential components of successful CDSS implementation across all specialties. The applications of Clinical Decision Support Systems span virtually every medical field, reinforcing clinical judgment, reducing variation in care, and enhancing patient safety. As healthcare systems worldwide continue to grapple with rising complexity, resource constraints, and the need for standardization, CDSS emerges as a cornerstone technology that bridges the gap between data and decision-making. This section explores how CDSS is being utilized in specific specialties—ranging from cardiology to dermatology—and highlights its transformative impact on modern clinical practice.

5.1 CARDIOLOGY

Cardiology is a demanding medical specialty characterized by its high stakes, complexity, and data intensity. Cardiovascular diseases (CVDs), including coronary artery disease, heart failure, arrhythmias, and valvular disorders, remain the leading cause of death and disability worldwide, imposing significant burdens on patients, healthcare systems, and societies. The management of these conditions requires precise, timely, and individualized interventions, which must be based on the best available scientific evidence. Given the vast amount of clinical data generated—from electrocardiograms (ECGs), laboratory results, imaging studies, to patient history and continuous monitoring—clinicians face the challenge of rapidly synthesizing this information to make optimal decisions. This complexity underscores the critical value of integrating Clinical Decision Support Systems (CDSS) into cardiology practice. CDSS harnesses advanced computational methods, including artificial intelligence and machine learning, to analyze large datasets and generate actionable insights tailored to the unique clinical context of each patient. By enhancing diagnostic accuracy, CDSS helps cardiologists identify subtle patterns of cardiac abnormalities that might be missed during routine assessments, thereby enabling earlier detection and intervention. These systems can automatically interpret ECGs, flag arrhythmias, detect ischemic changes, and integrate biomarkers like troponin levels to assist in diagnosing acute coronary syndromes. Beyond diagnosis, CDSS supports risk stratification and prognostication by embedding validated scoring systems—such as CHA_2DS_2-VASc, TIMI, and GRACE—that predict adverse events like stroke, sudden cardiac death, or heart failure exacerbations. This risk prediction empowers clinicians to prioritize care and tailor treatment strategies, improving patient outcomes. In treatment planning and management, CDSS ensures adherence to evolving clinical guidelines from leading cardiology organizations like the American Heart Association and

European Society of Cardiology. It recommends optimal medication regimens, flags potential drug interactions, and personalizes therapeutic approaches based on patient comorbidities and physiological parameters. Furthermore, CDSS plays a vital role in chronic disease monitoring by continuously tracking blood pressure, lipid profiles, weight fluctuations, and cardiac function, alerting clinicians to early signs of deterioration, which can prevent hospitalizations and improve quality of life.

Integration with remote patient monitoring technologies allows CDSS to analyze real-time patient data collected via wearable devices and home monitoring tools, facilitating timely clinical responses outside traditional care settings. In procedural cardiology, CDSS assists with imaging interpretation, guides the selection of diagnostic tests, and supports interventional decision-making by evaluating anatomical and functional data to optimize procedural outcomes and patient safety. Medication safety is another critical area where CDSS excels, helping manage complex pharmacotherapy regimens by providing dosing recommendations, monitoring for adverse drug reactions, and mitigating risks such as QT prolongation and bleeding complications. These functions are especially important given the prevalence of polypharmacy among cardiovascular patients, particularly the elderly.

Importantly, CDSS platforms are designed to integrate seamlessly with electronic health records (EHRs) and clinical workflows, ensuring that decision support is delivered in a non-intrusive manner that enhances clinician efficiency without causing alert fatigue. This integration fosters multidisciplinary collaboration and supports comprehensive care coordination across different providers and care settings. The evidence base supporting CDSS in cardiology is robust, demonstrating improvements in clinical outcomes, including reduced mortality, lower rehospitalization rates, improved medication adherence, and shorter time to critical interventions. Additionally, CDSS facilitates shared decision-making by providing patients with clear, data-driven explanations of their condition and treatment options, thereby enhancing patient engagement and satisfaction. The integration of Clinical Decision Support Systems into cardiology represents a significant advancement in the delivery of cardiovascular care. By leveraging technology to augment human expertise, CDSS empowers clinicians to navigate the complexity of cardiovascular disease with greater confidence, precision, and efficiency. This ultimately leads to better patient outcomes, improved safety, and optimized healthcare resource utilization, marking an essential step forward in the ongoing fight against cardiovascular disease worldwide. The integration of Clinical Decision Support Systems into cardiology has revolutionized the way cardiovascular care is delivered. From diagnostics to long-term disease management, CDSS empowers cardiologists with timely, accurate, and patient-specific information that enhances clinical decisions. As cardiology continues to advance with the integration of genomics, AI, and personalized care models, the role of CDSS will become even more critical in optimizing cardiovascular outcomes across diverse patient populations.

5.1.1 Diagnostic Support

One of the most pivotal roles of Clinical Decision Support Systems (CDSS) in cardiology lies in enhancing the accuracy and timeliness of diagnosis. Cardiovascular diseases often present with subtle or complex signs that can challenge even seasoned clinicians. CDSS tools, particularly those employing advanced machine learning and artificial intelligence, excel in interpreting electrocardiograms (ECGs) by automatically detecting nuanced abnormalities such as arrhythmias, myocardial infarctions, ischemia, and conduction disturbances. These algorithms are trained on extensive datasets, enabling the recognition of patterns that may be missed during manual interpretation. Beyond ECG analysis, modern CDSS platforms integrate multimodal clinical information—combining patient history, symptomatology, vital signs, laboratory biomarkers like troponin and natriuretic peptides, and imaging results from echocardiography or cardiac MRI. This integration facilitates comprehensive diagnostic suggestions, especially in complex presentations such as acute coronary syndrome (ACS), heart failure exacerbations, or valvular heart diseases. By offering probabilistic diagnostic pathways and highlighting differential diagnoses, CDSS acts as an indispensable adjunct that supports clinicians in making faster, more reliable decisions, thereby improving patient safety and reducing diagnostic errors. Furthermore, CDSS can stratify acute conditions by severity, prompting urgent interventions when needed and enabling early initiation of therapies. They also facilitate diagnostic standardization across institutions, improving overall care quality and enabling seamless communication between multidisciplinary teams. Ultimately, diagnostic support through CDSS not only accelerates clinical workflows but also promotes personalized and evidence-based care by leveraging the vast computational power to analyze data beyond human capability.

5.1.2 Risk Stratification and Prognostication

Clinical Decision Support Systems play a transformative role in risk stratification and prognostication in cardiology, helping clinicians identify patients at elevated risk for adverse cardiovascular events. Accurate risk assessment is vital in tailoring preventive strategies, optimizing resource allocation, and guiding the intensity of monitoring and treatment. CDSS tools embed validated risk scores such as the CHA_2DS_2-VASc score for stroke risk in atrial fibrillation, TIMI and GRACE scores for patients presenting with acute coronary syndromes, and risk calculators designed for heart failure progression or sudden cardiac death. By continuously analyzing real-time data from electronic health records (EHRs), including clinical variables, lab results, imaging findings, and patient demographics, CDSS systems dynamically update risk profiles. This ongoing risk evaluation supports proactive clinical decision-making—such as initiating anticoagulation in high-risk atrial fibrillation patients or prioritizing ICU admission for unstable ACS cases. The systems also help stratify patients according to long-term prognosis, guiding decisions on device implantation (e.g., ICDs) or more aggressive medical management. Moreover, prognostic tools within CDSS contribute to shared decision-making by quantifying risks and benefits clearly to patients and families, thereby improving adherence and satisfaction. By integrating predictive analytics, these platforms assist in identifying patients likely to benefit from novel therapies or clinical trials, ultimately fostering personalized medicine. The ability of CDSS to synthesize complex datasets into actionable risk categories significantly enhances clinical precision and patient outcomes.

5.1.3 Treatment Optimization

Optimizing treatment strategies is a cornerstone of cardiology CDSS, where adherence to evolving clinical guidelines and individual patient factors must be balanced meticulously. CDSS platforms facilitate this by embedding evidence-based protocols from authoritative bodies such as the American Heart Association (AHA) and European Society of Cardiology (ESC). In managing conditions like heart failure, CDSS ensures patients receive guideline-directed medical therapy (GDMT), recommending appropriate doses and combinations of beta-blockers, ACE inhibitors, angiotensin receptor-neprilysin inhibitors (ARNIs), mineralocorticoid receptor antagonists, and diuretics. These systems also incorporate drug safety modules that flag contraindications, potential drug-drug interactions, and patient-specific considerations such as renal impairment or electrolyte imbalances. This feature is critical given the frequent polypharmacy in cardiovascular patients, minimizing adverse effects and enhancing medication adherence. In interventional cardiology, CDSS supports treatment planning by analyzing angiographic findings, suggesting revascularization options, and optimizing antiplatelet therapy post-stent placement, thereby improving procedural outcomes. For arrhythmia management, CDSS assists in choosing between rate control and rhythm control strategies based on comprehensive clinical data, including symptom burden, echocardiographic parameters, and comorbidity profiles. By integrating predictive analytics, these systems can also anticipate treatment responses or complications, enabling timely therapy adjustments. Treatment optimization through CDSS ultimately elevates the standard of care by aligning therapies with the latest evidence while accounting for individual patient complexities.

5.1.4 Chronic Disease Monitoring

Chronic cardiovascular diseases demand vigilant long-term monitoring to prevent acute exacerbations and improve quality of life. CDSS enhances chronic disease management by continuously tracking essential clinical parameters such as blood pressure, LDL cholesterol levels, ejection fraction, and patient weight. These systems generate timely alerts when trends indicate potential clinical deterioration—for example, rapid weight gain in heart failure patients signaling fluid retention or elevated blood pressure readings suggesting inadequate control of hypertension. Integration with remote patient monitoring (RPM) devices, including Bluetooth-enabled blood pressure cuffs, weight scales, and ambulatory ECG patches, empowers clinicians to oversee patients in real-time without requiring frequent in-person visits. The automatic transmission and analysis of this data by CDSS enable earlier detection of adverse trends, facilitating prompt clinical interventions and reducing hospital admissions. This proactive approach is particularly valuable in managing high-risk populations such as elderly patients or those with multiple comorbidities. Additionally, CDSS platforms incorporate adherence monitoring by analyzing prescription refill data and patient-reported outcomes, supporting tailored counseling and behavioral interventions. Through automated reminders and education modules, these systems promote patient engagement and self-management. The seamless integration of chronic disease monitoring within clinical workflows ensures that providers can deliver personalized, continuous care that mitigates risks, improves outcomes, and reduces healthcare costs.

5.1.5 Procedural and Imaging Decision Support

Clinical Decision Support Systems play an increasingly critical role in procedural planning and diagnostic imaging interpretation in cardiology. Selecting the most appropriate imaging modality tailored to the clinical question—such as deciding between coronary CT angiography, stress echocardiography, or cardiac MRI—is facilitated by CDSS, which weighs patient-specific factors including pre-test probability, contraindications, and previous test results. By guiding imaging choices, these systems help avoid unnecessary procedures, reduce costs, and minimize patient risk. Once imaging data is obtained, CDSS assists with structured interpretation by automatically detecting and quantifying abnormalities—such as left ventricular dysfunction, valvular pathologies, myocardial scarring, or perfusion defects—and correlating findings with clinical and laboratory data. This standardized analysis reduces inter-observer variability and enhances diagnostic accuracy. In advanced applications, AI-powered algorithms can generate detailed reports highlighting critical findings, thus expediting clinical decision-making. For interventional procedures like transcatheter valve replacement or device implantation (e.g., pacemakers, ICDs), CDSS integrates anatomical imaging, functional assessment, and clinical risk factors to optimize patient selection and timing. The systems can simulate procedural outcomes, assess risks, and recommend peri-procedural management strategies. By streamlining procedural workflows and improving diagnostic precision, CDSS contributes to safer interventions and better patient outcomes.

5.1.6 Medication Management and Safety

Cardiac pharmacotherapy is often complex and fraught with risks, especially given the frequent use of anticoagulants, antiplatelet agents, and polypharmacy in elderly patients. CDSS is indispensable in promoting medication safety by providing evidence-based prescribing support, dose adjustments, and interaction alerts. For example, when initiating anticoagulation therapy such as warfarin or direct oral anticoagulants (DOACs), CDSS evaluates renal function, bleeding risk, and concomitant medications, offering real-time dosage recommendations and monitoring guidance, including INR tracking for warfarin. Additionally, these systems detect potential risks such as QT interval prolongation when multiple QT-prolonging drugs are prescribed concurrently, thus preventing life-threatening arrhythmias. CDSS also flags contraindications, allergy alerts, and duplicative therapies, significantly reducing adverse drug events. In complex regimens, particularly in elderly patients with multiple comorbidities, CDSS facilitates medication reconciliation, enhancing overall treatment adherence and safety. By integrating clinical guidelines and patient-specific data, CDSS enables personalized pharmacotherapy, minimizing toxicity while maximizing therapeutic efficacy. These tools also support clinicians in navigating rapidly evolving pharmaceutical landscapes and emerging drug safety data, ensuring that cardiac medication management is both current and patient-centered.

5.1.7 Integration with Clinical Workflows

Successful implementation of cardiology CDSS hinges on seamless integration into existing clinical workflows and electronic health records (EHRs). Modern CDSS platforms are designed to function as embedded tools within EHR systems, ensuring that clinicians receive timely decision support without disrupting their usual routines. This integration includes features such as embedded alerts for critical findings, smart order sets tailored to specific diagnoses, and prompts for documentation that enhance compliance with quality metrics. Such integration minimizes alert fatigue by prioritizing high-impact notifications and providing actionable recommendations rather than mere warnings. Furthermore, CDSS supports care coordination by enabling multidisciplinary teams—including cardiologists, primary care providers, pharmacists, and nurses—to share data and clinical insights efficiently. This interconnectedness improves continuity of care and reduces fragmentation, particularly important for chronic cardiac patients who often require complex, coordinated management. By aligning decision support with clinical workflows, CDSS fosters clinician acceptance and utilization, thereby maximizing its benefits. It also facilitates audit and feedback processes, allowing institutions to monitor adherence to guidelines and identify areas for quality improvement. Ultimately, well-integrated CDSS platforms enhance clinical efficiency, reduce errors, and support high-quality, patient-centered cardiovascular care.

5.1.8 Outcomes and Benefits

Extensive evidence underscores the substantial impact of Clinical Decision Support Systems in cardiology on improving patient outcomes and healthcare delivery. Numerous studies have demonstrated that CDSS enhances adherence to evidence-based therapies, such as timely administration of reperfusion in myocardial infarction and appropriate anticoagulation in atrial fibrillation, resulting in reduced morbidity and mortality. These systems have also been shown to lower hospital readmission rates by enabling proactive management of heart failure and other chronic cardiac conditions. CDSS improves medication safety by reducing prescription errors, drug interactions, and adverse events, particularly in complex cases involving polypharmacy. It shortens time to treatment in acute care scenarios through real-time alerts and streamlined protocols, contributing to faster recovery and improved survival rates. Additionally, by promoting shared decision-making and patient engagement through transparent risk communication, CDSS enhances patient satisfaction and adherence to therapy. Beyond clinical outcomes, CDSS contributes to healthcare system efficiency by optimizing resource utilization, reducing unnecessary testing and hospitalizations, and supporting population health management. As technology advances, continuous refinement of CDSS algorithms and integration with emerging data sources promise further gains. In sum, the widespread adoption of CDSS in cardiology represents a crucial step toward safer, more effective, and personalized cardiovascular care.

5.1.9 Remote ECG and Arrhythmia Monitoring

Remote ECG and Arrhythmia Monitoring represents a cutting-edge advancement in cardiac care, transforming how clinicians detect, diagnose, and manage cardiac rhythm disorders beyond the traditional hospital setting (Fig. 2). Arrhythmias, such as atrial fibrillation, ventricular tachycardia, and premature ventricular contractions, can be intermittent and asymptomatic, making timely detection challenging with conventional in-office ECGs alone. Remote monitoring technologies overcome these limitations by enabling continuous or frequent ambulatory ECG recording through wearable devices, patches, or implantable loop recorders that transmit data wirelessly to healthcare providers. This continuous stream of real-time cardiac electrical activity allows for early identification of arrhythmia episodes, often before symptoms arise, thus facilitating prompt clinical intervention and potentially preventing serious complications like stroke or sudden cardiac death. The integration of Clinical Decision Support Systems (CDSS) with remote ECG monitoring platforms enhances the diagnostic yield and clinical utility of these data streams. Advanced algorithms analyze vast amounts of ECG signals to detect subtle, complex arrhythmias and differentiate benign variations from clinically significant events. Machine learning models improve accuracy by reducing false positives and providing detailed arrhythmia classification, enabling cardiologists to focus on patients who require immediate attention. This automated interpretation not only accelerates diagnosis but also supports longitudinal rhythm trend analysis, helping clinicians understand arrhythmia burden and triggers over time. Remote arrhythmia monitoring is particularly valuable for patients with paroxysmal atrial fibrillation who are at risk for thromboembolic events but may be asymptomatic or unaware of their arrhythmia episodes. Early detection through continuous monitoring allows timely initiation or adjustment of anticoagulation therapy, reducing stroke risk. Similarly, patients with syncope, cryptogenic stroke, or unexplained palpitations benefit from remote monitoring by uncovering previously undiagnosed arrhythmias that guide further diagnostic and therapeutic decisions. Moreover, remote ECG monitoring fosters patient empowerment and engagement by involving them actively in their own care through user-friendly mobile apps and platforms. Patients receive feedback, reminders, and education that promote adherence to treatment plans and lifestyle modifications. From a healthcare system perspective, remote monitoring reduces the need for frequent outpatient visits, decreases hospitalization rates, and enables resource optimization by focusing attention on high-risk patients.

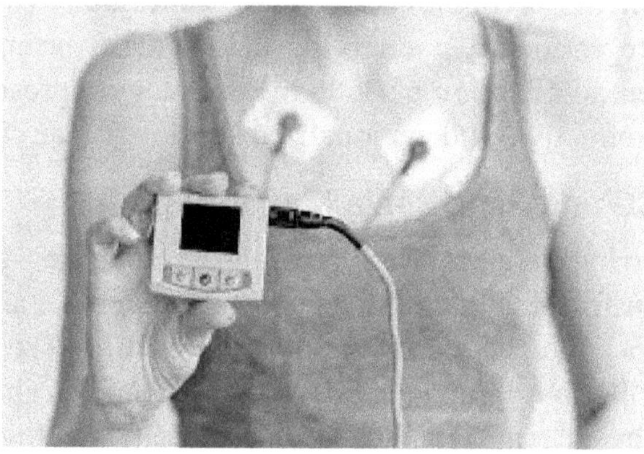

Fig. 2 Remote Arrhythmia Monitoring.

Challenges such as data privacy, device interoperability, and integration with electronic health records are being addressed through evolving standards and regulatory frameworks, ensuring secure and seamless information flow.

Additionally, advances in battery technology and miniaturization have improved device comfort and usability, supporting long-term patient compliance. Remote ECG and arrhythmia monitoring, coupled with intelligent decision support, represents a paradigm shift in cardiac rhythm management. This approach enables earlier, more accurate detection of arrhythmias, optimizes individualized treatment, reduces adverse outcomes, and enhances patient quality of life. As technology continues to evolve, remote monitoring will increasingly become an integral part of comprehensive cardiovascular care, bridging the gap between patients and clinicians and enabling a proactive rather than reactive model of care delivery.

5.2 ENDOCRINOLOGY

Endocrinology is a specialized field of medicine that focuses on the study, diagnosis, and treatment of disorders involving the endocrine system—a complex and highly coordinated network of glands and organs responsible for the production, regulation, and secretion of hormones. These biochemical messengers are released directly into the bloodstream and act on distant tissues and organs to maintain internal stability, known as homeostasis. The endocrine system plays a fundamental role in regulating numerous essential physiological processes, including metabolism, growth and development, sexual differentiation, reproductive health, immune responses, sleep-wake cycles, blood pressure, electrolyte balance, and mood regulation. The primary glands in the endocrine system include the pituitary gland, often referred to as the "master gland"; the hypothalamus, which acts as a critical interface between the nervous and endocrine systems; the thyroid and parathyroid glands, which govern metabolism and calcium homeostasis; the adrenal glands, responsible for stress response and fluid balance; the pancreas, which regulates glucose metabolism; and the gonads (testes and ovaries), which control reproductive function and secondary sexual characteristics. Each of these glands produces specific hormones that influence target tissues in finely tuned feedback loops, primarily governed by signals from the hypothalamic-pituitary axis. What distinguishes endocrinology from many other medical specialties is the system-wide influence that hormones exert. Even subtle hormonal imbalances can produce widespread and often nonspecific symptoms, ranging from fatigue, weight changes, and mood disturbances to infertility, growth disorders, or life-threatening emergencies like adrenal crisis or thyroid storm. As a result, endocrinologists must possess deep expertise in biochemistry, physiology, and systems biology to accurately interpret complex hormone interactions and arrive at precise diagnoses.

Endocrinology's interdisciplinary nature means it overlaps with several medical domains, including cardiology (in diabetes and hypertension), nephrology (in electrolyte disorders), gynecology (in menstrual and fertility issues), oncology (in endocrine tumors), and psychiatry (in mood and behavioral changes due to hormonal shifts). This integrative role positions endocrinologists at the center of collaborative, patient-centered care. In recent decades, the burden of endocrine disorders has risen sharply, driven by the global epidemics of diabetes mellitus, obesity, thyroid dysfunction, and metabolic syndrome. These conditions have not only increased in prevalence but also grown in complexity, with new genetic, autoimmune, and environmental contributors being identified. Advances in laboratory diagnostics, imaging techniques, and molecular biology have significantly expanded our understanding of endocrine pathophysiology and enabled earlier detection of endocrine diseases. Moreover, the digital transformation of healthcare has empowered endocrinologists with innovative tools such as Clinical Decision Support Systems (CDSS), continuous glucose monitors (CGMs), and smart insulin pumps, allowing for highly personalized, data-driven treatment strategies. Artificial intelligence and machine learning models are now being used to predict disease progression, optimize therapy, and enhance patient engagement through real-time feedback and telemedicine platforms. Ultimately, endocrinology is a dynamic and intellectually demanding specialty that combines analytical precision with holistic patient care. Endocrinologists are not only tasked with treating hormonal imbalances but also with restoring systemic equilibrium, improving quality of life, and preventing long-term complications through careful monitoring and evidence-based interventions. As the science of hormones continues to evolve, endocrinology remains at the forefront of medical innovation, shaping the future of personalized and preventive medicine.

5.2.1 Major Endocrine Glands and Hormones

The endocrine system is composed of a network of specialized glands that produce and release hormones—chemical messengers that regulate key physiological processes throughout the body. These glands operate in a tightly coordinated manner, often through feedback loops, to maintain homeostasis and ensure proper functioning of metabolism, growth, reproduction, mood, and other vital functions. Each gland secretes one or more hormones that target specific organs or tissues, influencing everything from energy production to sexual development. The major endocrine glands include the hypothalamus, which links the nervous and endocrine systems; the pituitary gland, often referred to as the "master gland" due to its role in controlling other glands; the thyroid and parathyroid glands, which regulate metabolism and calcium balance; the adrenal glands, which manage stress response and electrolyte levels; the pancreas, critical in blood glucose regulation; and the gonads (ovaries and testes), which control reproductive hormones and functions. Each of these glands plays a distinct but interdependent role in hormonal balance. Understanding the anatomy, physiology, and hormone outputs of each gland is essential for diagnosing and managing endocrine disorders. Even slight dysfunctions in hormone secretion can have wide-reaching effects, highlighting the need for precise regulation and monitoring.

Components of the endocrine system include:

- **Hypothalamus:** The hypothalamus is the central coordinating structure of the endocrine system, linking the nervous system to hormonal control. It produces releasing and inhibiting hormones that regulate the anterior pituitary gland's activity. These include TRH (thyrotropin-releasing hormone), CRH (corticotropin-releasing hormone), GnRH (gonadotropin-releasing hormone), and others. It also produces oxytocin and vasopressin (ADH), which are stored and released by the posterior pituitary. Through these actions, the hypothalamus governs temperature regulation, hunger, thirst, circadian rhythms, and stress responses. It is often considered the master regulator of endocrine and autonomic functions.
- **Pituitary Gland:** The pituitary gland, nestled at the base of the brain, is known as the "master gland" because it secretes hormones that control most other endocrine glands. It has two distinct parts: the anterior and posterior pituitary. The anterior pituitary secretes TSH, ACTH, GH, LH, FSH, and prolactin, each targeting specific organs like the thyroid, adrenal glands, and gonads. The posterior pituitary releases ADH and oxytocin, produced by the hypothalamus. Pituitary dysfunction can result in hormonal excess or deficiency syndromes, such as acromegaly, Cushing's disease, or hypopituitarism. Its central role makes it critical in maintaining hormonal balance throughout the body.
- **Thyroid Gland:** Located in the neck, the thyroid gland produces the hormones triiodothyronine (T3) and thyroxine (T4), which regulate metabolic rate, energy production, and thermoregulation. These hormones influence nearly every cell in the body, affecting heart rate, digestion, and neural function. The thyroid is controlled by TSH from the pituitary, forming a vital feedback loop. Disorders of the thyroid include hypothyroidism, hyperthyroidism, thyroid nodules, and cancer. Adequate iodine intake is crucial for normal thyroid function. Its role in developmental growth and metabolic stability underscores its importance in both pediatric and adult health.
- **Parathyroid Glands:** The parathyroid glands are four small structures located behind the thyroid gland, and they play a crucial role in calcium and phosphorus homeostasis. They secrete parathyroid hormone (PTH), which increases blood calcium levels by stimulating bone resorption, enhancing calcium reabsorption in the kidneys, and activating vitamin D

to increase intestinal absorption. Proper calcium balance is essential for muscle function, nerve conduction, and bone integrity. Disorders such as hyperparathyroidism can lead to osteoporosis, kidney stones, and neuromuscular symptoms. Despite their small size, these glands are vital for skeletal and mineral health.

- **Adrenal Glands:** Sitting atop the kidneys, the adrenal glands consist of two regions: the cortex and the medulla. The cortex secretes cortisol (stress hormone), aldosterone (fluid and electrolyte balance), and androgens, while the medulla produces catecholamines like epinephrine and norepinephrine (fight-or-flight response). These hormones help regulate blood pressure, glucose metabolism, immune response, and stress adaptation. Adrenal dysfunction can result in serious conditions like Addison's disease, Cushing's syndrome, or pheochromocytoma. The adrenal glands are essential for surviving both acute and chronic physiological stress.
- **Pancreas (Endocrine Portion):** The pancreas has both exocrine and endocrine functions; its endocrine role is centered in the islets of Langerhans. These clusters of cells secrete insulin (by beta cells), glucagon (by alpha cells), somatostatin, and pancreatic polypeptide to regulate blood glucose levels. Insulin lowers blood sugar, while glucagon raises it, ensuring tight glucose control. Endocrine dysfunction in the pancreas is the hallmark of diabetes mellitus, particularly type 1 and type 2. Proper pancreatic hormone balance is essential for energy metabolism and overall systemic stability. It plays a central role in digestion and metabolic homeostasis.
- **Gonads (Ovaries/Testes):** The gonads are the primary reproductive organs—ovaries in females and testes in males—that produce sex hormones and gametes. The ovaries secrete estrogen and progesterone, regulating the menstrual cycle, pregnancy, and secondary sexual characteristics. The testes produce testosterone, which governs sperm production, libido, and male secondary sex traits. These glands are regulated by LH and FSH from the pituitary gland. Disorders can lead to infertility, hormonal imbalances, or delayed puberty. Beyond reproduction, sex hormones also affect bone density, mood, and cardiovascular health.

5.2.2 Diabetes Mellitus

Diabetes Mellitus is the most common and impactful endocrine disorder worldwide, characterized by chronic hyperglycemia resulting from defects in insulin secretion, insulin action, or both. It significantly increases the risk of cardiovascular disease, kidney failure, blindness, and neuropathy, making it a major cause of morbidity and mortality globally. The condition is broadly categorized into Type 1 diabetes,

Type 2 diabetes, and gestational diabetes, each with distinct pathophysiological mechanisms and treatment approaches. Type 1 diabetes is an autoimmune condition leading to absolute insulin deficiency, while Type 2 diabetes arises from insulin resistance combined with progressive beta-cell dysfunction. Gestational diabetes develops during pregnancy and poses long-term health risks for both mother and child. Advances in glucose monitoring, pharmacotherapy, and lifestyle interventions have improved management outcomes, but prevention and early diagnosis remain critical. Endocrinologists play a central role in comprehensive diabetes care, emphasizing glycemic control, complication screening, and patient education.

Diabetes is the most prevalent endocrine disorder globally:

- **Type 1 Diabetes**– Autoimmune destruction of insulin-producing beta cells; requires lifelong insulin.
- **Type 2 Diabetes**– Insulin resistance and beta-cell dysfunction; managed with lifestyle, oral agents, and sometimes insulin.
- **Gestational Diabetes**– Occurs during pregnancy and increases future risk of type 2 diabetes.

Endocrinologists manage glycemic control using insulin therapy, oral hypoglycemics, CGMs (Continuous Glucose Monitors), insulin pumps, and integrated CDSS platforms.

5.2.3 Thyroid Disorders

Thyroid disorders are among the most common endocrine conditions and can significantly affect overall health due to the thyroid gland's central role in regulating metabolism. Located in the neck, the thyroid produces triiodothyronine (T3) and thyroxine (T4), hormones that influence body temperature, energy expenditure, heart rate, and cognitive function. These hormones are tightly controlled by thyroid-stimulating hormone (TSH) from the pituitary gland. Disorders may include hypothyroidism (underactive thyroid), hyperthyroidism (overactive thyroid), thyroid nodules, goiter, and thyroid cancer. Autoimmune conditions like Hashimoto's thyroiditis and Graves' disease are common causes. Symptoms can range from fatigue and weight changes to palpitations and mood disturbances. Diagnosis involves hormone assays, antibody tests, and imaging. Effective treatments, including hormone replacement or antithyroid therapy, are widely available, making early detection crucial for long-term health.

Thyroid disease is common and affects metabolic regulation:

- **Hypothyroidism** – Often due to Hashimoto's thyroiditis; symptoms include fatigue, weight gain, and cold intolerance.

- **Hyperthyroidism** – Often due to Graves' disease or toxic nodules; presents with weight loss, heat intolerance, palpitations.
- **Thyroid Nodules & Cancer** – Require ultrasound, biopsy, and possibly radioactive iodine or surgery.

Diagnosis is made with TSH, Free T4, thyroid antibodies, and imaging (ultrasound, radioactive iodine scans).

5.2.4 Pituitary Disorders

Pituitary disorders involve dysfunction of the pituitary gland, a pea-sized structure located at the base of the brain, often referred to as the "master gland" due to its role in regulating other endocrine glands. It secretes critical hormones such as ACTH, TSH, GH, LH, FSH, prolactin, and stores ADH and oxytocin from the hypothalamus. Disorders may result from pituitary adenomas (benign tumors), inflammation, trauma, or genetic mutations, leading to hormone overproduction or deficiency. Common conditions include prolactinomas, acromegaly, Cushing's disease, and hypopituitarism. Symptoms vary widely and can include vision problems, menstrual irregularities, infertility, growth abnormalities, or fatigue. Diagnosis relies on hormonal assays and MRI imaging. Treatment options include medication, surgery, and radiation, depending on the nature and severity of the disorder. Early recognition is key to preventing long-term endocrine complications.

The pituitary gland affects numerous systems through hormone production:

- **Prolactinomas:** Prolactinomas are the most common type of functioning pituitary tumors, arising from lactotroph cells that produce prolactin. Excess prolactin leads to galactorrhea (inappropriate milk production), menstrual irregularities such as amenorrhea, and infertility in women. In men, symptoms may include decreased libido, erectile dysfunction, and, less commonly, gynecomastia. Elevated prolactin suppresses gonadotropin-releasing hormone (GnRH), reducing LH and FSH levels. Diagnosis is based on serum prolactin levels and MRI imaging of the pituitary. Dopamine agonists like cabergoline or bromocriptine are first-line treatments and often reduce tumor size and hormone levels effectively.
- **Growth Hormone Excess (Acromegaly/Gigantism):** Excess secretion of growth hormone (GH), typically from a GH-secreting pituitary adenoma, leads to acromegaly in adults and gigantism in children. Acromegaly is characterized by enlargement of the hands, feet, jaw, and facial features, along with joint pain, hypertension, insulin resistance, and sleep apnea. Gigantism causes abnormal linear growth due to open growth plates. Elevated IGF-1 levels confirm the diagnosis, along with failure to suppress GH during an oral glucose tolerance test. MRI reveals the tumor, and

transsphenoidal surgery is often the initial treatment, followed by medication (e.g., somatostatin analogs) or radiotherapy if needed.

- **ACTH-Producing Tumors (Cushing's Disease):** ACTH-producing pituitary adenomas cause Cushing's disease, a condition of excess cortisol due to overstimulation of the adrenal glands. Patients typically present with central obesity, facial rounding ("moon face"), purple striae, hypertension, diabetes, and osteoporosis. Psychiatric symptoms such as depression or cognitive changes are also common. Diagnosis involves elevated serum cortisol, loss of diurnal rhythm, and failure to suppress cortisol with dexamethasone. High ACTH levels and pituitary imaging confirm the source. Transsphenoidal surgery is the primary treatment, with medical therapy or radiation as adjuncts in persistent or recurrent cases.
- **Hypopituitarism:** Hypopituitarism refers to partial or complete deficiency of one or more pituitary hormones, resulting from causes such as pituitary tumors, trauma, infarction (e.g., Sheehan's syndrome), infections, or radiation therapy. The condition leads to secondary deficiencies of target gland hormones, affecting the thyroid, adrenal glands, gonads, and growth axis. Symptoms are often subtle and progressive, including fatigue, weight loss, amenorrhea, decreased libido, and hypotension. Diagnosis involves evaluating baseline and dynamic hormone levels. MRI may show an empty sella or structural damage. Lifelong hormone replacement therapy tailored to the deficient axes is the cornerstone of management.

Evaluation includes dynamic hormone testing and pituitary MRI, often followed by medical or surgical treatment.

5.2.5 Adrenal Gland Disorder

Adrenal gland disorders encompass a diverse group of conditions that result from either overproduction or underproduction of adrenal hormones. Located atop each kidney, the adrenal glands consist of the cortex, which produces cortisol, aldosterone, and androgens, and the medulla, which secretes catecholamines like epinephrine and norepinephrine. These hormones are vital for stress response, metabolism, fluid and electrolyte balance, and cardiovascular regulation. Disorders such as Addison's disease (adrenal insufficiency), Cushing's syndrome (excess cortisol), primary aldosteronism, and pheochromocytoma (tumor of the adrenal medulla) can lead to severe clinical consequences if not identified and managed promptly. Symptoms may include fatigue, hypertension, muscle weakness, weight changes, or acute crises. Diagnosis typically involves hormonal assays and imaging (CT/MRI). Endocrinologists play a key role in managing these disorders through medical therapy, hormonal replacement, or surgical intervention when necessary.

Adrenal conditions can be life-threatening if not identified early:

- **Addison's Disease:** Addison's disease is a form of primary adrenal insufficiency characterized by inadequate production of cortisol and often aldosterone. Patients typically present with fatigue, muscle weakness, weight loss, hypotension, and hyperpigmentation of the skin and mucous membranes due to elevated ACTH levels. Electrolyte imbalances such as hyponatremia and hyperkalemia are common. The condition can lead to life-threatening adrenal crises if untreated. Diagnosis is confirmed by low cortisol levels and a poor response to ACTH stimulation testing. Treatment requires lifelong glucocorticoid and often mineralocorticoid replacement. Early recognition and management are essential to prevent morbidity and mortality.
- **Cushing's Syndrome:** Cushing's syndrome results from chronic exposure to excess cortisol, either due to endogenous overproduction or exogenous steroid use. It is clinically characterized by central obesity, round "moon" face, buffalo hump, hypertension, glucose intolerance or diabetes, muscle weakness, and skin changes such as purple striae and easy bruising. Patients may also experience mood disturbances and osteoporosis. Diagnosis involves measuring elevated cortisol levels through 24-hour urine cortisol, late-night salivary cortisol, and dexamethasone suppression tests. Treatment depends on the underlying cause, including surgery for tumors, radiation, or medical therapy to inhibit cortisol synthesis.
- **Pheochromocytoma:** Pheochromocytoma is a rare catecholamine-secreting tumor originating from the adrenal medulla or extra-adrenal chromaffin cells. It causes episodic or sustained hypertension, often accompanied by headaches, palpitations, sweating, and anxiety due to sudden surges of epinephrine and norepinephrine. Diagnosis involves elevated plasma or urine metanephrines and imaging studies to localize the tumor. If untreated, pheochromocytoma can lead to hypertensive crises, arrhythmias, and stroke. Surgical removal is the definitive treatment, preceded by careful preoperative blood pressure control with alpha- and beta-blockers. Genetic testing is recommended due to familial associations.
- **Primary Aldosteronism:** Primary aldosteronism, also known as Conn's syndrome, is caused by excessive secretion of aldosterone from the adrenal cortex, leading to resistant hypertension and hypokalemia. Aldosterone promotes sodium retention and potassium excretion, resulting in fluid overload and muscle weakness. Patients may present with headaches, fatigue, and frequent urination. Screening includes measuring aldosterone-renin ratio, followed by confirmatory suppression tests. Imaging helps

identify adrenal adenomas or hyperplasia. Treatment options include mineralocorticoid receptor antagonists like spironolactone or surgical adrenalectomy if a unilateral adenoma is present. Early diagnosis improves cardiovascular outcomes by controlling blood pressure and correcting electrolyte disturbances.

Diagnosis often involves serum/urine hormone levels and imaging (CT/MRI).

5.2.6 Calcium and Bone Metabolism

Calcium and bone metabolism are tightly regulated processes essential for maintaining skeletal strength and numerous physiological functions. Calcium, the most abundant mineral in the body, is crucial for bone structure, muscle contraction, nerve transmission, and blood clotting. The balance of calcium levels is controlled primarily by the coordinated actions of parathyroid hormone (PTH), vitamin D, and calcitonin. PTH increases blood calcium by stimulating bone resorption, enhancing intestinal absorption via activated vitamin D, and reducing renal calcium excretion. Vitamin D promotes calcium absorption from the gut, while calcitonin lowers blood calcium by inhibiting bone breakdown. Disruptions in this regulation can lead to disorders such as osteoporosis, osteomalacia, rickets, and hyper- or hypocalcemia. Bone remodeling is a continuous process involving osteoclast-mediated resorption and osteoblast-driven formation, maintaining skeletal integrity. Proper calcium and bone metabolism is critical for growth, repair, and overall metabolic health.

Endocrinologists are key in managing bone health and mineral metabolism:

- **Osteoporosis:** Osteoporosis is a widespread metabolic bone disease characterized by decreased bone density and microarchitectural deterioration, leading to increased fracture risk. It is especially common in postmenopausal women due to estrogen deficiency, which accelerates bone loss. Aging also contributes by reducing bone formation and calcium absorption. Diagnosis primarily relies on DEXA (dual-energy X-ray absorptiometry) scans, which measure bone mineral density. Patients are often asymptomatic until fractures occur, most commonly in the hip, spine, or wrist. Prevention and treatment focus on calcium and vitamin D supplementation, weight-bearing exercise, and medications like bisphosphonates. Early detection is crucial to reduce morbidity and mortality associated with fragility fractures.
- **Hyperparathyroidism:** Hyperparathyroidism is a condition characterized by excessive secretion of parathyroid hormone (PTH), which leads to elevated blood calcium levels due to increased bone resorption, enhanced intestinal absorption, and reduced renal excretion of calcium.

Primary hyperparathyroidism is often caused by a parathyroid adenoma, while secondary forms result from chronic kidney disease or vitamin D deficiency. Clinically, it can cause bone pain, fractures, kidney stones, and neuropsychiatric symptoms. Diagnosis involves elevated serum calcium, high PTH levels, and imaging for adenoma localization. Treatment may include surgical removal of the overactive gland or medical management in mild cases. Proper management prevents complications like osteoporosis and nephrolithiasis.

- **Vitamin D Deficiency:** Vitamin D deficiency impairs calcium absorption in the intestines, leading to hypocalcemia and compensatory secondary hyperparathyroidism, which increases bone resorption. This deficiency contributes to bone fragility and conditions such as osteomalacia in adults and rickets in children, characterized by defective bone mineralization. Common causes include inadequate sunlight exposure, poor dietary intake, malabsorption syndromes, and chronic kidney disease. Symptoms may include bone pain, muscle weakness, and increased fracture risk. Diagnosis is based on low serum 25-hydroxyvitamin D levels. Treatment involves vitamin D supplementation and addressing underlying causes to restore normal bone metabolism and strength.
- **Paget's Disease:** Paget's disease of bone is a chronic disorder characterized by abnormal, excessive bone remodeling that leads to structurally disorganized and weakened bone. It typically affects older adults and may involve one or multiple bones, including the pelvis, spine, skull, and long bones. The disease manifests with bone pain, deformities, fractures, and in some cases, neurological complications due to nerve compression. Elevated alkaline phosphatase levels and characteristic radiographic findings aid in diagnosis. The exact cause is unknown but may involve genetic and viral factors. Treatment includes bisphosphonates to normalize bone turnover and alleviate symptoms. Early intervention helps prevent complications and improves quality of life.

Treatments include bisphosphonates, calcium, vitamin D, denosumab, and anabolic agents.

5.2.7 Reproductive Endocrinology

Reproductive endocrinology is the branch of medicine that focuses on the hormonal regulation of the reproductive system in both males and females. It involves the study and treatment of disorders related to fertility, menstrual cycles, puberty, and sexual development. Key hormones like gonadotropins (LH and FSH), estrogen, progesterone, and testosterone play central roles in reproductive function. This specialty addresses conditions such as polycystic ovary syndrome (PCOS), infertility, menstrual irregularities, and hypogonadism. It also manages complex issues like assisted reproductive technologies (ART) and hormone replacement therapies. Understanding the delicate hormonal balance is essential for optimizing reproductive health and outcomes.

Hormonal balance is vital in reproduction and sexual function:

- **PCOS (Polycystic Ovary Syndrome):** Polycystic Ovary Syndrome (PCOS) is a common endocrine disorder affecting women of reproductive age, characterized by irregular menstrual cycles, hyperandrogenism (excess male hormones causing symptoms like hirsutism and acne), and insulin resistance. It is a leading cause of infertility and metabolic complications such as type 2 diabetes and cardiovascular disease. The diagnosis is based on clinical features, hormone levels, and ultrasound findings showing polycystic ovaries. Management includes lifestyle modification, insulin-sensitizing agents, and hormonal therapies to regulate cycles and reduce androgen effects. Early diagnosis is crucial to prevent long-term metabolic and reproductive complications.
- **Hypogonadism:** Hypogonadism refers to diminished function of the gonads resulting in low production of sex hormones—testosterone in men and estrogen in women. It can be congenital, such as Klinefelter syndrome or Turner syndrome, or acquired due to trauma, infections, tumors, or systemic diseases. Symptoms vary from delayed puberty and infertility to decreased libido, muscle mass, and bone density. Diagnosis involves hormonal assays including LH, FSH, and sex steroid levels, along with imaging if needed. Treatment focuses on hormone replacement therapy to restore secondary sexual characteristics, improve quality of life, and prevent complications like osteoporosis.
- **Menstrual Disorders:** Menstrual disorders encompass a wide range of abnormalities in the menstrual cycle, including amenorrhea, oligomenorrhea, menorrhagia, and dysmenorrhea, often resulting from hormonal imbalances or pituitary dysfunction. Causes can include hypothalamic amenorrhea, polycystic ovary syndrome, thyroid disorders, hyperprolactinemia, or structural uterine abnormalities. These disorders may lead to infertility, anemia, and impaired quality of life. Diagnosis requires detailed history, physical examination, hormone evaluations, and sometimes imaging studies. Treatment is tailored according to the underlying cause and may involve hormonal therapy, lifestyle changes, or surgical interventions.
- **Infertility:** Infertility is defined as the inability to conceive after one year of unprotected intercourse and affects both men and women. Hormonal

evaluation plays a crucial role in diagnosing underlying endocrine causes, including ovulatory dysfunction, hypogonadism, or hyperprolactinemia. Assessment often includes measuring gonadotropins, sex steroids, thyroid function, and prolactin levels. Treatment depends on the specific diagnosis and may involve ovulation induction, assisted reproductive technologies (ART) like IVF, or hormone replacement. Early and thorough endocrine evaluation enhances the chances of successful conception and guides individualized treatment plans.

Management involves hormone replacement, ovulation induction, or assisted reproductive technologies.

5.2.8 Obesity and Metabolic Syndrome

Obesity is a complex, chronic condition characterized by excessive body fat accumulation that negatively impacts health. It is a major risk factor for developing metabolic syndrome, a cluster of conditions including central obesity, insulin resistance, hypertension, dyslipidemia, and pro-inflammatory states. Metabolic syndrome significantly increases the risk of type 2 diabetes, cardiovascular disease, and stroke. The interplay of genetic, environmental, and hormonal factors drives the pathophysiology of obesity and metabolic syndrome. Hormonal imbalances involving insulin, leptin, ghrelin, and adiponectin contribute to altered appetite regulation and energy metabolism. Effective management requires a multidisciplinary approach focusing on lifestyle modification, pharmacotherapy, and sometimes surgical interventions. Early identification and treatment are essential to prevent long-term complications.

Endocrinologists address obesity from a hormonal and metabolic lens:

- **Endocrine Causes of Obesity:** Endocrine disorders can significantly contribute to obesity by disrupting normal hormonal regulation of metabolism and appetite. Conditions like hypothyroidism reduce basal metabolic rate, leading to weight gain and fatigue. Cushing's syndrome, caused by excess cortisol, promotes central fat accumulation and muscle wasting. Polycystic Ovary Syndrome (PCOS) often features insulin resistance and hyperandrogenism, which exacerbate weight gain. Other endocrine causes include growth hormone deficiency and hypothalamic disorders. Recognizing these underlying conditions is crucial for effective treatment. Managing the primary endocrine disorder can lead to improved weight control and metabolic health.
- **Metabolic Syndrome:** Metabolic syndrome is a constellation of interrelated risk factors, including insulin resistance, central obesity, hypertension, and dyslipidemia, that collectively increase the risk of cardiovascular disease and type 2 diabetes. Central or visceral obesity plays a pivotal role

by releasing pro-inflammatory cytokines and adipokines, which worsen insulin sensitivity. The syndrome also involves elevated triglycerides, low HDL cholesterol, and increased blood pressure. Diagnosis is based on specific clinical criteria, and management requires lifestyle changes such as diet and exercise, alongside pharmacological treatment targeting individual components. Early identification and comprehensive care are essential to reduce morbidity and mortality associated with this condition.

Treatment includes lifestyle modification, pharmacotherapy (e.g., GLP-1 agonists), and bariatric surgery when appropriate.

5.2.9 Genetic and Syndromic Endocrinology

Genetic and syndromic endocrinology focuses on inherited and complex disorders that affect the endocrine system, often presenting with multiple hormonal imbalances and systemic features. Many endocrine diseases arise from mutations in genes regulating hormone synthesis, receptor function, or signaling pathways. Examples include congenital adrenal hyperplasia, multiple endocrine neoplasia (MEN) syndromes, and familial hypocalciuric hypercalcemia. These conditions frequently involve abnormalities in growth, metabolism, and reproductive function. Early genetic diagnosis allows for tailored management and screening of at-risk family members. Syndromic endocrinopathies often present with distinctive physical, metabolic, or neurological features alongside hormonal dysfunction. Advances in molecular genetics and personalized medicine have improved understanding and treatment of these disorders. Genetic counseling plays a key role in patient care and family planning. Integrating genetic insights with clinical endocrinology enhances disease prognosis and therapy effectiveness.

Some endocrine disorders are inherited and require genetic evaluation:

- **Multiple Endocrine Neoplasia (MEN 1 & 2):** Multiple Endocrine Neoplasia (MEN) syndromes are inherited disorders characterized by tumors arising in multiple endocrine glands. MEN type 1 primarily affects the parathyroids, pancreatic islets, and pituitary gland, often leading to hyperparathyroidism, gastrinomas, and pituitary adenomas. MEN type 2 is associated with medullary thyroid carcinoma, pheochromocytomas, and parathyroid hyperplasia. These syndromes result from mutations in specific genes, such as MEN1 and RET proto-oncogene. Early diagnosis through genetic testing is critical to manage tumor risk and initiate preventive interventions. Lifelong monitoring is essential to detect new tumors early and reduce morbidity. Treatment typically involves surgery, medical therapy, and genetic counseling for affected families.
- **Congenital Adrenal Hyperplasia (CAH):** Congenital Adrenal Hyperplasia (CAH) is a group of inherited enzyme deficiencies that impair cortisol

biosynthesis in the adrenal cortex. The most common form is 21-hydroxylase deficiency, leading to cortisol and aldosterone deficiency with excess androgen production. Clinical features range from salt-wasting crises in infancy to ambiguous genitalia and precocious puberty. Early diagnosis via newborn screening is essential to prevent life-threatening adrenal crises. Management involves lifelong glucocorticoid and mineralocorticoid replacement to restore hormone balance and suppress excess androgen production. Genetic counseling helps families understand inheritance patterns and risks. Advances in molecular genetics have improved diagnostic accuracy and personalized treatment approaches.

- **Familial Thyroid Cancer and Paraganglioma Syndromes:** Familial thyroid cancer syndromes, including medullary thyroid carcinoma, are often linked to germline mutations in the RET proto-oncogene, necessitating early detection and preventive thyroidectomy in mutation carriers. Paraganglioma syndromes are hereditary conditions characterized by tumors arising from extra-adrenal chromaffin cells and are associated with mutations in genes such as SDHx. These tumors can secrete catecholamines, causing hypertension and other symptoms. Genetic testing is vital for diagnosis, risk assessment, and screening of at-risk family members. Early identification improves outcomes through timely surgical intervention and surveillance. Genetic counseling supports patients and families in understanding inheritance patterns and making informed decisions about management and family planning.

Endocrinologists collaborate with geneticists to manage inherited conditions and provide family screening.

5.2.10 Endocrine Emergencies

Endocrine emergencies are acute, life-threatening conditions resulting from severe hormonal imbalances or dysfunctions within the endocrine system. These crises require prompt recognition and immediate intervention to prevent serious morbidity or mortality. Common endocrine emergencies include diabetic ketoacidosis, thyroid storm, adrenal crisis, and myxedema coma, each presenting with distinct clinical features. Rapid diagnosis is often challenging due to overlapping symptoms with other medical conditions. Understanding the underlying hormonal disturbances is crucial for targeted treatment. Timely management involves stabilization of vital signs, correction of metabolic abnormalities, and addressing the primary endocrine disorder. These emergencies can affect patients across all age groups, emphasizing the importance of awareness among healthcare providers. Early intervention can significantly improve outcomes and reduce complications. Collaboration among multidisciplinary teams is often necessary for comprehensive care. Recognizing endocrine emergencies is vital in acute medical settings to save lives and optimize patient recovery.

Endocrine emergencies are potentially life-threatening:

- **Thyroid Storm:** Thyroid storm is an acute, life-threatening exacerbation of hyperthyroidism characterized by a sudden and severe increase in thyroid hormone levels. It often occurs in patients with untreated or poorly controlled hyperthyroidism triggered by stressors such as infection, surgery, or trauma. Symptoms include high fever, tachycardia, hypertension, agitation, and delirium. Without rapid treatment, it can lead to heart failure, arrhythmias, and multiorgan failure. Diagnosis is clinical, supported by elevated thyroid hormones. Management focuses on controlling hypermetabolism, using antithyroid medications, beta-blockers, and supportive care. Early intervention significantly reduces mortality.
- **Myxedema Coma:** Myxedema coma is a rare but severe form of hypothyroidism that results in profound mental status changes including confusion, stupor, or coma. It is typically precipitated by infections, cold exposure, or medications in patients with longstanding untreated hypothyroidism. Clinical features include hypothermia, bradycardia, hypoventilation, and hypotension. The condition represents an extreme metabolic slowdown affecting multiple organ systems. Diagnosis is based on clinical presentation and low thyroid hormone levels. Treatment requires immediate thyroid hormone replacement and supportive measures such as warming and respiratory support. Prompt recognition is crucial to improve survival chances.
- **Adrenal Crisis:** Adrenal crisis occurs due to an acute deficiency of cortisol, often in patients with known adrenal insufficiency or unrecognized adrenal failure. It is frequently triggered by physiological stress such as infection, trauma, or surgery. Symptoms include severe hypotension, abdominal pain, vomiting, confusion, and shock. Without urgent treatment, adrenal crisis can rapidly progress to death. Diagnosis is clinical, confirmed by low cortisol levels and electrolyte disturbances like hyponatremia and hyperkalemia. Management involves immediate administration of intravenous hydrocortisone and aggressive fluid resuscitation. Early treatment is essential to prevent fatal outcomes.
- **Diabetic Ketoacidosis (DKA) and Hyperosmolar Hyperglycemic State (HHS):** DKA and HHS are acute metabolic emergencies in diabetes characterized by severe hyperglycemia and dehydration. DKA primarily occurs in type 1 diabetes due to insulin deficiency, leading to ketone

production and metabolic acidosis. HHS usually affects type 2 diabetics, with extreme hyperglycemia causing hyperosmolarity but minimal ketosis. Both conditions present with polyuria, polydipsia, altered consciousness, and electrolyte imbalances. Prompt diagnosis relies on blood glucose, ketone levels, and arterial blood gases. Treatment involves fluid replacement, insulin therapy, and correction of electrolyte abnormalities. Early intervention is critical to reduce morbidity and mortality.

5.2.11 Role of Technology and CDSS in Endocrinology

Technology and Clinical Decision Support Systems (CDSS) have revolutionized endocrinology by enhancing diagnostic accuracy, treatment personalization, and patient monitoring. Advanced imaging, wearable devices, and continuous glucose monitors provide real-time data, allowing clinicians to track hormonal levels and metabolic changes closely. CDSS integrates patient data with evidence-based guidelines to assist endocrinologists in making timely and precise decisions, reducing errors and improving outcomes. These systems help in managing complex endocrine disorders such as diabetes, thyroid diseases, and adrenal dysfunction by suggesting tailored treatment plans. Telemedicine platforms enable remote consultations, expanding access to specialized care. Moreover, artificial intelligence and machine learning algorithms are increasingly used to predict disease progression and optimize therapies. Technology streamlines data management, facilitating research and enhancing clinical workflows. Overall, the synergy between technology and CDSS supports proactive, patient-centered endocrinology care, improving quality and efficiency.

Modern endocrinology benefits from digital tools and data analytics:

- **Clinical Decision Support Systems (CDSS):** Clinical Decision Support Systems (CDSS) play a critical role in endocrinology by assisting clinicians with complex decision-making processes. These systems use algorithms and patient data to provide recommendations for insulin dosing, ensuring safer and more effective diabetes management. CDSS also supports thyroid disorder treatment by helping tailor medication doses based on lab results and clinical symptoms. Additionally, they assist in predicting the risk of bone fractures by integrating patient history, bone density scores, and other risk factors. By reducing human error and standardizing care, CDSS improves patient outcomes and treatment consistency. The systems often incorporate updated clinical guidelines, keeping healthcare providers informed of best practices. Overall, CDSS enhances precision and efficiency in managing endocrine diseases.
- **Wearables and Continuous Glucose Monitors (CGMs):** Wearable devices and Continuous Glucose Monitors (CGMs) have transformed

diabetes care by providing real-time glucose monitoring. These tools allow patients and clinicians to observe glucose trends continuously, enabling rapid adjustments in insulin therapy and lifestyle. CGMs help detect hypoglycemia and hyperglycemia episodes early, reducing the risk of complications. Wearables also improve patient engagement and adherence by delivering alerts and feedback directly to smartphones or smartwatches. Beyond glucose monitoring, some devices track physical activity, heart rate, and sleep, offering a comprehensive view of health. The data generated facilitates personalized treatment plans and supports telemedicine consultations. This technology empowers patients to manage their condition proactively and improves long-term outcomes.

- **Electronic Health Record (EHR) Integration:** Integration of Endocrinology care with Electronic Health Records (EHR) enables seamless longitudinal tracking of patients' hormonal levels, medications, and clinical progress. EHR systems store comprehensive medical histories, lab results, and imaging, allowing endocrinologists to monitor disease progression over time. Automated alerts within EHR can notify clinicians about abnormal hormone levels or potential medication side effects, enhancing patient safety. This integration also supports multidisciplinary collaboration by providing all healthcare providers with access to updated patient information. EHR facilitates data analytics for research and quality improvement in endocrine care. It simplifies prescription management and ensures adherence to clinical guidelines. Ultimately, EHR integration leads to more coordinated, efficient, and personalized endocrinology care.

These technologies improve outcomes, reduce errors, and support personalized care.

Endocrinology is a comprehensive specialty that spans metabolic, hormonal, reproductive, and skeletal health. It requires a deep understanding of biochemistry, pathophysiology, and system-wide integration. With the increasing prevalence of endocrine disorders and the rise of technology-driven care, endocrinologists play a vital role in both acute and chronic disease management. Their expertise improves patient quality of life, prevents complications, and supports holistic health through precision medicine.

5.2.12 Continuous Glucose Monitoring (CGM) in Diabetes

Continuous Glucose Monitoring (CGM) has revolutionized the management of diabetes by providing real-time, dynamic glucose data throughout the day and night. Unlike traditional fingerstick glucose tests, which offer only intermittent snapshots, CGM devices continuously measure glucose levels in the interstitial fluid, offering detailed insights into glucose trends and fluctuations. This technology empowers both patients and healthcare providers with comprehensive glucose profiles, enabling more precise adjustments in insulin dosing, diet, and physical activity. CGM is particularly valuable for individuals with type 1 diabetes but is increasingly used in type 2 diabetes as well, especially for those requiring intensive insulin therapy. The devices typically consist of a small sensor inserted under the skin, a transmitter, and a receiver or smartphone app that displays glucose data and trends. Many modern CGMs also offer alerts for hypoglycemia (low blood sugar) and hyperglycemia (high blood sugar), providing early warnings that help prevent dangerous episodes. This real-time feedback helps reduce severe hypoglycemic events and improves overall glycemic control by allowing users to respond promptly to glucose changes (Fig. 3).

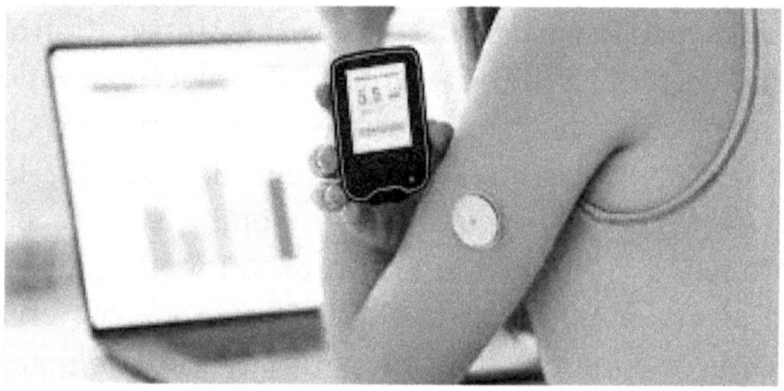

Fig. 3 Continuous Glucose Monitoring (CGM)

The detailed glucose data from CGM helps clinicians tailor individualized treatment plans based on actual glucose patterns rather than isolated readings. This personalized approach can improve HbA1c levels, a key marker of long-term glucose control, while minimizing glucose variability, which is linked to diabetes complications. Furthermore, CGM supports behavioral changes by increasing patient awareness of how meals, exercise, stress, and medications affect glucose levels. For pediatric patients, CGM usage enhances safety and allows parents to monitor glucose remotely. Integration with insulin pumps in hybrid closed-loop systems (also called artificial pancreas systems) is advancing diabetes care by automating insulin delivery based on CGM readings, reducing the burden of diabetes management.

Despite its many benefits, CGM technology faces challenges such as cost, insurance coverage, and the need for patient education to interpret and act on the data correctly. Sensor accuracy has improved significantly over the years, but occasional calibration with fingerstick tests may still be necessary depending on the device. The psychological impact of continuous data can be mixed, with some patients feeling more empowered, while others may experience data overload or anxiety. Nonetheless, ongoing advancements aim to make CGM devices smaller, more accurate, and more user-friendly. The future of diabetes care increasingly depends on CGM technology, which supports proactive, data-driven management strategies and enhances quality of life. As research continues, CGM is also being explored for use in prediabetes and gestational diabetes, expanding its potential impact. Overall, CGM represents a major step forward in diabetes management, offering the promise of improved clinical outcomes and greater patient autonomy.

5.3 PULMONOLOGY

Pulmonology is a specialized branch of medicine dedicated to the comprehensive diagnosis, treatment, and management of diseases that affect the respiratory system, which includes the lungs, airways, pleura, and associated structures responsible for ventilation and gas exchange. The respiratory system plays a vital role in sustaining life by facilitating the exchange of oxygen and carbon dioxide between the environment and the bloodstream. Pulmonology addresses a wide range of conditions that disrupt normal breathing and impair oxygen delivery to tissues, which can result in severe health consequences if left untreated. Pulmonologists are experts trained to evaluate and manage both acute respiratory crises, such as pneumonia or pulmonary embolism, and chronic disorders including asthma, chronic obstructive pulmonary disease (COPD), and interstitial lung diseases (ILD). These specialists work collaboratively with other medical disciplines, such as critical care medicine, allergy and immunology, infectious diseases, thoracic surgery, and oncology, to provide holistic care tailored to individual patient needs.

The field of pulmonology encompasses a diverse spectrum of diseases ranging from common conditions like asthma and COPD to rare and complex disorders such as idiopathic pulmonary fibrosis and pulmonary hypertension. Pulmonary infections, which can be caused by bacteria, viruses, fungi, or mycobacteria (as in tuberculosis), represent a significant clinical challenge worldwide, especially with rising antimicrobial resistance. Lung cancers, both primary and metastatic, are another major focus of pulmonology, requiring integration of diagnostic imaging, biopsy techniques, and multidisciplinary oncologic management. The pleura, the double-layered membrane surrounding the lungs, can also be affected by diseases such as pleuritis, pleural effusions, and malignancies, which fall under the pulmonologist's purview.

The practice of pulmonology has evolved significantly due to advances in diagnostic technologies. Tools such as high-resolution computed tomography (HRCT), pulmonary function tests (PFTs), bronchoscopy, and arterial blood gas (ABG) analysis have revolutionized the ability to detect and characterize respiratory diseases at early stages, enabling timely intervention. Additionally, innovations in minimally invasive procedures allow pulmonologists to obtain tissue biopsies and perform therapeutic interventions with reduced patient discomfort and risk. The integration of molecular diagnostics and biomarkers into clinical practice has further refined disease classification and treatment personalization, particularly in lung cancer and interstitial lung disease.

Treatment modalities in pulmonology are varied and tailored to disease severity and patient-specific factors. Pharmacological therapies include bronchodilators, corticosteroids, antibiotics, antifibrotic agents, anticoagulants, and novel biologic medications targeting specific inflammatory pathways. Oxygen therapy remains a cornerstone for managing chronic hypoxemia in advanced lung diseases, improving survival and quality of life. Pulmonary rehabilitation programs, combining physical exercise, education, and psychological support, have been shown to enhance functional capacity and reduce hospitalizations. For severe cases, mechanical ventilation—both invasive and non-invasive—provides vital respiratory support in intensive care settings. Surgical interventions, including lung volume reduction surgery and lung transplantation, offer life-saving options for selected patients with end-stage lung disease.

Pulmonologists also play a critical role in managing respiratory complications arising in systemic illnesses such as autoimmune diseases, heart failure, and critical illnesses like acute respiratory distress syndrome (ARDS). Their expertise is indispensable in evaluating unexplained respiratory symptoms, guiding multidisciplinary care, and supporting patients through chronic disease management. The emphasis on preventive care, smoking cessation, vaccination, and environmental risk reduction reflects pulmonology's holistic approach to respiratory health.

Recent years have witnessed tremendous growth in pulmonology research, focusing on understanding the molecular and genetic basis of respiratory diseases to develop targeted therapies. The advent of precision medicine, artificial intelligence in imaging interpretation, and telemedicine platforms has expanded the scope and accessibility of pulmonology services. Pulmonologists increasingly employ wearable technology and remote monitoring tools to track patient status and intervene promptly, particularly in chronic diseases like asthma and COPD.

In summary, pulmonology is a dynamic and rapidly evolving medical specialty that addresses a broad range of respiratory conditions crucial for maintaining adequate oxygenation and overall health. Through the integration of advanced diagnostics, personalized therapeutics, multidisciplinary collaboration, and patient-centered care, pulmonology continues to improve outcomes and quality of life for millions of patients worldwide. The ongoing commitment to research, education, and innovation ensures that pulmonologists remain at the forefront of combating respiratory diseases in an ever-changing healthcare landscape.

5.3.1 Anatomy and Physiology of the Respiratory System

The respiratory system is a complex network of structures responsible for the critical function of gas exchange, ensuring that oxygen is delivered to the body while removing carbon dioxide, a metabolic waste product. It is broadly divided into the upper airway and the lower airway, each with distinct roles in the respiratory process. The upper airway includes the nose, which filters, warms, and humidifies incoming air; the pharynx, a muscular passageway shared with the digestive system; and the larynx, which houses the vocal cords and protects the lower airway during swallowing. The lower airway begins with the trachea, a rigid tube reinforced by cartilaginous rings, which divides into the two primary bronchi—each entering a lung. These bronchi further branch into smaller bronchioles, creating a vast network of airways that culminate in the alveoli, tiny sac-like structures where gas exchange occurs. The alveoli are lined by a thin layer of epithelial cells and surrounded by a dense network of capillaries. Their large surface area and thin walls facilitate the efficient diffusion of oxygen into the bloodstream and the removal of carbon dioxide from blood into the alveolar air to be exhaled. The lungs themselves are divided into lobes—three on the right and two on the left—each separated by fissures. The lungs are enveloped by the pleura, two thin serous membranes that create a lubricated space allowing the lungs to move smoothly within the chest cavity during breathing, minimizing friction.

Pulmonary circulation is a unique circulatory loop where deoxygenated blood is transported from the right ventricle of the heart via the pulmonary arteries to the lungs for oxygenation. Oxygen-rich blood then returns to the left atrium through the pulmonary veins to be pumped systemically. This efficient system ensures that oxygenated blood reaches all tissues, maintaining cellular metabolism. Breathing, or ventilation, is a mechanical process driven by the coordinated action of respiratory muscles and controlled by the central nervous system. The diaphragm, the primary muscle of respiration, contracts and flattens to increase thoracic volume during inspiration, while accessory muscles assist during heavy breathing. The intercostal muscles between ribs aid in expanding and contracting the chest wall. Respiratory centers in the brainstem continuously monitor blood levels of carbon dioxide and oxygen via chemoreceptors, adjusting the rate and depth of breathing accordingly to maintain homeostasis. Understanding this detailed anatomy and physiology is crucial for clinicians to diagnose respiratory diseases accurately and tailor treatments. Disruptions at any level—whether airway obstruction, alveolar damage, pleural disease, or circulatory impairment—can lead to impaired gas exchange and respiratory distress. Hence, a thorough knowledge of normal respiratory function forms the foundation for managing a wide array of pulmonary disorders effectively.

5.3.2 Common Respiratory Diseases

- **Asthma:** Asthma is a chronic inflammatory disorder of the airways characterized by airway hyperresponsiveness, episodic bronchoconstriction, and reversible airflow obstruction. The inflammation leads to swelling and mucus production, narrowing the airways and making breathing difficult. Patients typically experience recurrent episodes of wheezing, coughing—especially at night or early morning—shortness of breath, and chest tightness. Triggers include allergens, respiratory infections, exercise, cold air, and irritants like smoke or pollution. The underlying immune response involves activation of eosinophils, mast cells, and T-helper 2 lymphocytes. Asthma severity ranges from mild intermittent symptoms to severe persistent disease requiring aggressive management. Treatment focuses on controlling inflammation with inhaled corticosteroids and relieving bronchospasm with bronchodilators. Early diagnosis and proper treatment can significantly reduce exacerbations and improve quality of life. Patient education on trigger avoidance and inhaler technique is essential for optimal disease control.
- **Chronic Obstructive Pulmonary Disease (COPD):** Chronic Obstructive Pulmonary Disease (COPD) is a progressive respiratory disorder characterized by irreversible airflow limitation, primarily due to emphysema and chronic bronchitis. The disease predominantly affects smokers and those exposed to environmental pollutants, though genetic factors like alpha-1 antitrypsin deficiency may contribute. Emphysema involves destruction of alveolar walls, reducing gas exchange surface area, while chronic bronchitis leads to excessive mucus production and airway inflammation. Patients present with chronic cough, sputum production, and progressive breathlessness, often worsening over time. COPD exacerbations, commonly triggered by infections or pollutants, can cause acute respiratory failure. Diagnosis relies on spirometry showing reduced FEV1/FVC ratio. Management includes smoking cessation, bronchodilators, corticosteroids, pulmonary rehabilitation, and oxygen therapy for advanced disease. Preventing exacerbations and improving functional capacity are central to care.
- **Pneumonia:** Pneumonia is an acute infection of the lung parenchyma that leads to inflammation and consolidation of alveolar spaces, impairing oxygen exchange. It can be caused by bacteria, viruses, fungi, or other pathogens, with bacterial pneumonia being the most common. Patients typically present with fever, productive cough, chest pain, dyspnea, and fatigue. The infection triggers an immune response, resulting in accumulation of fluid, immune cells, and fibrin in the alveoli, which appear

as areas of consolidation on chest imaging. Severity ranges from mild illness treated outpatient to severe pneumonia requiring hospitalization or intensive care. Risk factors include advanced age, immunosuppression, smoking, and chronic illnesses. Diagnosis is based on clinical presentation, chest X-rays, and microbiological studies. Treatment involves appropriate antimicrobial therapy tailored to the suspected or confirmed pathogen and supportive care. Vaccination against common pathogens like Streptococcus pneumoniae and influenza is crucial for prevention.

- **Interstitial Lung Disease (ILD):** Interstitial Lung Disease (ILD) refers to a diverse group of disorders characterized by inflammation and fibrosis of the lung interstitium, the supportive tissue surrounding alveoli. This fibrosis thickens the interstitial space, leading to stiff, less compliant lungs and impaired gas exchange. Patients typically experience progressive exertional dyspnea, a dry cough, and fatigue. Causes of ILD include idiopathic pulmonary fibrosis, connective tissue diseases, occupational exposures (such as asbestos), and drug toxicities. Diagnosis involves high-resolution CT scanning, pulmonary function tests demonstrating restrictive patterns, and sometimes lung biopsy. The prognosis varies widely, with some forms responding to immunosuppressive therapy while others, like idiopathic pulmonary fibrosis, have a poor prognosis. Management focuses on controlling inflammation, slowing fibrosis progression, and supporting lung function through oxygen therapy and rehabilitation. Lung transplantation may be an option for advanced cases.
- **Pulmonary Embolism (PE):** Pulmonary Embolism (PE) is an acute and potentially life-threatening condition caused by the obstruction of one or more pulmonary arteries by thrombi, most commonly originating from deep veins of the legs. This blockage disrupts normal blood flow, causing ventilation-perfusion mismatch and leading to hypoxia. Symptoms vary widely but often include sudden onset dyspnea, chest pain (often pleuritic), tachypnea, and sometimes hemoptysis. Risk factors include prolonged immobility, surgery, malignancy, pregnancy, and inherited clotting disorders. Diagnosis is based on clinical assessment, D-dimer testing, and imaging modalities such as CT pulmonary angiography or ventilation-perfusion scans. Prompt treatment with anticoagulation is essential to prevent clot propagation and recurrence. In severe cases, thrombolytic therapy or surgical embolectomy may be required. Early recognition and intervention reduce mortality and complications like pulmonary hypertension.

5.3.3 Diagnostic Modalities in Pulmonology

- **Pulmonary Function Tests (PFTs):** Pulmonary Function Tests (PFTs) are essential non-invasive assessments that measure lung volumes, capacities, and airflow rates to evaluate respiratory health. These tests help distinguish between obstructive lung diseases, such as asthma and COPD, where airflow is impeded, and restrictive diseases, like pulmonary fibrosis, where lung expansion is limited. Common components include spirometry, which measures forced expiratory volume in one second (FEV1) and forced vital capacity (FVC), lung volume measurements, and diffusion capacity for carbon monoxide (DLCO) to assess gas exchange efficiency. PFTs aid in diagnosing the severity and progression of lung disorders, guiding treatment decisions, and monitoring response to therapy. They also play a crucial role in preoperative evaluations and occupational health assessments. Accurate technique and patient cooperation are vital for reliable results. Repeated testing can track disease course over time, making PFTs indispensable in pulmonology practice.
- **Chest X-Ray and CT Scan:** Chest X-rays are the most commonly used imaging modality in pulmonology, providing a quick overview of lung fields, airways, heart, and pleura. They help detect infections, tumors, pleural effusions, pneumothorax, and structural abnormalities. However, their resolution limits detection of subtle or early lung diseases. Computed Tomography (CT) scans offer detailed cross-sectional images with superior resolution, enabling visualization of lung parenchyma, interstitial changes, small nodules, and vascular structures. High-resolution CT (HRCT) is particularly valuable for diagnosing interstitial lung diseases and characterizing patterns of fibrosis. CT scans also assist in lung cancer staging and guiding biopsies. Both imaging techniques are crucial in acute and chronic respiratory disease evaluation, influencing diagnosis, prognosis, and management strategies. Advances in imaging technology continue to improve diagnostic accuracy and patient outcomes.
- **Bronchoscopy:** Bronchoscopy is a minimally invasive endoscopic procedure that allows direct visualization of the tracheobronchial tree using a flexible or rigid bronchoscope. It is invaluable for diagnosing airway abnormalities, infections, tumors, and inflammatory conditions. The procedure permits biopsy of suspicious lesions, collection of bronchoalveolar lavage fluid for microbiological analysis, and removal of mucus plugs, foreign bodies, or blood clots obstructing the airways. Bronchoscopy is also used therapeutically to place stents or perform laser therapy in obstructive tumors. It requires skilled operators and is generally performed under sedation or anesthesia. Complications are rare but can include bleeding,

infection, or pneumothorax. Bronchoscopy has transformed pulmonary diagnostics by enabling direct tissue sampling and targeted treatment, especially in complex respiratory cases.

- **Arterial Blood Gas (ABG) Analysis:** Arterial Blood Gas (ABG) analysis is a critical diagnostic test that measures the partial pressures of oxygen (PaO2) and carbon dioxide (PaCO2) in arterial blood, as well as blood pH and bicarbonate levels. It provides vital information about a patient's oxygenation status, ventilation efficiency, and acid-base balance. ABG is essential in managing critically ill patients with respiratory failure, metabolic disorders, or mixed acid-base abnormalities. It helps differentiate between hypoxemia caused by lung disease, ventilation-perfusion mismatch, or impaired diffusion. ABG results guide the administration of oxygen therapy, ventilator settings, and other interventions. The procedure involves arterial puncture, which requires technical skill and carries risks like bleeding or arterial injury. Despite these, ABG remains a cornerstone in pulmonary and critical care medicine due to its rapid and precise diagnostic value.
- **Sleep Studies:** Sleep studies, or polysomnography, are diagnostic tests designed to evaluate sleep disorders, particularly obstructive sleep apnea (OSA), central sleep apnea, and other breathing-related disturbances during sleep. These studies record multiple physiological parameters such as airflow, respiratory effort, oxygen saturation, brain activity (EEG), eye movements, and muscle activity. Sleep apnea is characterized by repeated episodes of airway obstruction leading to intermittent hypoxia, fragmented sleep, and excessive daytime sleepiness. Untreated sleep apnea is associated with hypertension, cardiovascular disease, stroke, and impaired quality of life. Sleep studies help quantify the severity of apnea, differentiate types of sleep-disordered breathing, and guide treatment decisions like Continuous Positive Airway Pressure (CPAP) therapy. Advances in home-based sleep monitoring devices have increased accessibility and patient compliance. Sleep studies are essential for comprehensive respiratory and neurological assessment in patients with unexplained fatigue, snoring, or cardiovascular complications.

5.3.4 Pulmonary Therapeutics

- **Pharmacological Treatments:** Pharmacological treatments form the cornerstone of managing many pulmonary diseases and are carefully tailored to each condition. Bronchodilators, such as beta-agonists and anticholinergics, relax airway smooth muscle, providing rapid relief in obstructive diseases like asthma and COPD. Corticosteroids reduce airway inflammation and prevent exacerbations. Antibiotics are essential in treating bacterial infections like pneumonia or COPD exacerbations. Antifibrotic agents help slow progression in diseases such as idiopathic pulmonary fibrosis. Anticoagulants prevent and treat thromboembolic events like pulmonary embolism. Immunomodulators are used in autoimmune-related lung diseases to control immune response. Combination therapies improve efficacy and reduce side effects. Proper medication adherence and monitoring are vital for optimal outcomes. Ongoing research continues to expand therapeutic options with targeted biologics and novel agents.

- **Oxygen Therapy:** Oxygen therapy is vital for patients experiencing hypoxemia to maintain adequate tissue oxygenation and prevent organ dysfunction. It can be administered via nasal cannula, face masks, or high-flow systems depending on the severity of oxygen deficiency. Chronic lung diseases such as COPD often require long-term oxygen therapy to improve survival and quality of life. Acute conditions like pneumonia, pulmonary embolism, or respiratory failure also benefit from supplemental oxygen. Careful monitoring is necessary to avoid complications such as oxygen toxicity or carbon dioxide retention in susceptible patients. Pulse oximetry and arterial blood gases guide oxygen dosing and adjustments. Advances include portable oxygen concentrators, enhancing mobility and patient independence. Oxygen therapy is an essential supportive treatment integrated into comprehensive pulmonary care plans.
- **Mechanical Ventilation:** Mechanical ventilation supports breathing in patients with respiratory failure who cannot maintain adequate gas exchange independently. It can be delivered invasively via an endotracheal tube or tracheostomy or non-invasively through masks (NIV). Indications include acute respiratory distress syndrome (ARDS), severe COPD exacerbations, neuromuscular weakness, or airway obstruction. Ventilators control parameters such as tidal volume, respiratory rate, and oxygen concentration, allowing precise respiratory support tailored to the patient's needs. Complications include ventilator-associated pneumonia, barotrauma, and muscle weakness, necessitating careful monitoring and weaning strategies. Advances in ventilator technology and modes have improved patient outcomes. Multidisciplinary care involving pulmonologists, intensivists, respiratory therapists, and nurses is crucial for optimal management.
- **Pulmonary Rehabilitation:** Pulmonary rehabilitation is a multidisciplinary program designed to improve lung function, exercise capacity, and overall quality of life in patients with chronic respiratory diseases. It

combines supervised exercise training, education on disease management, nutritional counseling, and psychological support. Pulmonary rehab helps reduce symptoms like dyspnea, decrease hospitalizations, and enhance daily functioning. Techniques include aerobic exercise, strength training, breathing exercises, and energy conservation strategies. Patient education focuses on medication adherence, smoking cessation, and coping mechanisms. Behavioral interventions aim to improve motivation and adherence to lifestyle changes. Pulmonary rehabilitation is especially beneficial for COPD, interstitial lung disease, and post-acute respiratory failure patients. It represents an essential non-pharmacological component of comprehensive respiratory care.

- **Surgical Interventions:** Surgical interventions are considered for selected pulmonary patients when medical therapy is insufficient or when anatomical abnormalities require correction. Lung resection, including lobectomy or pneumonectomy, is commonly performed for lung cancer or localized infections. Lung volume reduction surgery (LVRS) is a therapeutic option for severe emphysema, removing diseased lung tissue to improve respiratory mechanics. Lung transplantation offers a life-saving option for end-stage lung diseases unresponsive to other treatments, such as idiopathic pulmonary fibrosis or cystic fibrosis. Surgical procedures require careful patient selection, preoperative evaluation, and postoperative care. Advances in minimally invasive thoracic surgery, like video-assisted thoracoscopic surgery (VATS), have reduced morbidity. Multidisciplinary teams involving surgeons, pulmonologists, and anesthesiologists optimize outcomes. Surgical options continue to evolve, improving survival and quality of life for patients with advanced respiratory diseases.

5.3.5 Critical Care in Pulmonology

Critical Care in Pulmonology involves the specialized management of patients with severe respiratory conditions requiring intensive monitoring and advanced life support. Pulmonologists are integral members of the ICU team, providing expert care for critically ill patients suffering from acute respiratory distress syndrome (ARDS), respiratory failure, ventilator-associated pneumonia (VAP), and other life-threatening pulmonary complications. ARDS, characterized by diffuse alveolar damage and severe hypoxemia, demands precise ventilatory support using lung-protective strategies that minimize barotrauma and volutrauma while optimizing oxygenation. Pulmonologists tailor ventilator settings such as tidal volume, positive end-expiratory pressure (PEEP), and FiO_2 to balance oxygen delivery with the risk of ventilator-induced lung injury. In addition to mechanical ventilation, critical care pulmonologists manage sedation and analgesia to ensure patient comfort, reduce anxiety, and facilitate synchrony with the ventilator. Weaning protocols are carefully implemented to assess readiness for liberation from ventilatory support, minimizing the risk of prolonged intubation or premature extubation, which can lead to complications like ventilator-associated pneumonia or respiratory muscle weakness. Pulmonologists also play a key role in diagnosing and treating ventilator-associated pneumonia, a common ICU infection that increases morbidity and mortality. This includes selecting appropriate antimicrobial therapy guided by microbiological data and preventing infection through strict adherence to ventilator care bundles.

Management of sepsis-induced lung injury is another critical aspect, as systemic infections frequently precipitate or worsen respiratory failure. Pulmonologists coordinate with intensivists to optimize hemodynamic support, maintain adequate tissue perfusion, and manage multi-organ dysfunction. Continuous monitoring of respiratory mechanics, blood gases, and hemodynamic parameters helps guide therapeutic decisions in this fragile population.

The care of critically ill respiratory patients requires a multidisciplinary approach. Pulmonologists collaborate closely with respiratory therapists, nurses, infectious disease specialists, pharmacists, and nutritionists to deliver comprehensive care. They oversee protocols for deep vein thrombosis prophylaxis, stress ulcer prevention, and nutritional support, which are essential to reduce ICU-related complications. In addition, advanced diagnostic tools such as bedside ultrasound, bronchoscopy, and hemodynamic monitoring devices aid pulmonologists in rapidly identifying complications, guiding interventions, and assessing response to therapy. Bronchoscopy is often performed in the ICU to clear secretions, obtain diagnostic samples, and manage airway obstructions. Pulmonology critical care also encompasses the management of special populations, including patients with chronic respiratory diseases exacerbated by acute illness, immunocompromised patients with opportunistic infections, and those requiring extracorporeal membrane oxygenation (ECMO) for refractory respiratory failure. Pulmonologists are involved in evaluating indications for ECMO and managing its complex care requirements. Ethical considerations and communication with patients' families are also integral, as critical care often involves decisions about the goals of care, limitations of life support, and end-of-life management. Pulmonologists provide compassionate guidance and support during these difficult discussions. Continuous education, research, and protocol development in critical care pulmonology contribute to improving patient outcomes and advancing the field. Innovations such as precision ventilation modes, sedation protocols, and infection control measures have significantly enhanced survival and quality of life for critically ill patients. Overall, critical care in pulmonology is a demanding, multidisciplinary specialty requiring advanced clinical skills, thorough knowledge of respiratory pathophysiology, and the ability to make rapid, informed decisions under pressure. Pulmonologists' expertise is essential in optimizing respiratory function, preventing complications, and supporting recovery in the ICU setting, ultimately saving lives and improving outcomes for some of the most vulnerable patients.

5.3.6 Emerging Trends and Research in Pulmonology

Recent advances in pulmonology have revolutionized the diagnosis and management of respiratory diseases, offering new hope for patients with previously difficult-to-treat conditions. Biologic therapies have emerged as a breakthrough for severe asthma, targeting specific inflammatory pathways such as IgE, IL-5, and IL-4/13 to reduce exacerbations and improve lung function with fewer side effects compared to traditional corticosteroids. Similarly, targeted antifibrotic treatments, including pirfenidone and nintedanib, have shown promise in slowing the progression of lung fibrosis, especially idiopathic pulmonary fibrosis, transforming the outlook for patients with this otherwise fatal disease. In lung cancer care, immunotherapy has dramatically changed the therapeutic landscape by harnessing the body's immune system to recognize and destroy tumor cells. Checkpoint inhibitors and other immune modulators are now integral to treatment protocols, improving survival rates and offering personalized options based on tumor genetics and patient immune profiles. Technological innovations are also reshaping pulmonology practice. Minimally invasive bronchoscopic techniques, such as endobronchial ultrasound (EBUS) and navigational bronchoscopy, enable precise biopsy and staging of lung lesions with reduced patient risk and faster recovery. Wearable respiratory monitors allow continuous, real time tracking of lung function and symptoms outside clinical settings, enabling proactive management and personalized care plans. Artificial intelligence (AI) is increasingly applied in imaging interpretation, enhancing the accuracy and speed of detecting lung nodules, fibrosis, and other pathologies on chest X-rays and CT scans.

Cutting-edge research is focused on understanding the genetic and molecular mechanisms underlying respiratory diseases. This growing knowledge base is paving the way for personalized medicine approaches, where treatments are tailored to individual patient's genetic profiles and disease phenotypes, optimizing efficacy and minimizing adverse effects. Gene editing technologies, novel biomarkers, and advanced drug delivery systems are among the promising tools under investigation. Together, these advances represent a paradigm shift toward more precise, effective, and patient-centered pulmonology care, with ongoing research and innovation continually expanding the boundaries of what is possible in respiratory medicine.

Remote Spirometry and Sleep Apnea Monitoring

Remote spirometry is an innovative approach that enables patients to perform lung function tests outside the traditional clinical environment, such as in the comfort of their own homes or local community centers. This method utilizes compact, portable spirometry devices that measure key respiratory parameters, including Forced Expiratory Volume in one second (FEV1), Forced Vital Capacity (FVC), and Peak Expiratory Flow Rate (PEFR). These parameters provide crucial insights into lung function and help clinicians assess the severity and progression of respiratory diseases. The primary aim of remote spirometry is to facilitate continuous monitoring of chronic respiratory conditions like asthma, chronic obstructive pulmonary disease (COPD), and interstitial lung diseases, which often require frequent evaluation to prevent exacerbations and manage symptoms effectively.

By enabling patients to conduct spirometry tests independently, remote spirometry empowers them to take a more active role in their disease management. The data collected is transmitted securely through digital platforms, often integrated with smartphone apps or cloud-based systems, allowing healthcare providers to access real-time information and promptly identify any decline in lung function. Early detection of worsening symptoms can lead to timely interventions, such as medication adjustments or clinical visits, reducing the risk of severe exacerbations, hospitalizations, and overall healthcare costs. Moreover, remote spirometry offers the advantage of convenience and accessibility, particularly for patients living in remote areas or those with mobility limitations who may face challenges attending frequent clinic appointments. This technology also proves invaluable during public health crises, such as pandemics, where minimizing hospital visits is critical. Additionally, longitudinal tracking of lung function through remote spirometry provides a rich dataset, helping physicians tailor personalized treatment plans and monitor the effectiveness of therapies over time. Despite its benefits, successful implementation of remote spirometry requires patient education to ensure proper technique and reliable test results. Furthermore, healthcare systems must address challenges related to data security, device calibration, and standardization to maintain accuracy and patient privacy. As technology advances, the integration of artificial intelligence and machine learning with remote spirometry holds promise to further enhance diagnostic precision and predictive analytics in respiratory care. Overall, remote spirometry represents a significant leap forward in chronic respiratory disease management, combining technology with patient-centered care to improve outcomes and quality of life.

Technology and Devices: Modern remote spirometers are designed to be highly compact and user-friendly, making them accessible for patients of all ages and technical abilities. These devices often connect seamlessly to smartphones, tablets, or computers via Bluetooth or Wi-Fi, enabling effortless data transfer and real-time interaction. Equipped with clear digital displays, they guide users through proper test maneuvers and provide immediate feedback to ensure accurate and reliable lung function measurements. Many of these spirometers integrate with sophisticated cloud-based platforms that securely store and transmit patient data directly to healthcare providers. This instant connectivity facilitates timely clinical review, enabling physicians to monitor disease progression and adjust treatments without the need for in-person visits. Additionally, built-in algorithms help detect suboptimal effort or technical errors, further enhancing data quality. The portability and ease of use empower patients to engage actively in their respiratory care. Advances in software also allow trend analysis and personalized alerts, improving disease management. Overall, these innovations in remote spirometry technology are transforming how respiratory diseases are monitored and treated in real-world settings.

Clinical Applications: Remote spirometry plays a crucial role in the continuous monitoring of patients with chronic respiratory conditions by enabling healthcare providers to detect early signs of lung function decline. This timely identification allows for prompt medical interventions that can prevent severe exacerbations and reduce the need for emergency hospital visits or prolonged inpatient care. By providing real-time data, remote spirometry facilitates personalized treatment adjustments tailored to each patient's changing condition, improving overall disease management and quality of life. This approach is particularly advantageous during public health crises, such as pandemics, when minimizing in-person clinic visits is essential to reduce exposure risks. Additionally, it greatly benefits patients living in remote or underserved areas with limited access to specialized healthcare, ensuring they receive consistent monitoring and care without the burden of frequent travel. Ultimately, remote spirometry empowers patients and clinicians alike, fostering proactive and efficient respiratory disease management.

Advantages:

- Increases patient engagement and self-management.
- Facilitates early identification of disease exacerbations.
- Reduces the burden on healthcare systems.
- Provides longitudinal lung function data for trend analysis.

Challenges and Limitations:

- Requires patient training for accurate technique.
- Data interpretation depends on device calibration and standardization.

- Limited by patient compliance and technological literacy.
- Privacy and data security concerns must be addressed.

Sleep Apnea Monitoring

Sleep apnea monitoring is a critical diagnostic process that assesses abnormal breathing patterns during sleep, with the primary goal of identifying disorders such as obstructive sleep apnea (OSA) and central sleep apnea (CSA). These conditions involve repeated episodes where breathing either partially or completely stops, leading to disrupted sleep and decreased oxygen levels. Monitoring typically involves measuring key parameters, including the apnea-hypopnea index (AHI), which quantifies the number of breathing interruptions per hour of sleep, and oxygen saturation levels that indicate how effectively oxygen is being delivered to the body during these events. In addition, respiratory effort sensors track chest and abdominal movements to differentiate between obstructive and central apnea types. Sleep architecture—the structure and pattern of sleep stages—is also analyzed to understand how apnea impacts overall sleep quality. The data collected helps clinicians assess the severity of sleep apnea, guiding treatment decisions such as the use of continuous positive airway pressure (CPAP) devices or alternative therapies. Modern monitoring techniques include in-lab polysomnography (PSG), the gold standard, as well as portable home sleep apnea testing (HSAT) devices, which increase accessibility and comfort for patients. These technologies utilize a combination of airflow sensors, pulse oximetry, and sometimes electroencephalography (EEG) to provide comprehensive insight into the patient's sleep and respiratory health. By accurately diagnosing sleep apnea, clinicians can prevent associated complications such as hypertension, cardiovascular disease, and daytime fatigue, significantly improving patient outcomes and quality of life.

Types of Monitoring

- **Polysomnography (PSG):** Polysomnography (PSG) is considered the gold standard for diagnosing sleep apnea and other sleep disorders. Conducted overnight in specialized sleep laboratories, PSG involves comprehensive monitoring of multiple physiological parameters throughout the sleep cycle. This includes brain waves via electroencephalography (EEG) to assess sleep stages, eye movements (EOG) to detect REM sleep, and muscle activity (EMG) to identify muscle tone and movements. In addition, airflow sensors measure breathing patterns, while respiratory effort belts track chest and abdominal movements to distinguish between obstructive and central apneas. Pulse oximetry continuously monitors oxygen saturation levels, highlighting episodes of oxygen desaturation. Heart rate and rhythm are recorded using electrocardiography (ECG) to detect cardiac arrhythmias related to sleep apnea events. This extensive data collection allows for detailed evaluation of sleep architecture and the severity of breathing disruptions. PSG's comprehensive nature makes it invaluable for complex or unclear cases but requires an overnight stay, specialized equipment, and trained personnel, which can limit accessibility and increase cost.

- **Home Sleep Apnea Testing (HSAT):** Home Sleep Apnea Testing (HSAT) offers a convenient and cost-effective alternative to in-lab polysomnography for diagnosing obstructive sleep apnea in patients with a high pretest probability and without significant comorbidities. HSAT utilizes portable monitoring devices that patients can easily use in their own homes, allowing sleep evaluation in a natural, familiar environment. These devices typically record essential parameters such as airflow through nasal cannulas or thermistors, oxygen saturation via pulse oximetry, and respiratory effort through belts placed around the chest and abdomen. Some models also monitor snoring and body position to provide additional diagnostic insights. Although HSAT captures fewer physiological signals compared to PSG and does not measure brain activity or sleep stages, it reliably detects apneas and hypopneas to calculate the apnea-hypopnea index (AHI). This enables timely diagnosis and initiation of treatment for many patients, reducing the need for costly and less accessible sleep lab studies. However, HSAT is not recommended for patients with complex sleep disorders or significant comorbid conditions, where in-lab testing remains necessary for comprehensive evaluation.

Technology and Devices:

Advances include wireless, wearable sensors that track multiple parameters without cumbersome wiring. Some devices integrate smartphone apps for data collection and patient feedback. Cloud platforms allow remote data transmission to sleep specialists for interpretation.

Clinical Applications:

Sleep apnea monitoring is critical for diagnosing and managing OSA, which is linked to cardiovascular disease, hypertension, daytime sleepiness, and impaired quality of life. Monitoring guides therapy decisions such as continuous positive airway pressure (CPAP) usage, oral appliances, or surgical interventions.

Advantages:

- Enables convenient, at-home evaluation.
- Improves patient comfort and compliance.
- Facilitates early diagnosis and treatment initiation.

- Supports longitudinal assessment to gauge treatment effectiveness.

Challenges and Limitations:

- Home testing may miss complex sleep disorders requiring full PSG.
- Device accuracy and reliability vary across products.
- Interpretation requires expertise to avoid misdiagnosis.
- Patient factors such as comorbidities can complicate data analysis.

5.4 NEUROLOGY

Neurology is the branch of medicine that focuses on the diagnosis, treatment, and management of disorders affecting the nervous system, which includes the brain, spinal cord, peripheral nerves, and muscles. It is a complex and rapidly evolving field that plays a critical role in maintaining and restoring neurological function, addressing both acute emergencies and chronic, debilitating conditions. Neurologists are trained to manage a wide spectrum of disorders ranging from common headaches and epilepsy to life-threatening strokes, neurodegenerative diseases, neuromuscular syndromes, and central nervous system infections. The nervous system is central to nearly every bodily function—controlling movement, sensation, cognition, emotion, memory, and autonomic processes. As such, neurological disorders often present with diverse and overlapping symptoms like weakness, numbness, seizures, speech disturbances, confusion, visual changes, or altered consciousness. The complexity of the nervous system requires careful clinical evaluation supported by advanced diagnostic tools. Among the most common neurological conditions is stroke, a leading cause of disability and death worldwide. Rapid identification and intervention, including thrombolysis or mechanical thrombectomy, are crucial for minimizing brain damage. Epilepsy, characterized by recurrent unprovoked seizures, affects people across all age groups and requires long-term antiepileptic therapy and lifestyle management. Parkinson's disease, a progressive movement disorder, and Alzheimer's disease, the most common form of dementia, are examples of chronic, age-related neurodegenerative disorders that significantly impact quality of life.

Neurology also encompasses multiple sclerosis (MS), an autoimmune condition that causes demyelination of neurons, leading to varied neurological deficits. Peripheral neuropathies, often caused by diabetes, toxins, or infections, result in tingling, pain, and weakness in the limbs. Neuromuscular disorders, including myasthenia gravis and amyotrophic lateral sclerosis (ALS), impair muscle function due to nerve-muscle communication failure or motor neuron loss.

The diagnostic approach in neurology relies on a detailed clinical history, neurological examination, and specialized tests. Neuroimaging—such as MRI and

CT scans—provides detailed visualization of brain and spinal cord structures, identifying strokes, tumors, inflammation, and structural abnormalities. Electroencephalography (EEG) is essential for diagnosing seizure disorders and altered consciousness, while nerve conduction studies and electromyography (EMG) assess peripheral nerve and muscle function. In acute care, neurologists are central in managing emergencies like status epilepticus, intracerebral hemorrhage, and traumatic brain injury, often working alongside intensivists in neurocritical care settings. Rapid decision-making, familiarity with evolving protocols, and multidisciplinary coordination are vital in such scenarios. In contrast, chronic neurological care emphasizes symptom management, rehabilitation, and supportive therapy, often involving occupational therapists, physiotherapists, speech therapists, and psychologists. Treatment strategies in neurology are both pharmacological and non-pharmacological. Medications include antiepileptics, antiplatelets, dopaminergic agents, immunomodulators, and neuroprotective drugs. Surgical interventions such as deep brain stimulation (DBS) for Parkinson's disease or epilepsy surgery are considered when medications are insufficient. Physical rehabilitation, cognitive therapy, and palliative care also form integral components of patient-centered neurological care.

Neurology has seen remarkable technological and therapeutic advances in recent years. Genomic medicine and molecular diagnostics are shedding light on inherited neurological disorders, enabling earlier diagnosis and targeted therapies. Biologic drugs and monoclonal antibodies are revolutionizing the treatment of conditions like MS and migraines. Artificial intelligence (AI) is being integrated into neuroimaging and predictive modeling to assist in early detection and outcome forecasting. Tele-neurology has expanded access to care in remote areas, especially useful for follow-up and chronic disease management. Neurological research continues to evolve, focusing on understanding the brain's complexity, repairing damaged neural circuits, and identifying biomarkers for early disease detection. Clinical trials are exploring promising therapies such as stem cell treatments, gene therapy, and brain-computer interfaces for conditions previously deemed untreatable. The integration of neuroscience with disciplines like psychiatry, rehabilitation, and robotics highlights the interdisciplinary nature of modern neurology. Neurology is a dynamic and intellectually demanding field that lies at the intersection of basic neuroscience and clinical medicine. Its impact on public health is profound, as neurological disorders account for a significant portion of global morbidity and disability. As the population ages and diagnostic capabilities expand, the demand for neurological expertise continues to grow. With continued innovation and a holistic, patient-centered approach, neurology holds immense promise for improving lives affected by complex and often devastating nervous system disorders.

5.4.1 Epilepsy Detection

Epilepsy detection has significantly evolved with advancements in neurotechnology, enabling earlier diagnosis, improved monitoring, and better management of seizures. Epilepsy is a chronic neurological condition characterized by recurrent, unprovoked seizures resulting from abnormal electrical activity in the brain. Early and accurate detection is crucial for initiating treatment and reducing risks associated with uncontrolled seizures, such as injury, cognitive impairment, and sudden unexpected death in epilepsy (SUDEP). Traditional diagnostic methods primarily rely on electroencephalography (EEG), which records electrical signals in the brain to identify abnormal patterns indicative of seizure activity. Video-EEG monitoring, often performed in inpatient settings, is the gold standard for confirming diagnosis and localizing seizure foci, especially in patients with drug-resistant epilepsy. Recent advances have introduced portable and ambulatory EEG devices that allow prolonged monitoring in outpatient or home settings, capturing events that may not occur during short hospital stays. These devices enhance diagnostic yield and reduce the need for inpatient admissions. Furthermore, wearable seizure detection devices using sensors like accelerometers, gyroscopes, and heart rate monitors can detect physical manifestations of seizures, such as tonic-clonic movements, and alert caregivers in real time. Machine learning algorithms are being developed to interpret large volumes of EEG and sensor data, identifying subtle pre-seizure patterns and predicting seizures before they happen. This has opened the door to personalized alert systems and even closed-loop neurostimulation devices that intervene before a clinical seizure occurs. Neuroimaging techniques such as MRI and PET scans complement EEG findings, especially in patients being evaluated for epilepsy surgery. Functional imaging helps identify structural or metabolic abnormalities associated with seizure onset zones. Invasive techniques, including stereo-EEG, are used in refractory epilepsy cases to pinpoint deeper seizure foci not captured by scalp EEG. Advanced detection technologies are crucial for tailoring individualized treatment plans, ranging from medication to surgery and neurostimulation therapies like vagus nerve stimulation (VNS) and responsive neurostimulation (RNS). As technology continues to evolve, the integration of AI, real-time analytics, and mobile platforms is transforming epilepsy care, making it more accessible, proactive, and precise.

5.4.2 Parkinson's Tracking

Parkinson's disease is a progressive neurodegenerative disorder characterized by tremors, rigidity, bradykinesia (slowness of movement), and postural instability. Effective tracking of Parkinson's symptoms over time is critical for tailoring treatment, monitoring disease progression, and improving patient outcomes. Traditionally, neurologists rely on clinical examinations and patient-reported symptoms to assess disease status. However, these methods can be subjective and limited by variability in symptom reporting or the episodic nature of clinical visits. This has led to a growing interest in objective, technology-based tools for continuous Parkinson's tracking. Wearable sensors are at the forefront of Parkinson's monitoring. These devices, often worn on the wrist, ankle, or chest, track motor symptoms such as tremors, gait disturbances, and movement speed in real-time. Accelerometers, gyroscopes, and inertial measurement units (IMUs) embedded in wearables provide continuous data on mobility and balance, enabling accurate quantification of symptoms across daily activities. Smartphone apps linked to these devices allow patients to record symptoms, medication intake, and quality-of-life parameters, creating a comprehensive, digital disease diary that informs treatment decisions. In addition to physical symptoms, non-motor aspects of Parkinson's—such as sleep disturbances, mood changes, and cognitive decline—are increasingly being monitored through digital tools and behavioral assessments. Voice analysis, facial expression recognition, and typing patterns are also being explored as non-invasive digital biomarkers. These tools help detect subtle symptom changes that might not be evident during clinic visits but are essential for early intervention. Continuous tracking allows for better evaluation of treatment responses, particularly in patients using levodopa or undergoing deep brain stimulation (DBS), where timing and effectiveness of therapy must be finely adjusted. Artificial intelligence and machine learning models analyze vast datasets generated from wearable sensors to detect disease trends, predict symptom fluctuations, and guide personalized care. These algorithms can flag early signs of deterioration or motor complications, prompting timely adjustments in medication or therapy. Telemedicine platforms integrated with Parkinson's tracking tools have further expanded access to care, allowing remote consultations and enabling neurologists to review real-time symptom data. Overall, continuous and objective tracking of Parkinson's symptoms represents a major advancement in disease management, offering clinicians a more detailed picture of disease behavior and empowering patients to take an active role in their care journey.

5.4.3 EEG Wearables

EEG wearables represent a transformative development in neurotechnology, enabling continuous, non-invasive monitoring of brain activity in real-world settings. Electroencephalography (EEG) is a diagnostic tool used to measure electrical signals generated by neuronal activity in the brain, commonly employed to assess conditions such as epilepsy, sleep disorders, traumatic brain injuries, and cognitive dysfunction. Traditional EEG systems are bulky, require specialized facilities, and are limited to brief recordings within clinical settings. EEG wearables address these limitations by offering compact, user-friendly, wireless devices that can be worn comfortably for extended periods. Modern EEG wearables are designed with flexible, lightweight headbands or caps containing dry or minimally conductive electrodes that capture high-resolution brain signals. These devices transmit data wirelessly to smartphones, tablets, or cloud platforms, enabling real-time monitoring and remote data analysis. The ease of use and portability allow for naturalistic monitoring during daily activities, sleep, or exercise—offering a more complete understanding of brain function outside controlled environments. This has significant implications for diagnosing intermittent neurological conditions like seizures or monitoring cognitive decline in neurodegenerative diseases. One of the key applications of EEG wearables is in epilepsy detection and seizure forecasting. By enabling long-term data collection, these devices help identify subtle changes in brainwave patterns that may precede seizures, allowing for timely alerts and potential interventions. In mental health, EEG wearables are being explored for detecting mood disorders, attention deficits, and stress levels by analyzing specific EEG frequency bands linked to emotional and cognitive states. In sleep medicine, these wearables help diagnose insomnia, sleep apnea, and other sleep disorders by tracking brain activity during various sleep stages. Researchers and clinicians are increasingly using EEG wearables in brain-computer interface (BCI) development, enabling individuals with severe disabilities to control external devices using brain signals. This opens new frontiers in assistive technology and neurorehabilitation. Machine learning algorithms applied to wearable EEG data are also enhancing pattern recognition, improving diagnostic accuracy, and enabling personalized therapy in neuropsychiatric care. Despite some limitations—such as signal noise, electrode placement variability, and lower spatial resolution compared to traditional EEG—ongoing advances in sensor technology, materials, and AI-driven analysis continue to improve performance.

Overall, EEG wearables are revolutionizing how we study and manage brain function, shifting from hospital-based diagnostics to real-time, patient-centered neuro-monitoring. Their potential to enhance early diagnosis, continuous assessment, and personalized treatment makes them a cornerstone in the future of digital neurology.

5.5 ONCOLOGY

Oncology is the branch of medicine dedicated to the study, diagnosis, treatment, and prevention of cancer. Cancer is a group of diseases characterized by the uncontrolled growth and spread of abnormal cells, which can invade nearby tissues and, in advanced stages, metastasize to distant organs. Oncology plays a critical role in public health, as cancer is one of the leading causes of death globally. The field encompasses medical oncology (systemic therapies like chemotherapy and targeted agents), surgical oncology (tumor removal), and radiation oncology (therapeutic use of ionizing radiation). Oncologists work as part of multidisciplinary teams that may include pathologists, radiologists, surgeons, radiation therapists, palliative care specialists, and nurses to offer comprehensive care. Cancer can affect virtually any part of the body, with some of the most common types being breast, lung, prostate, colorectal, and cervical cancer. Hematological malignancies such as leukemia, lymphoma, and multiple myeloma also fall under oncology's domain. Early detection significantly improves outcomes, and screening programs for cancers like breast, cervical, and colorectal have become essential tools in reducing mortality. Common symptoms of cancer may include unexplained weight loss, fatigue, persistent pain, lumps, or changes in bodily functions, although many cancers remain asymptomatic until advanced stages. Diagnosis involves a combination of imaging studies (X-rays, CT scans, MRI, PET scans), laboratory tests (tumor markers), and most importantly, tissue biopsy for histopathological evaluation. Advances in molecular diagnostics, including immunohistochemistry, gene expression profiling, and next-generation sequencing, have revolutionized the way cancers are classified and treated. These techniques help identify specific mutations, hormone receptor status, and genetic aberrations, enabling personalized treatment strategies based on tumor biology rather than location alone.

Cancer treatment has seen a transformative shift from one-size-fits-all approaches to precision oncology. Traditional modalities like chemotherapy remain widely used, particularly in rapidly dividing cancers, but often come with significant side effects. Radiation therapy is highly targeted and often used in combination with surgery or chemotherapy. Targeted therapies, which block specific molecules involved in tumor growth (e.g., HER2 in breast cancer, EGFR in lung cancer), have greatly improved outcomes with fewer side effects. Immunotherapy, which activates the patient's immune system to recognize and attack cancer cells, has been a groundbreaking advancement, particularly in melanoma, lung, and bladder cancers. Hormone therapy is used in cancers like breast and prostate, where hormones play a role in tumor growth. Bone marrow transplantation is essential in some blood cancers. Surgery remains vital for localized tumors, either for curative intent or palliation. Minimally invasive surgical techniques, such as laparoscopic or robotic-assisted surgery, have reduced recovery times and complications. In advanced or metastatic cancers, palliative care becomes central to symptom management and quality of life. The psychosocial impact of cancer is profound, affecting not only the patient but also caregivers and families. Supportive care—including nutritional support, pain management, psychological counseling, and rehabilitation—is an integral part of oncology. Survivorship care is another emerging focus, ensuring long-term monitoring for recurrence, secondary cancers, and managing treatment-related complications.

Oncology is also at the forefront of medical research. Cancer genomics and liquid biopsy technologies are enhancing early detection and treatment monitoring. CAR-T cell therapy, a form of immunotherapy using engineered T-cells, is showing remarkable results in certain leukemias and lymphomas. Artificial intelligence is improving cancer imaging, diagnosis, and even predicting treatment responses. Personalized vaccines, nanotechnology-based drug delivery, and tumor microenvironment targeting are active areas of investigation. Despite progress, cancer care still faces numerous challenges. Late diagnoses, limited access to specialized care, drug resistance, and the high cost of newer therapies are ongoing concerns, particularly in low- and middle-income countries. Preventive strategies—such as tobacco cessation, vaccination (HPV, hepatitis B), healthy lifestyles, and occupational safety—remain crucial in reducing cancer incidence. Oncology is a dynamic, multidisciplinary field that continues to evolve with scientific advancements. With increasing understanding of tumor biology, technological innovation, and a shift toward patient-centered care, oncology is not only saving more lives but also improving the quality of life for millions of patients worldwide. As research accelerates, the future of oncology holds immense promise in making cancer more treatable—and, in many cases, curable.

5.5.1 Symptoms

Cancer symptoms vary widely depending on the type, location, and stage of the disease, but they often reflect the disruption of normal body function caused by abnormal cell growth. Common general symptoms include unexplained weight loss, persistent fatigue, fever, night sweats, and loss of appetite. Localized symptoms may involve pain, lumps or swellings, bleeding, or organ-specific dysfunctions, such as difficulty swallowing (esophageal cancer), chronic cough (lung cancer), or changes in bowel habits (colorectal cancer). Skin changes like discoloration, sores that don't heal, or mole alterations may signal skin cancers like melanoma. Some cancers present silently and only become apparent at advanced stages, highlighting the importance of routine screening and awareness of subtle symptoms. Neurological symptoms such as headaches, seizures, or vision changes may indicate brain tumors, while bone pain could suggest metastasis. Hematological malignancies often present with anemia, frequent infections, or easy bruising due to bone marrow involvement. Recognizing symptoms early allows for timely diagnosis, treatment, and improved prognosis. It's also crucial to differentiate between benign and malignant causes, which requires a thorough medical evaluation. Patient-reported symptoms, even if vague, should never be ignored, especially if persistent or worsening over time. In some cancers, paraneoplastic syndromes may occur, where immune responses to cancer cells cause distant, systemic symptoms. Educating the public and primary care providers about early warning signs plays a critical role in cancer prevention and early detection efforts globally.

5.5.2 Monitoring

Monitoring in oncology refers to the ongoing assessment of a patient's disease status during and after treatment to evaluate response, detect recurrence, and manage complications. It plays a pivotal role in personalized cancer care, ensuring that therapies remain effective and timely adjustments are made when needed. Monitoring starts with baseline assessments using imaging (e.g., CT, MRI, PET scans), blood tests (e.g., tumor markers), and biopsy results. During treatment, regular imaging and lab tests help determine tumor shrinkage, stability, or progression. Tools like RECIST criteria guide clinicians in quantifying tumor response in solid cancers. Monitoring also includes tracking side effects, organ function (e.g., liver, kidney, cardiac), and patient-reported outcomes. In hematologic cancers, bone marrow biopsies and flow cytometry are used to assess remission or relapse. After treatment, surveillance continues to detect recurrence early, which is critical for curative potential in some cancers. Surveillance intervals depend on the cancer type, stage, and treatment modality. Advances such as liquid biopsy, which detects circulating tumor DNA (ctDNA), are transforming post-treatment monitoring, allowing for earlier detection of microscopic recurrence. Digital health tools and wearable devices now enable remote monitoring of symptoms, activity levels, and physiological parameters. Monitoring is also essential for assessing long-term effects of treatment and for survivorship planning. Regular follow-up builds patient confidence, ensures prompt management of any new issues, and supports ongoing care coordination. Thus, cancer monitoring is a continuous, dynamic process integral to both acute care and long-term survivorship.

5.5.3 Chemotherapy

Chemotherapy is a cornerstone of cancer treatment involving the use of cytotoxic drugs to kill rapidly dividing cancer cells. It is used for curative, adjuvant, neoadjuvant, or palliative purposes depending on the cancer type, stage, and individual patient profile. Chemotherapy works by interfering with cell division, DNA replication, or cellular metabolism, targeting both primary tumors and metastatic cells. It may be given intravenously, orally, or directly into body cavities. Often, it is used in combination with surgery, radiation, or targeted therapies to enhance efficacy. Chemotherapy regimens vary in drug combinations, cycles, and intensity, carefully tailored to maximize tumor control while minimizing harm to normal cells. However, due to its systemic nature, chemotherapy affects rapidly dividing healthy cells such as those in the bone marrow, gastrointestinal tract, and hair follicles, leading to common side effects. Drug resistance, cumulative toxicity, and immunosuppression are significant concerns in long-term or high-dose regimens. Oncologists use performance status scores and lab evaluations to determine a patient's ability to tolerate treatment. Advances in chemotherapy include liposomal drug formulations, antibody-drug conjugates, and personalized dosing based on genetic metabolism profiles. Pre-medications like antiemetics, growth factors, and hydration protocols are used to reduce toxicity. Monitoring response through imaging and tumor markers is crucial during treatment. Patient education about adherence, expected side effects, and self-monitoring enhances outcomes. Despite newer therapies like immunotherapy and targeted agents, chemotherapy remains a mainstay in many cancers and continues to evolve with better delivery and precision.

5.5.4 Side Effect Tracking

Tracking side effects in oncology is essential for ensuring patient safety, treatment continuity, and quality of life. Chemotherapy, radiation, targeted therapy, and immunotherapy can cause a wide range of adverse effects, both acute and chronic. Side effect tracking involves systematically monitoring symptoms such as nausea, fatigue, pain, neuropathy, mucositis, diarrhea, and hematological abnormalities. Oncology teams use standardized tools like the Common Terminology Criteria for Adverse Events (CTCAE) to classify and grade the severity of toxicities. Regular blood tests assess for neutropenia, anaemia, liver or kidney dysfunction, and electrolyte imbalances. Technology is increasingly being used to track side effects in real-time; mobile apps and patient portals allow patients to report symptoms remotely, enabling early intervention. Wearables can monitor heart rate, temperature, and activity levels, which may reflect early signs of complications like infection or dehydration. Effective side effect tracking helps guide supportive care measures, such as antiemetics for nausea, growth factors for bone marrow suppression, or dose adjustments when toxicities become unmanageable. It also improves communication between patients and clinicians, fostering shared decision-making. Tracking cognitive side effects ("chemo brain"), emotional distress, and sleep disturbances is vital in holistic cancer care. Psychological side effects like anxiety, depression, and fear of recurrence are common and need to be addressed alongside physical symptoms. Consistent tracking empowers patients to be proactive in managing their symptoms, reduces emergency visits, and improves adherence to therapy. In the era of personalized medicine, side effect profiling is also helping predict individual risk and tailor treatments accordingly.

5.6 MENTAL HEALTH

Mental health refers to a person's emotional, psychological, and social well-being. It influences how individuals think, feel, and act, and it plays a central role in how they handle stress, relate to others, and make decisions. Mental health is more than the absence of mental illness—it is a dynamic state of internal equilibrium that enables individuals to use their abilities in harmony with universal values of society. Good mental health allows people to realize their potential, cope with the normal stresses of life, work productively, and contribute meaningfully to their communities.

Mental health affects people across all stages of life, from childhood and adolescence through adulthood and aging. It is influenced by a wide range of social, psychological, and biological factors. Early life experiences—such as trauma, abuse, neglect, or loss—can increase the risk of mental health challenges later in life. Other factors include genetics, brain chemistry, chronic medical conditions, and social determinants like poverty, discrimination, isolation, and exposure to violence. Mental health is also shaped by one's environment, including family relationships, education, employment, housing, and access to healthcare. Mental health conditions are common and varied, ranging from mild to severe. They include mood disorders (such as depression and bipolar disorder), anxiety disorders, schizophrenia, personality disorders, obsessive-compulsive disorder (OCD), post-traumatic stress disorder (PTSD), and neurodevelopmental conditions like autism and ADHD. Substance use disorders and behavioral addictions are also closely tied to mental health. These conditions can significantly impair an individual's daily functioning, relationships, and quality of life if left untreated.

Globally, mental health disorders are among the leading causes of disability, contributing to a significant burden on individuals, families, and healthcare systems. Despite their prevalence, mental illnesses are often underdiagnosed and undertreated, largely due to stigma, lack of awareness, and limited access to mental health services. Cultural beliefs and misconceptions frequently contribute to the marginalization of people with mental illnesses, preventing them from seeking help. In many low- and middle-income countries, mental health care is under-resourced and integrated poorly into primary care systems. Modern mental healthcare encompasses a wide spectrum of interventions. Psychotherapy (such as cognitive behavioral therapy, psychodynamic therapy, and counseling), pharmacological treatments (antidepressants, mood stabilizers, antipsychotics), lifestyle interventions, and community support services all play a vital role in treatment and recovery. Emerging therapies, such as digital mental health tools, telepsychiatry, and neuromodulation techniques (like TMS and ECT), are broadening the scope of intervention. Prevention strategies—such as school-based programs, workplace mental health policies, and early intervention initiatives—are also gaining traction. Mental health promotion is increasingly recognized as a public health priority. Global initiatives led by the World Health Organization (WHO) and other health bodies aim to integrate mental health into universal healthcare, reduce stigma, and protect the rights of those living with mental illnesses. Creating supportive environments that foster resilience, reduce stressors, and encourage social inclusion is essential. Mental health literacy—awareness of symptoms, coping strategies, and resources—must be cultivated across all age groups to empower individuals and reduce treatment gaps. The COVID-19 pandemic further highlighted the importance of mental health, with a global rise in anxiety, depression, grief, and burnout. It underscored the need for scalable, accessible mental health care and the importance of emotional well-being in times of crisis. Mental health is not only an individual concern—it affects families, workplaces, schools, and societies at large. Investing in mental health yields economic, social, and humanitarian benefits by improving productivity, reducing healthcare costs, and enhancing quality of life. Mental health is a fundamental aspect of overall health and well-being. As awareness grows and stigma gradually diminishes, there is a collective responsibility to build more compassionate, accessible, and comprehensive mental health systems. Addressing mental health with the same urgency and respect as physical health is key to achieving holistic and sustainable healthcare for all.

5.6.1 Digital CBT (Cognitive Behavioral Therapy)

Digital Cognitive Behavioral Therapy (Digital CBT) is the modern, technology-enabled adaptation of traditional CBT, one of the most evidence-based psychotherapeutic approaches for treating mental health disorders such as depression, anxiety, stress, and insomnia. Digital CBT programs are delivered via mobile apps, web platforms, or virtual therapy interfaces, offering structured modules that guide users through cognitive restructuring, behavioral activation, and mindfulness exercises. These platforms often incorporate interactive features like mood tracking, journaling, goal setting, and cognitive distortion identification. The core principles of CBT—challenging negative thought patterns and modifying unhelpful behaviors—are preserved, but delivered in a user-friendly, on-demand digital format that increases accessibility. One of the major advantages of digital CBT is its scalability. It allows people in remote areas, or those reluctant to seek face-to-face therapy due to stigma or time constraints, to receive support in a private and convenient manner. Many digital CBT platforms include self-guided modules, though some also offer therapist support via text or video, making the approach hybrid in nature. These tools often integrate artificial intelligence to personalize content and monitor progress, enhancing user engagement. Clinical trials have shown that digital CBT can be as effective as traditional therapy for mild to moderate mental health issues. Digital CBT is also cost-effective and ideal for managing long-term or recurring mental health conditions. It plays a vital role in school-based mental health programs, workplace wellness initiatives, and chronic disease management. However, challenges remain, including digital literacy barriers, data privacy concerns, and the need for proper clinical oversight. Regulatory approvals and clinical validation are essential to ensure safety and efficacy. As mental health needs continue to rise globally, digital CBT stands out as a powerful, adaptable, and innovative solution for expanding access to psychological care.

5.6.2 Anxiety and Depression Monitoring

Anxiety and depression monitoring is an essential aspect of mental health care, enabling early detection, real-time tracking, and tailored interventions. As two of the most prevalent mental health disorders worldwide, anxiety and depression impact millions of individuals across all age groups. Ongoing monitoring helps evaluate symptom severity, response to treatment, and overall mental well-being. Traditionally, assessment relied on clinical interviews and self-reported scales like the PHQ-9 (for depression) and GAD-7 (for anxiety). However, with technological advancements, digital tools are now central to continuous and unobtrusive mental health monitoring. Smartphone apps, wearable devices, and online platforms allow users to log mood changes, sleep patterns, physical activity, heart rate variability, and social behavior—all potential indicators of mental health status. These systems use algorithms and machine learning to identify patterns suggestive of worsening symptoms or treatment non-responsiveness. Some tools even prompt users to complete brief daily assessments and provide feedback or coping strategies based on real-time data. Clinicians can remotely review patient-reported outcomes and make timely adjustments to medications or therapy plans. Mental health monitoring is particularly valuable for individuals at risk of relapse, those undergoing treatment changes, or people in high-stress environments such as healthcare workers or students. It also supports preventive mental health by identifying subclinical symptoms before they escalate. Remote monitoring reduces the frequency of in-person visits while maintaining continuity of care, especially in underserved or rural populations. Ethical considerations, including data privacy, user consent, and equitable access, must be addressed to build trust and ensure inclusivity. As awareness grows and stigma decreases, integrating anxiety and depression monitoring into primary care and digital health ecosystems will be key to delivering timely, person-centered mental health support.

6 Chapter | DATA PRIVACY, SECURITY, AND ETHICAL CONCERNS

6.0 INTRODUCTION: AN OVERVIEW

In today's digital age, the unprecedented growth of data—particularly personal, medical, and behavioral data—has brought data privacy, security, and ethical concerns to the forefront of societal, technological, and regulatory discourse. As industries become more data-driven and technologies such as artificial intelligence (AI), machine learning, cloud computing, and the Internet of Things (IoT) integrate into everyday life, the collection, storage, analysis, and sharing of sensitive information have grown exponentially. While this digital transformation has enhanced efficiency, personalization, and accessibility, it has also introduced significant risks that can compromise individual rights and societal trust. Data privacy refers to the right of individuals to control how their personal information is collected, used, and shared. It is deeply rooted in human rights and autonomy, ensuring individuals have agency over their digital footprint. Privacy is not just about secrecy but about informed consent, purpose limitation, and transparency. In sectors such as healthcare, finance, education, and public administration, maintaining data privacy is not only a legal obligation but also a moral imperative. Unauthorized access to sensitive information can lead to identity theft, financial loss, reputational damage, and psychological harm (Fig. 1).

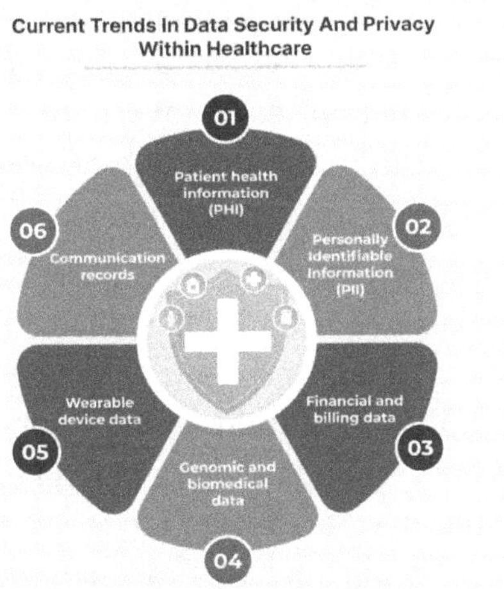

Fig. 1 Current Trends in Data Security and Privacy within Healthcare

Data security, on the other hand, involves protecting data from unauthorized access, corruption, theft, or loss. It encompasses a wide range of technical and administrative measures including encryption, authentication protocols, access controls, firewalls, and data backup systems. As cyber threats grow in sophistication—ranging from phishing and ransomware to insider threats and data breaches—organizations must adopt a proactive, layered defense strategy. Data security is essential not only for protecting privacy but also for maintaining operational continuity, stakeholder trust, and regulatory compliance. Ethical concerns go beyond the technical and legal aspects of data handling and delve into broader questions of fairness, accountability, transparency, and societal impact. Who owns the data? How is consent obtained and respected? Are data-driven decisions perpetuating bias or discrimination? The use of algorithms in sensitive domains like criminal justice, employment, lending, and healthcare can inadvertently reinforce inequalities if not designed and tested ethically. Moreover, the commodification of personal data by big tech companies raises issues of digital exploitation and power asymmetry. The ethical use of artificial intelligence and big data analytics has become a key topic of debate. Predictive systems, while efficient, often function as black boxes, making it difficult for users to understand how decisions are made or contest outcomes. This opaqueness can erode accountability and trust. Algorithmic bias—stemming from unrepresentative training data or flawed design—can disproportionately harm marginalized communities, leading to outcomes that are neither fair nor accurate. As AI begins to make or assist in decisions about hiring, diagnosis, parole, or insurance, the need for transparent, explainable, and ethically governed systems becomes more urgent.

The regulatory landscape is evolving to address these concerns. Laws such as the General Data Protection Regulation (GDPR) in Europe, the Health Insurance Portability and Accountability Act (HIPAA) in the U.S., and India's Digital Personal Data Protection Act (DPDPA) establish standards for data handling, user consent, breach notification, and cross-border data transfer. Compliance with these frameworks is now a critical part of data governance. However, regulatory gaps still exist, particularly in emerging domains such as biometric surveillance, genetic data, and AI-driven profiling.

In sectors like healthcare, where data is highly personal and impacts life-altering decisions, the stakes are even higher. Electronic health records (EHRs), telemedicine, wearable devices, and genomic databases pose complex challenges regarding data ownership, interoperability, and secondary use. Patients must be assured that their health data will be used ethically, kept secure, and not misused for commercial, discriminatory, or surveillance purposes. Ethics committees, data protection officers, and robust consent mechanisms are crucial in navigating this landscape. The global nature of the internet also introduces jurisdictional complexities, with data often crossing borders into regions with differing privacy standards. This raises concerns about sovereignty, data localization, and international cooperation in cybercrime investigations. Furthermore, the digital divide means that marginalized populations may not have the digital literacy or legal protection necessary to safeguard their own data.

As our world becomes increasingly digitized, protecting data privacy, ensuring cybersecurity, and upholding ethical standards are not just technological challenges—they are social, legal, and philosophical imperatives. The future of innovation depends not only on how much data we can harness, but also on how responsibly we manage, secure, and respect that data. Trust, once broken, is difficult to rebuild; therefore, embedding ethics, security, and privacy at the core of digital design and policy is essential for creating an equitable, safe, and sustainable digital society.

6.1 HIPAA, GDPR, AND OTHER REGULATORY FRAMEWORKS

In an era where data is generated, stored, and shared across digital platforms at an unprecedented pace, the importance of regulatory frameworks to safeguard personal and sensitive information has never been greater. Governments and international bodies have introduced robust legal systems to ensure that individuals' privacy rights are respected, data is processed securely, and organizations are held accountable for how they handle information. Among the most prominent of these frameworks are the Health Insurance Portability and Accountability Act (HIPAA) in the United States and the General Data Protection Regulation (GDPR) in the European Union. These regulations, though region-specific, have had a far-reaching influence on global data governance standards.

HIPAA, enacted in 1996, was designed to modernize the flow of healthcare information, protect patients from fraud and abuse, and secure protected health information (PHI). It mandates strict controls over who can access health records, how they are shared, and what security measures must be in place. Covered entities and their business associates are required to ensure confidentiality, integrity, and availability of health data through administrative, physical, and technical safeguards.

Meanwhile, GDPR, implemented in 2018, is widely regarded as one of the most comprehensive data protection laws in the world. It gives EU citizens enhanced rights over their personal data, including the right to access, correct, delete, and restrict processing. GDPR imposes strict conditions on consent, mandates breach notifications, and enforces transparency in data usage (Fig. 2).

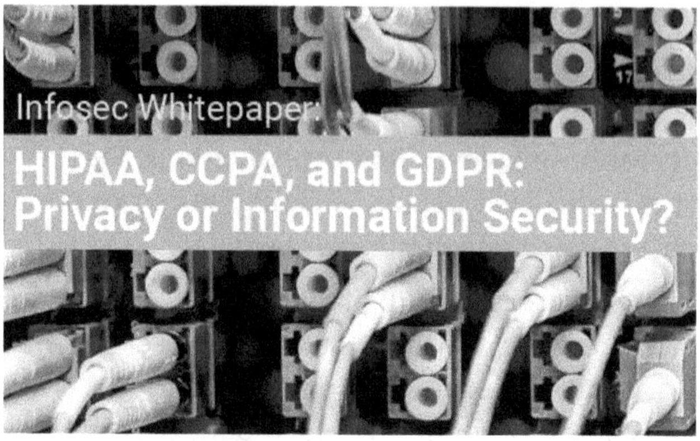

Fig. 2 HIPAA, CCPA, and GDPR: Privacy or Information Security

Its extraterritorial scope means that any organization, regardless of location, must comply when handling the data of EU residents. Beyond HIPAA and GDPR, numerous other national and regional regulations have emerged, such as India's Digital Personal Data Protection Act (DPDPA), Canada's Personal Information Protection and Electronic Documents Act (PIPEDA), and California's Consumer Privacy Act (CCPA). These frameworks vary in scope but share common principles: individual rights, lawful processing, security measures, and accountability. Together, these regulations are shaping a new era of data ethics and compliance. Organizations must now balance innovation with legal responsibility, and integrate privacy-by-design principles into their systems and services. The rise of AI, biometrics, and cloud computing poses fresh regulatory challenges, calling for dynamic legal responses and stronger global cooperation. Ultimately, these regulatory frameworks aim not only to protect personal data but also to build trust—trust in systems, service providers, and governments. In a digital society where data is currency, ensuring privacy and ethical stewardship is no longer optional—it is a fundamental requirement.

6.1.1 Health Insurance Portability and Accountability Act (HIPAA)

The Health Insurance Portability and Accountability Act (HIPAA), enacted in the United States in 1996, is a federal law that established national standards for the protection of individually identifiable health information, also known as Protected Health Information (PHI). HIPAA was designed to improve the efficiency and effectiveness of the healthcare system by encouraging the use of electronic data interchange while ensuring the privacy and security of patient data. The Privacy Rule, implemented in 2003, sets limits on the use and disclosure of PHI without patient consent and grants patients rights over their health information, such as the right to access, amend, or receive a copy of their medical records. Components defining the HIPAA compliance framework is depicted in Fig. 3.

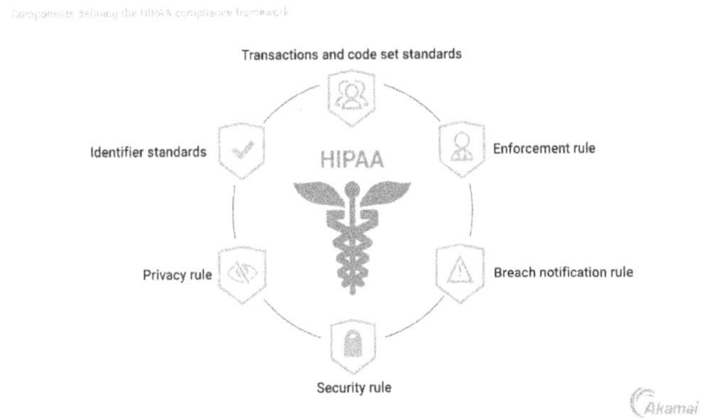

Fig. 3 Components defining the HIPAA compliance framework

HIPAA also includes the Security Rule, which mandates that covered entities—such as healthcare providers, health plans, and healthcare clearinghouses—and their business associates implement administrative, physical, and technical safeguards to protect electronic PHI (ePHI). These include access controls, encryption, audit trails, and regular risk assessments. Violations of HIPAA can result in significant financial penalties and legal consequences, especially in cases of willful neglect or breaches involving large volumes of data.

In recent years, the growing use of telehealth, electronic health records (EHRs), and mobile health apps has posed new compliance challenges. The HITECH Act (Health Information Technology for Economic and Clinical Health), introduced in 2009, expanded HIPAA's enforcement and breach notification requirements. While HIPAA is considered a strong privacy framework, it is U.S.-centric and primarily healthcare-focused, making it less adaptable to other sectors. Nevertheless, HIPAA remains a cornerstone of health data protection, aiming to balance innovation and privacy in a rapidly evolving digital health landscape.

6.1.2 General Data Protection Regulation (GDPR)

The General Data Protection Regulation (GDPR), enacted by the European Union and effective since May 2018, is one of the world's most comprehensive and stringent data protection laws. It applies to all organizations that process the personal data of EU citizens, regardless of where the organization is based. GDPR's primary goal is to empower individuals with greater control over their personal information and ensure that data is collected, stored, and used lawfully, transparently, and for specific purposes. Key principles of GDPR include data minimization, accuracy, accountability, storage limitation, integrity, and confidentiality.

One of GDPR's most impactful features is its extraterritorial scope, which means that even non-EU organizations must comply if they offer goods, services, or monitor behavior of EU residents. The regulation mandates clear and affirmative consent mechanisms, and individuals have enhanced rights such as the right to access, rectify, erase (the "right to be forgotten"), restrict processing, and data portability. GDPR also requires organizations to implement Data Protection Impact Assessments (DPIAs) for high-risk data processing and appoint Data Protection Officers (DPOs) in certain cases. Types of data compliance regulations and standards is given in Fig.4.

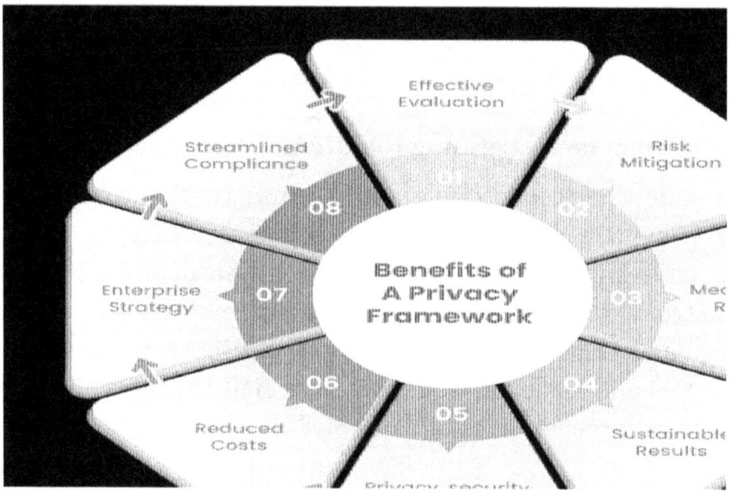

Fig. 4 Types of Data Compliance Regulations and Standards

GDPR imposes strict breach notification rules, requiring that data breaches be reported to supervisory authorities within 72 hours and, in some cases, to the affected individuals. Non-compliance can lead to heavy fines—up to €20 million or 4% of global annual turnover, whichever is higher. The regulation has set a global benchmark, influencing privacy laws in other jurisdictions such as Brazil's LGPD and India's DPDPA. GDPR underscores the shift toward a human-centered approach to data, where privacy is seen as a fundamental right, not just a compliance checkbox.

6.1.3 Other Regulatory Frameworks

Beyond HIPAA and GDPR, a variety of national and regional data protection frameworks have emerged to address the challenges of modern data ecosystems. In India, the Digital Personal Data Protection Act (DPDPA), enacted in 2023, provides a legal framework for processing digital personal data. It emphasizes user consent, purpose limitation, and data minimization, while also establishing a Data Protection Board to enforce compliance. Brazil's LGPD (Lei Geral de Proteção de Dados), closely modeled on GDPR, applies to all sectors and promotes transparency, accountability, and user rights. In Canada, the Personal Information Protection and Electronic Documents Act (PIPEDA) governs how private sector organizations collect, use, and disclose personal information. It requires meaningful consent, fair practices, and protection of personal data, with a focus on balancing individual privacy and business needs. Meanwhile, the California Consumer Privacy Act (CCPA) and its extension, the California Privacy Rights Act (CPRA), provide residents of California with rights similar to those under GDPR, including the right to know what data is collected and the right to opt out of data sales.

Asia-Pacific countries, including Japan, South Korea, Singapore, and Australia, have also adopted robust privacy laws with varying levels of enforcement and alignment with global standards. For example, Singapore's Personal Data Protection Act (PDPA) focuses on both organizational accountability and consumer trust. These frameworks reflect growing global awareness of data rights and a collective effort to regulate the digital economy. However, the lack of global harmonization creates compliance complexities for multinational organizations Benefits of a privacy framework is given in Fig. 5.

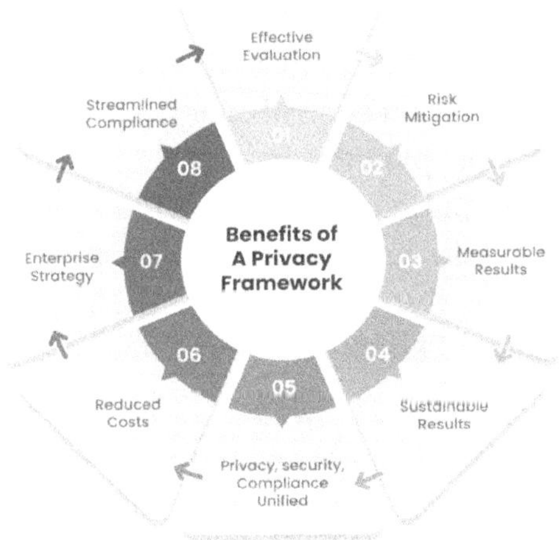

Fig.5 Benefits of a Privacy Framework

Together, these regulatory frameworks form a patchwork of data governance systems aimed at protecting personal data, ensuring ethical use, and fostering digital trust. As data becomes increasingly borderless, future efforts may focus on developing interoperable global standards and enhancing cross-border cooperation to address emerging threats in AI, biometrics, and digital surveillance.

6.2 INFORMED CONSENT IN DIGITAL HEALTH MONITORING

Informed consent is a foundational principle of healthcare ethics and legal practice, rooted in the idea that every individual has the right to make autonomous decisions about their own body and personal information. Traditionally applied in clinical settings, informed consent has long served to ensure that patients understand and voluntarily agree to medical procedures, treatments, or participation in research. However, in the modern era of digital health monitoring, this concept must be adapted to address new technologies, evolving data ecosystems, and complex ethical scenarios. Digital health tools such as wearable devices, remote sensors, mobile health applications, AI-powered diagnostics, and telemedicine platforms collect vast amounts of health-related data—often passively and continuously—raising profound implications for privacy, security, and consent. In this context, informed consent is not merely a regulatory formality but a dynamic ethical process. It involves ensuring that users are fully aware of what data is being collected, how it will be used, who will access it, and for what purposes. This includes both direct uses—such as providing health insights or alerts—and secondary uses, like data sharing with researchers, insurance providers, or third-party analytics firms. Individuals must be informed about potential risks, including data breaches, misuse, unintended profiling, or algorithmic discrimination. They also need to be aware of the benefits, such as personalized healthcare, early diagnosis, and improved treatment adherence, so they can make truly informed decisions.

One of the key goals of informed consent in digital health is to respect individual autonomy, enabling users to retain control over their personal health information. It also aims to promote transparency in data handling practices, encouraging organizations to clearly communicate what they do with user data. This builds trust—an essential element in user adoption and long-term engagement with digital health technologies. Without trust, even the most advanced systems may fail to deliver their intended benefits, as users may choose to withhold data or abandon platforms entirely.

However, implementing effective informed consent in digital health is far from simple. Unlike traditional clinical interactions, digital platforms often present consent as a static, one-time checkbox—usually buried in lengthy and complex terms of service or privacy policies. Users may not read or understand what they're agreeing to, and the consent they provide may be too broad, bundled, or ambiguous to meet ethical standards. There is also a concern about digital literacy, especially among vulnerable populations such as the elderly, individuals with disabilities, or those from low-resource settings who may struggle to comprehend or exercise their data rights.

Moreover, digital health tools often collect data continuously and evolve over time, introducing new features, partnerships, or data uses without re-engaging users for fresh consent. This undermines the principle of ongoing, informed participation. To address this, experts advocate for dynamic consent models—interactive, user-centered systems that provide updates, allow granular choices, and let users modify or withdraw their consent easily at any point. Such systems reinforce ethical practice by making consent meaningful, revocable, and user-controlled.

Legal frameworks like the General Data Protection Regulation (GDPR) in Europe and HIPAA in the U.S. reinforce the importance of informed consent, requiring clear and specific user permission before collecting or processing personal data. Yet, the ethical responsibility goes beyond legal compliance. Developers, healthcare providers, and technology companies must collaborate to design privacy-aware interfaces, use plain language, avoid coercive "dark patterns," and make privacy a visible and integral part of the user experience. Ultimately, informed consent in digital health monitoring is not a checkbox—it is a continuous dialogue between users and the technologies they engage with. As artificial intelligence, remote care, and data-driven personalization become more widespread, the ethical obligation to ensure truly informed, voluntary, and contextual consent becomes more urgent. Achieving this requires not only better policies but also thoughtful design, robust user education, transparent communication, and a shared commitment to upholding the dignity and rights of every individual in the digital health ecosystem.

6.2.1 Components of Informed Consent

In the context of digital health monitoring, informed consent must go beyond simple agreement and instead provide clear, comprehensive, and accessible information to users. As technologies such as wearable devices, mobile health apps, and AI-based diagnostics become more prevalent, the scope of data being collected and processed has widened significantly. To ensure ethical and legal compliance, consent must be detailed and structured around specific components that empower users to make informed choices. A fundamental element is the purpose of data collection—users should understand whether their data is being used for clinical care, research, performance tracking, or commercial analytics. The types of data collected must also be transparently listed, whether physiological (e.g., heart rate, sleep patterns), behavioral, or geolocation-based. Data access is another critical factor, as users must know exactly who has access to their data—healthcare providers, app developers, insurers, or third-party partners. Furthermore, informed consent must disclose data sharing policies, particularly if data is transferred across organizations or borders. Users should be informed about the retention period of their data—how long it will be stored—and the protocols for secure deletion. The consent process should clearly highlight potential risks, such as cybersecurity threats, unauthorized access, or re-identification. Finally, it must uphold and explain user rights, including the ability to withdraw consent, request data deletion, or access their information at any time. By addressing these components thoroughly, digital health platforms can foster transparency, autonomy, and trust in the evolving healthcare landscape(Table- 1).

In the digital setting, consent must include:

- **Purpose of Data Collection:** Informed consent must clearly state the specific reasons data is being collected—whether for medical diagnosis, health tracking, treatment personalization, or research purposes. Users should understand how the data supports clinical care or analytics. Consent should differentiate between core healthcare functions and secondary uses. Clarity about commercial or non-clinical uses is also essential. This empowers users to make decisions aligned with their comfort level.
- **Types of Data Collected:** Consent should provide a transparent list of all data types being gathered, such as biometric (heart rate, respiratory rate), behavioral (activity level, sleep patterns), and environmental (location, time). Users must be made aware of both direct and indirect data. Differentiating between identifiable and anonymized data enhances trust. The scope of data should match the stated purpose. Any changes in data types collected over time should trigger updated consent.
- **Data Access:** Users must be informed about who can view, use, or process their health data—this includes clinicians, app developers, researchers, insurers, or cloud storage partners. Clear identification of all stakeholders involved in data access ensures transparency. Role-based access permissions should be disclosed. The extent of human vs. automated access should also be clarified. Secure and auditable access management builds user confidence.
- **Data Sharing:** Consent must explicitly address if and how data will be shared with third parties, including external researchers, marketing firms, or partner platforms. Whether data is shared in identifiable or anonymized form should be clearly stated. Cross-border data transfer and international access must be disclosed. Opt-in or opt-out mechanisms should be provided. Users should retain the ability to revoke sharing permission at any time.
- **Data Retention Period and Deletion Policies:** The duration for which user data will be stored must be communicated in simple terms. Consent should cover whether data will be kept indefinitely, for a fixed term, or until the user revokes it. Policies on secure deletion, archiving, or de-identification must be clear. Mechanisms for users to request deletion should be straightforward. Transparent retention practices support ethical compliance and data minimization.
- **Potential Risks:** Users should be informed of potential risks such as data breaches, unauthorized access, re-identification of anonymized data, and misuse by third parties. Transparency about cybersecurity practices and breach notification policies is critical. Risks should be described

realistically—not alarmist but honest. Consent should include how these risks are mitigated. Proactively informing users of threats supports informed decision-making.

- **User Rights:** Informed consent must emphasize the user's rights over their data, including the ability to withdraw consent, access data, request corrections, or demand deletion. Users should also have the right to request data portability or object to specific data uses. These rights must be executable with simple, accessible tools. Compliance with regional laws like GDPR or HIPAA should be referenced. Upholding user rights is essential to ethical digital health.

Table 1 : The summary of the Components of Informed Consent in tabular form

Component	Summary Description
Purpose of Data Collection	Clearly explains why data is being collected—e.g., for clinical care, health tracking, research, or commercial use. Differentiates between primary healthcare use and secondary purposes. Empowers informed decision-making.
Types of Data Collected	Lists all data types collected—biometric (e.g., heart rate), behavioral (e.g., sleep), and environmental (e.g., location). Distinguishes identifiable vs. anonymized data. Scope should match intended use and be updated as necessary.
Data Access	Identifies who can access or process the data—clinicians, developers, insurers, etc. Clarifies role-based access and human vs. automated access. Emphasizes transparency and secure access management.
Data Sharing	Specifies whether and how data will be shared with third parties (e.g., researchers, marketers). States if data is shared in identifiable or anonymized form. Includes opt-in/opt-out choices and revocation rights.
Data Retention & Deletion Policies	Communicates how long data is stored (fixed, indefinite, or user-controlled). Outlines deletion policies, secure disposal, and user rights to request deletion. Supports ethical and compliant data retention practices.
Potential Risks	Discloses risks like data breaches, unauthorized access, and data misuse. Describes risk mitigation strategies (e.g., encryption, audits). Promotes realistic, non-alarmist transparency to help users make informed choices.
User Rights	Emphasizes rights to withdraw consent, access/correct/delete data, and request data portability. Must be easily actionable. References compliance with laws like GDPR or HIPAA. Protects user autonomy and control.

6.2.2 Digital vs. Traditional Consent

Traditional informed consent typically occurs in person, allowing for real-time explanation, dialogue, and clarification between healthcare providers and patients. In contrast, digital health monitoring relies heavily on remote, asynchronous methods—often through app-based or online platforms. This shift introduces challenges such as users overlooking lengthy policy texts, misinterpreting vague language, or passively agreeing to bundled terms. The lack of human interaction can hinder comprehension and reduce engagement. Consent in digital settings may lack granularity, offering limited control over specific data uses. Therefore, modern approaches must prioritize dynamic, clear, and ongoing consent mechanisms. These should be user-friendly, transparent, and adaptable to evolving technologies.

This introduces new challenges:

- Users may skip or ignore long policy texts
- Interfaces may not clearly communicate implications
- Consent may be bundled or not granular (e.g., "agree to all")

Hence, a shift toward dynamic, ongoing, and informed digital consent is critical.

6.2.3 Granularity and Specificity

Modern informed consent in digital health must prioritize granularity and specificity, empowering users to make precise choices about their data. Rather than accepting blanket agreements, users should be able to select which types of data they wish to share, such as heart rate, location, or sleep patterns. They should also have control over which app features are enabled, especially those involving sensitive monitoring. Furthermore, opting in or out of research participation should be presented clearly and separately. This level of detail enhances transparency and autonomy, ensuring ethical standards are met. Granular consent also reduces the risk of data misuse or overreach.

Modern informed consent should be granular, allowing users to:

- Choose which data to share
- Select which features to enable
- Opt-in or out of research uses This enhances user control and reduces misuse. Blanket consent (i.e., "agree to all") is increasingly seen as ethically inadequate.

6.2.4 Consent in Vulnerable Populations

In the digital health landscape, special attention must be given to vulnerable populations such as children, the elderly, individuals with cognitive impairments, and those with limited digital literacy. These groups may face significant barriers in understanding complex consent forms or app interfaces. Therefore, simplified language, visual aids, and interactive formats are essential. Where appropriate, guardians or legal representatives should be involved in the consent process. Additional safeguards must be built in to prevent manipulation, confusion, or data misuse. Ethical digital health design should focus on accessibility, clarity, and user protection at every stage.

Digital health tools are used by children, elderly, mentally impaired individuals, and populations with low digital literacy. For these groups:

- Consent must be simplified
- Guardians or legal representatives may be involved
- Additional protections are needed to avoid exploitation

Ethical digital design must prioritize accessibility and clarity.

6.2.5 Withdrawal of Consent

Informed consent is an ongoing process, and users should have the right to withdraw their consent at any time without facing any penalties or loss of services. Clear, simple instructions must be provided to guide users through the withdrawal process. Upon withdrawal, previously collected data should be securely deleted or anonymized as per user requests. This principle respects user autonomy and control over personal information. Ensuring easy withdrawal aligns with legal standards such as the GDPR and reinforces ethical responsibility in digital health. Such transparency builds trust between users and technology providers.

Informed consent is not a one-time event. Users must be able to withdraw consent at any time, with:

- Clear instructions
- No penalties for withdrawal
- Deletion of previously collected data upon request

This aligns with legal frameworks like GDPR and strengthens ethical practice.

6.2.6 Challenges in Implementation

Despite its vital importance, digital informed consent faces several key hurdles. Privacy policies are often overly complex, making it difficult for users to fully understand what they are consenting to. Dark patterns—design elements that manipulate or coerce users into giving consent—undermine genuine choice and autonomy. There is also a lack of standardization across different platforms, leading to inconsistent and confusing consent experiences. Furthermore, regulatory enforcement remains inadequate in many regions, weakening protections for users. To overcome these challenges, developers, healthcare providers, and regulators must collaborate closely to design and implement user-centered, transparent consent models that truly respect individual rights.

Despite its importance, digital informed consent faces hurdles:

- Overly complex privacy policies

- Dark patterns (designs that manipulate consent)
- Lack of standardization across platforms
- Inadequate regulatory enforcement in many regions

Developers, healthcare providers, and regulators must collaborate to improve user-centered consent models.

6.2.7 Legal and Ethical Considerations

Regulations like HIPAA, GDPR, and newer laws such as India's Digital Personal Data Protection Act (DPDPA) mandate that digital health platforms obtain consent that is freely given, specific, informed, and unambiguous. These laws emphasize transparency and user autonomy, ensuring individuals have full control over how their personal health data is collected, used, and shared. Ethically, informed consent upholds respect for persons, safeguarding their dignity and autonomy while promoting accountability among data handlers. Failure to comply with these regulations can result in significant legal penalties, financial fines, damage to organizational reputation, and a loss of user trust. Therefore, adherence to both legal and ethical standards is essential for the responsible and sustainable development of digital health technologies.

6.2.8 Role of Technology in Enhancing Consent

In today's data-driven world, obtaining meaningful consent is more important—and more complex—than ever before. Traditional consent forms, often lengthy and filled with legal jargon, can leave users confused and disengaged. However, technology is stepping in to bridge this gap, transforming the way individuals understand and give consent. Interactive consent forms now use visuals and videos to simplify key concepts, while real-time prompts keep users informed whenever new data is collected. Blockchain ensures transparent and tamper-proof records of consent, and AI assistants help break down complicated terms into plain, accessible language. These innovations are making consent not only more informed but also more user-centric. By empowering individuals through clarity and control, technology is reshaping consent into a dynamic, transparent process.

Innovative solutions are emerging to make consent more meaningful:

- Interactive consent forms with visuals or videos
- Real-time prompts when new data is collected
- Blockchain to record consent transparently
- AI assistants to explain terms in plain language

These advances promote transparency and user engagement.

6.2.9 Future Directions

Looking ahead, the future of informed consent in digital health is set to become more dynamic, adaptive, and user-focused. Personalized consent pathways will tailor information and choices to individual needs, making the process more relevant and understandable. Continuous consent mechanisms—such as periodic reaffirmations—will ensure that users remain engaged and aware as their health data continues to be used or shared. Integration with digital identity systems will streamline consent across platforms, improving security and efficiency. Additionally, as healthcare becomes increasingly global, the development of universal standards for consent will be crucial to protect user rights across borders. Ultimately, informed consent will evolve into a continuous, interactive relationship—far beyond the traditional one-time checkbox approach.

The future of informed consent in digital health will likely involve:

- Personalized consent pathways
- Continuous consent mechanisms (e.g., periodic reaffirmation)
- Integration with digital identity systems
- Global standards for consent in cross-border digital health solutions

As digital health evolves, informed consent must be treated as an active, ongoing relationship—not a one-time checkbox.

6.3 DATA OWNERSHIP AND ACCESS CONTROL

In the digital age, where data is a powerful asset, clearly defining data ownership and access control has become a fundamental requirement for any organization. Data ownership refers to the legal rights and full control over a set of data, while access control governs who can view, modify, or distribute that data. Together, these concepts ensure that sensitive information is managed responsibly, securely, and ethically. Establishing data ownership means identifying who within an organization—or outside it—has the authority over specific datasets. This could be the individual who generated the data, the organization that collected it, or in some cases, a combination of stakeholders. Clearly defined ownership is essential for accountability, decision-making, and compliance with regulatory requirements such as GDPR, HIPAA, or data localization laws. Equally important is the implementation of robust access control mechanisms. These determine which users or systems can access particular datasets, under what circumstances, and at what level of permission (e.g., read-only, edit, share). Role-based access control (RBAC), attribute-based access control (ABAC), and least-privilege principles are commonly used strategies to limit access to only those who truly need it. Organizations must also ensure that access rights are continuously reviewed and updated. As roles, projects, and organizational structures change, outdated permissions can pose security and compliance risks. Automated tools and identity management systems can assist in dynamically adjusting access levels based on real-time conditions and user behaviour. Additionally, transparency is critical. Users should be aware of who owns their data, how it is stored, and who has access to it. Mechanisms like audit trails and data access logs help organizations maintain visibility and accountability, providing a record of when data is accessed and by whom.

Data ownership also comes with responsibilities. Owners must safeguard the data, maintain its integrity, and ensure that it is used in alignment with both internal policies and external regulations. They are also typically responsible for managing data lifecycle activities—such as retention, archiving, or deletion. Furthermore, empowering individuals with control over their own data—especially in sectors like healthcare, finance, and education—has become a key ethical and legal priority. User-centric models such as personal data vaults and consent dashboards are emerging to give individuals more visibility and control over how their data is used. Data ownership and access control are not just technical or legal challenges—they are strategic imperatives. Organizations that define clear data governance frameworks, enforce strict access controls, and respect user rights will be better positioned to build trust, protect data, and innovate responsibly in a data-driven future.

6.3.1 Data Ownership

Data ownership refers to the responsibility and authority assigned to individuals, departments, or entities over specific datasets within an organization. It defines who is accountable for the accuracy, integrity, security, and proper use of the data. A data owner has the authority to set policies on how data is accessed, shared, and maintained, ensuring compliance with internal standards and external regulations. This role also involves overseeing data quality and lifecycle management, from creation to deletion. Clear data ownership promotes accountability and reduces risks associated with data misuse or breaches. It also supports better decision-making by assigning stewardship to those most familiar with the data's context. In complex organizations, data ownership helps avoid duplication and ensures consistency across departments. Establishing data owners is essential for effective data governance frameworks. Ultimately, well-defined ownership ensures that data is treated as a strategic asset, aligning with organizational goals and ethical standards.

- **Role of Data Owners:** Data owners play a critical role in the effective management and governance of organizational data. They are entrusted with the responsibility of overseeing specific datasets to ensure their accuracy, integrity, and confidentiality. As key decision-makers, data owners have the authority to approve or restrict access based on business needs and compliance requirements. One of their core duties is to classify data according to its sensitivity, risk level, and value to the organization, ensuring appropriate protection measures are applied. They also serve as custodians of compliance, making sure that data handling practices align with laws and regulations such as GDPR, HIPAA, or industry-specific mandates. By enforcing data standards and policies, data owners help maintain trust, security, and operational efficiency. Their involvement is crucial in mitigating risks associated with data breaches, misuse, or loss. In essence, data owners act as both gatekeepers and stewards of data assets. Their role is foundational to strong data governance and organizational accountability.

- Ensure data accuracy, integrity, and confidentiality.
- Approve access to the data.
- Classify data according to sensitivity and business value.
- Ensure compliance with relevant regulations (e.g., GDPR, HIPAA, etc.).

◉ **Assignment of Ownership:** In any organization, assigning ownership of data is a critical aspect of effective data governance. Clear ownership ensures accountability, proper data stewardship, and improved data quality across departments. Typically, data owners are individuals in key roles such as business unit heads, department managers, or designated data stewards. These roles are responsible for overseeing the accuracy, integrity, and security of data within their domain. Formally documenting ownership helps establish clear lines of responsibility and supports compliance with internal policies and external regulations. Moreover, this documentation is not static; it must be reviewed and updated periodically to reflect organizational or operational changes. By doing so, organizations maintain control over their data assets and reduce the risks of data misuse or mismanagement. Proper assignment of ownership fosters a culture of data accountability and supports strategic decision-making. It also ensures that any issues or anomalies can be swiftly addressed by the appropriate individuals. Ultimately, a structured ownership framework is a foundational pillar in managing enterprise data effectively.

- Data owners are typically business unit heads, data stewards, or department managers.
- Ownership is formally documented and reviewed periodically.

Responsibilities of Data Owners: Data owners play a crucial role in ensuring that data within their domain is properly managed, secured, and utilized. Their responsibilities extend beyond mere oversight—they are actively involved in key processes that uphold the integrity and availability of data. One of their primary duties is to approve access requests, ensuring that only authorized personnel can interact with sensitive or critical data. In addition, they are responsible for monitoring and auditing data usage to detect anomalies, ensure compliance, and identify potential risks. Data owners must also define backup and recovery requirements to safeguard information against loss or system failure. In the event of a data breach, they are tasked with initiating and managing the reporting process, working with relevant teams to contain and assess the impact. These responsibilities are central to maintaining data security, supporting business continuity, and aligning data practices with organizational goals and regulatory standards.

- Approve access requests.
- Monitor and audit data usage.
- Define backup and recovery requirements.
- Handle breach reporting for their data assets.

6.3.2 Data Custodianship

Data custodianship involves the technical management and safeguarding of data based on the guidelines set by data owners. Data custodians are typically IT professionals or system administrators who handle the day-to-day tasks related to data storage, maintenance, and protection. Their role includes implementing security measures, performing regular backups, and ensuring data availability and integrity. They also manage data access controls, applying the permissions approved by data owners. While data owners set the policies and define how data should be used, data custodians ensure those policies are executed effectively through technical means. This collaboration between data owners and custodians is essential to maintaining a secure and well-governed data environment. Data custodians play a critical role in preventing data loss, unauthorized access, and ensuring that data systems operate smoothly. Through their efforts, organizations can trust that their data assets are both protected and accessible when needed.

Responsibilities:

- Implement and maintain security measures.
- Manage data storage, backup, and access systems.
- Ensure data availability and system performance.
- Collaborate with data owners to enforce access policies.

6.3.3 Access Control Principles

Access control principles are fundamental to protecting sensitive data and ensuring that users only interact with information appropriate to their responsibilities. The

Need-to-Know Basis means users are granted access solely to the data necessary for performing their specific job functions, reducing the risk of unauthorized exposure. The Least Privilege Principle further enforces security by limiting users to the minimal level of access required, preventing excessive permissions that could lead to misuse or data breaches. Role-Based Access Control (RBAC) assigns access rights based on predefined job roles rather than individual identities, simplifying management and ensuring consistency. Finally, the Segregation of Duties principle helps avoid conflicts of interest and fraud by dividing critical tasks among multiple individuals—for example, separating approval authority from execution responsibilities. Together, these principles form a strong framework to maintain data security, accountability, and operational integrity within organizations.

- **Need-to-Know Basis:** The Need-to-Know principle ensures that users access only the information essential for their specific job functions. This minimizes unnecessary exposure of sensitive data and reduces the risk of accidental or intentional misuse. By restricting access, organizations can better protect confidential information and comply with privacy regulations. It encourages a focused approach to data sharing, allowing only relevant personnel to view or modify data. Ultimately, it strengthens overall data security by limiting data availability strictly to those who truly need it.
- **Least Privilege Principle:** The Least Privilege Principle requires that users have the minimum level of access necessary to perform their tasks. This helps to prevent over-permissioning, which can increase the risk of security breaches or data leaks. By restricting access rights, the principle limits potential damage from compromised accounts or insider threats. It also promotes disciplined access management and regular reviews to ensure permissions remain appropriate. Implementing least privilege helps maintain tighter control over sensitive systems and data.
- **Role-Based Access Control (RBAC):** Role-Based Access Control assigns access permissions based on a user's job role rather than their individual identity. This simplifies access management by grouping users with similar responsibilities under predefined roles. It ensures consistency in access rights and reduces administrative overhead, especially in large organizations. RBAC supports scalability and helps enforce organizational policies effectively. By focusing on roles, it also makes audits and compliance checks more straightforward.
- **Segregation of Duties:** Segregation of Duties (SoD) is a key control to prevent conflicts of interest and reduce fraud risks. It divides critical tasks among multiple individuals so that no single person has control over all

parts of a process. For example, the roles of approval and execution are kept separate to maintain checks and balances. SoD enhances accountability and transparency within business processes. This principle is vital for maintaining trust and integrity in organizational operations.

6.3.4 Access Authorization

Access authorization is a vital component of an organization's data security framework, ensuring that only authorized individuals can gain access to sensitive information and systems. The process begins with a formal request workflow, where access requests must be submitted and approved by designated data owners. These approvals are then reviewed by security or administrative teams to maintain proper oversight and compliance. A robust approval mechanism requires that all access grants be logged and auditable, providing a clear trail for accountability and future reference. Additionally, temporary access permissions should have defined expiry dates to minimize risks associated with prolonged or unnecessary access. User onboarding processes include provisioning access rights based on job requirements, while offboarding or role changes must trigger the immediate revocation of access to prevent unauthorized use. Together, these measures help safeguard organizational data, reduce the risk of breaches, and support regulatory compliance. Effective access authorization balances operational needs with strong security controls, maintaining trust and protecting valuable data assets.

- **Request Process:** Access requests should follow a clearly defined and formal workflow to ensure consistency and accountability. This process begins when a user submits a request specifying the data or systems they need access to and the purpose for it. Data owners are responsible for reviewing and approving these requests based on relevance and necessity. Additionally, security or administrative teams conduct a secondary review to verify compliance with policies and to assess potential risks. A structured request process helps prevent unauthorized access and ensures that every request is properly evaluated before approval.
- **Approval Mechanism:** The approval mechanism must include detailed logging of every access request and decision to maintain transparency. All approvals should be auditable, allowing organizations to track who granted access, when, and for what purpose. This documentation is critical for internal audits, regulatory compliance, and forensic investigations in case of security incidents. Furthermore, temporary access permissions should always have predefined expiry dates to limit the duration of access. Implementing these controls strengthens governance and reduces the risk of lingering access that could be exploited.

- **User Onboarding and Offboarding:** During user onboarding, access provisioning must be carefully aligned with the employee's role, ensuring they receive the appropriate permissions from day one. This helps employees perform their duties effectively while minimizing unnecessary exposure to sensitive data. Equally important is the offboarding process, where access rights must be promptly revoked when an employee leaves or changes roles within the organization. Delays or oversights in revoking access can lead to security vulnerabilities or data breaches. A well-managed onboarding and offboarding process supports both operational efficiency and security integrity.

6.3.5 Authentication and Access Mechanisms

Authentication and access mechanisms are essential elements in securing organizational data and systems from unauthorized use. Authentication methods verify the identity of users before granting access, using techniques such as password-based logins, multi-factor authentication (MFA), and biometric verification. These methods add layers of security to ensure that only legitimate users can access sensitive resources. Access is typically provided through defined channels, including web portals, virtual private networks (VPNs), and cloud management dashboards, all equipped with logging to track user activity. Continuous monitoring of access is crucial, involving regular reviews of access logs to detect any irregularities or unauthorized attempts. Automated alerts can notify security teams of unusual access patterns, enabling quick responses to potential threats. Together, these mechanisms form a robust defense against cyberattacks and data breaches, helping organizations maintain control over their critical assets while supporting secure and efficient user access. Implementing strong authentication and vigilant access monitoring is vital for protecting both business operations and sensitive information.

- **Authentication Methods:** Authentication methods are the first line of defense in verifying a user's identity before granting access to systems or data. Traditional password-based authentication remains common, but it is often supplemented with more secure options like multi-factor authentication (MFA), which requires additional verification steps such as a one-time code or biometric scan. Biometric methods, including fingerprint or facial recognition, add another layer of security by using unique physical traits. Combining these methods enhances protection against unauthorized access and reduces the risk of credential theft. Organizations should adopt strong authentication strategies tailored to their security needs and risk levels.

- **Access Channels:** Access channels refer to the specific platforms or entry points through which users connect to organizational systems and data. These channels include web portals, virtual private networks (VPNs), cloud management dashboards, and other authorized interfaces. It is crucial that these channels are well-defined and secured, with comprehensive logging enabled to capture detailed records of user activity. Proper control and monitoring of access channels help prevent unauthorized entry and provide visibility into how data and resources are being used. Ensuring secure and logged access channels is fundamental to maintaining a secure IT environment.
- **Monitoring Access:** Monitoring access involves the continuous oversight of who is accessing systems and data, when, and how. Regular reviews of access logs are essential to identify any anomalies, such as unexpected login times or access from unusual locations. This proactive monitoring helps detect potential security breaches early and supports compliance with regulatory requirements. Automated alert systems can notify security teams of suspicious or unauthorized activities, allowing for swift investigation and response. Effective access monitoring ensures ongoing protection and reinforces accountability within the organization.

6.3.6 Data Access Reviews and Audits

Data access reviews and audits are essential components of a robust data governance strategy, ensuring that sensitive information is protected from unauthorized use or exposure. Regularly scheduled reviews—whether quarterly or bi-annual—help organizations verify that only authorized personnel have access to critical data. These periodic assessments allow for timely updates to access permissions, reducing the risk of data breaches and misuse. Complementing these reviews, audit trails serve as comprehensive logs that record all data access activities, providing transparency and accountability. Maintaining these logs is crucial not only for internal security but also for meeting regulatory compliance requirements. Additionally, managing third-party access through strict contracts and data-sharing agreements ensures external entities adhere to the same standards of data protection. Together, these practices create a structured framework that safeguards sensitive data while supporting organizational compliance and operational integrity.

- **Periodic Review:** Periodic reviews, conducted quarterly or bi-annually, are vital for maintaining strict control over access to sensitive data. These reviews ensure that only authorized individuals retain access privileges and help identify any outdated or unnecessary permissions. By regularly assessing who can view or modify sensitive information, organizations can minimize the risk of unauthorized data exposure. Access permissions are promptly updated during these reviews to reflect changes in roles or employment status. This process strengthens data security and supports compliance with regulatory requirements. Ultimately, periodic reviews help maintain a dynamic and secure data access environment.

- **Audit Trails:** Audit trails play a crucial role in tracking and monitoring data access activities within an organization. By maintaining detailed logs of who accessed sensitive or critical data, when, and what actions were taken, audit trails enhance transparency and accountability. These records are indispensable for investigating security incidents or unauthorized access attempts. Additionally, retaining audit logs for specified periods is often a regulatory requirement, ensuring that organizations can demonstrate compliance during audits. Proper management and protection of audit logs further secure the integrity of access records. Overall, audit trails serve as a foundational tool in safeguarding sensitive data.
- **Third-Party Access:** Managing third-party access to sensitive data requires stringent controls to mitigate risks associated with external entities. Access is regulated through formal contracts and data-sharing agreements that clearly outline the responsibilities and security expectations of third parties. These agreements ensure that third-party access complies with the organization's internal policies and relevant legal requirements. Regular reviews and audits of third-party access help confirm ongoing adherence to security protocols. By enforcing these measures, organizations can protect sensitive information while collaborating with external partners. This approach balances operational needs with data security imperatives.

6.3.7 Policy Enforcement and Violations

Policy enforcement and handling violations are critical aspects of maintaining a secure and compliant data environment. Effective enforcement mechanisms ensure that access restrictions are consistently applied and that any deviations are promptly identified and addressed. Automated tools play a significant role in enforcing policies by continuously monitoring access permissions and flagging unauthorized activities in real time. However, manual oversight remains essential to provide context, perform detailed reviews, and generate reports for management and compliance purposes. Together, these enforcement approaches create a balanced system that promotes adherence to security protocols. When violations occur, it is important to have clear consequences to deter non-compliance and reinforce the seriousness of data protection. Disciplinary actions, aligned with company HR and IT security policies, may include warnings, suspension, or termination depending on the severity of the breach. In addition to internal consequences, legal ramifications can arise if violations involve breaches of regulatory laws, potentially leading to fines, penalties, or legal action against individuals or the organization. Establishing and communicating these enforcement and consequence frameworks encourages a culture of accountability and vigilance. This structured approach not only protects sensitive data but also supports regulatory compliance and helps maintain stakeholder trust.

- **Enforcement Mechanisms:** Enforcement mechanisms are essential to ensure that data access policies are consistently followed and violations are promptly detected. Automated tools play a critical role by continuously monitoring user activities and enforcing access restrictions in real time, reducing the chances of human error or oversight. These tools can instantly block unauthorized attempts, generate alerts, and provide detailed logs for further analysis. However, automated systems alone are not sufficient; manual oversight is necessary to interpret complex cases, conduct thorough investigations, and verify compliance through periodic reviews. Reporting mechanisms, both automated and manual, enable transparent communication of enforcement activities to management and compliance teams. Together, automation and human intervention create a comprehensive enforcement framework that balances efficiency with accuracy. This dual approach strengthens the organization's ability to protect sensitive data effectively and respond quickly to potential breaches.
- **Consequences of Violation:** Clear and enforceable consequences for policy violations are vital to maintaining a secure and compliant data environment. Disciplinary actions, aligned with company HR and IT security policies, serve as a deterrent against non-compliance and can range from formal warnings to suspension or termination, depending on the severity and intent behind the violation. These actions ensure that employees understand the seriousness of protecting sensitive data and adhering to access protocols. Beyond internal disciplinary measures, legal consequences can arise if violations breach regulatory laws, potentially exposing individuals and organizations to fines, penalties, or legal proceedings. Regulatory bodies often mandate strict enforcement to uphold data privacy and security standards, emphasizing the importance of compliance. By clearly communicating these consequences, organizations foster a culture of accountability and responsibility, reinforcing the critical importance of data protection across all levels of the workforce.

6.4 CYBERSECURITY RISKS AND SOLUTIONS

Cybersecurity risks have become one of the most pressing challenges for organizations in today's increasingly digital world. As businesses rely more heavily on technology and store vast amounts of sensitive data online, they become attractive targets for cybercriminals. These risks encompass a wide range of threats, including malware, ransomware, phishing attacks, insider threats, and vulnerabilities in software or hardware systems. The consequences of successful cyberattacks can be severe, leading to data breaches, financial losses, operational disruptions, and damage to an organization's reputation. In addition, regulatory bodies are imposing stricter requirements to protect data privacy and security, making it imperative for organizations to adopt comprehensive cybersecurity strategies. Addressing cybersecurity risks involves not only identifying and understanding potential threats but also implementing robust solutions that can prevent, detect, and respond to attacks effectively. Preventive measures such as firewalls, encryption, and multi-factor authentication help reduce vulnerabilities, while continuous monitoring tools enable early detection of suspicious activities. When incidents do occur, having a well-defined response and recovery plan minimizes damage and ensures business continuity. Furthermore, governance and compliance frameworks guide organizations in maintaining strong security postures and meeting legal obligations. By integrating risk management with technological defenses and policy enforcement, organizations can better protect their critical assets and build resilience against evolving cyber threats. Ultimately, a proactive and layered approach to cybersecurity is essential in safeguarding information and sustaining trust in the digital age (Table-2).

6.4.1 Cybersecurity Risks

Cybersecurity risks refer to potential threats or vulnerabilities that can compromise the confidentiality, integrity, and availability of digital information and systems. These risks can arise from various sources, including malicious attacks like malware, ransomware, phishing, or insider threats such as negligent or malicious employees. Other risks include system vulnerabilities, weak access controls, outdated software, and inadequate security policies. The growing sophistication of cyberattacks, combined with the increasing amount of sensitive data stored and transmitted digitally, heightens the risk exposure for organizations. Cybersecurity risks can lead to data breaches, financial losses, reputational damage, and legal penalties, making proactive risk identification and management essential for any business.

6.4.2 Types of Cybersecurity Risks

Cybersecurity risks can be categorized into several types, each requiring specific attention. Common risks include malware infections that disrupt or damage systems, phishing attacks aimed at stealing credentials, ransomware that encrypts data for ransom, and denial-of-service attacks that overload systems to cause downtime. Insider threats, whether intentional or accidental, can lead to unauthorized access or data leaks. Additionally, vulnerabilities in software or hardware can be exploited by attackers to gain control or access sensitive information. Understanding these diverse risks helps organizations tailor their defenses and response strategies effectively.

6.4.3 Preventive Solutions

Preventive solutions focus on minimizing vulnerabilities and blocking threats before they cause harm. This includes deploying firewalls, antivirus software, and intrusion detection systems to guard against external attacks. Regular software updates and patch management close security gaps in applications and operating systems. Strong access controls, including multi-factor authentication, ensure that only authorized users can access sensitive systems and data. Employee training and awareness programs are also critical to prevent social engineering attacks such as phishing. Together, these proactive measures build a solid first line of defense against cybersecurity threats.

6.4.4 Detection and Monitoring Solutions

Early detection of cybersecurity incidents is crucial to limit damage and respond swiftly. Continuous monitoring tools, such as security information and event management (SIEM) systems, collect and analyze data from across the network to identify suspicious activities or anomalies. Endpoint detection and response (EDR) solutions monitor devices for signs of compromise. Automated alerts help security teams react promptly to potential threats. Additionally, regular security audits and vulnerability assessments uncover hidden weaknesses that attackers might exploit. These detection and monitoring efforts enable organizations to maintain situational awareness and strengthen their security posture.

6.4.5 Response and Recovery Solutions

Even with strong defenses, cybersecurity incidents can occur, so having a clear response and recovery plan is vital. Incident response teams must be prepared to contain and mitigate attacks quickly to prevent escalation. This includes isolating affected systems, eradicating malware, and restoring data from secure backups. Recovery solutions focus on returning to normal operations with minimal downtime and data loss. Post-incident analysis helps organizations learn from breaches and improve their defenses. Communication plans ensure timely updates to stakeholders, regulators, and affected parties, maintaining transparency and trust.

6.4.6 Governance and Compliance Solutions

Governance and compliance play a key role in managing cybersecurity risks through policies, standards, and regulatory adherence. Organizations need to establish clear cybersecurity policies that define roles, responsibilities, and acceptable use. Compliance with regulations such as GDPR, HIPAA, or industry-specific standards ensures that security measures meet legal requirements. Regular audits and assessments verify that controls are effective and identify gaps for improvement. Governance frameworks promote accountability and continuous risk management, aligning cybersecurity efforts with overall business objectives and regulatory expectations.

Table - 2 Summary of Cyber Security Risks and Solutions

Risks/ Solution	Description
Cybersecurity Risks	Potential threats compromising confidentiality, integrity, and availability of data, including malware, phishing, insider threats, weak controls, and outdated systems. Risks lead to breaches, financial loss, reputational damage, and legal penalties.
Types of Cybersecurity Risks	Categories include malware, phishing, ransomware, denial-of-service attacks, insider threats, and software/hardware vulnerabilities. Understanding these helps tailor defense strategies.
Preventive Solutions	Measures to minimize vulnerabilities: firewalls, antivirus, intrusion detection, patch management, strong access controls (MFA), and employee training to prevent social engineering.
Detection and Monitoring Solutions	Continuous monitoring tools (SIEM, EDR), automated alerts, security audits, and vulnerability assessments for early threat detection and maintaining security posture.
Response and Recovery Solutions	Incident response plans to contain attacks, isolate systems, remove malware, restore backups, and conduct post-incident reviews. Communication ensures transparency with stakeholders.
Governance and Compliance Solutions	Establishing cybersecurity policies, roles, and responsibilities. Ensuring compliance with laws (e.g., GDPR, HIPAA). Regular audits promote accountability and continuous risk management aligned with business goals.

6.5 ETHICAL USE OF AI IN HEALTH MONITORING

The ethical use of Artificial Intelligence (AI) in health monitoring has become a critical focus as AI technologies increasingly influence how healthcare is delivered, monitored, and managed. From wearable devices tracking vital signs to predictive algorithms identifying disease risks, AI offers immense benefits in improving patient outcomes, enhancing early diagnosis, and optimizing care delivery. However, alongside these advancements come serious ethical concerns that must be carefully addressed to ensure responsible use. Issues such as patient privacy, data security, algorithmic bias, and the transparency of AI decision-making processes are at the forefront of these concerns. As AI systems handle sensitive health data, maintaining strict confidentiality and obtaining informed patient consent are essential. Patients must also have the right to understand how their data is used and how AI-generated decisions are made (Fig. 6).

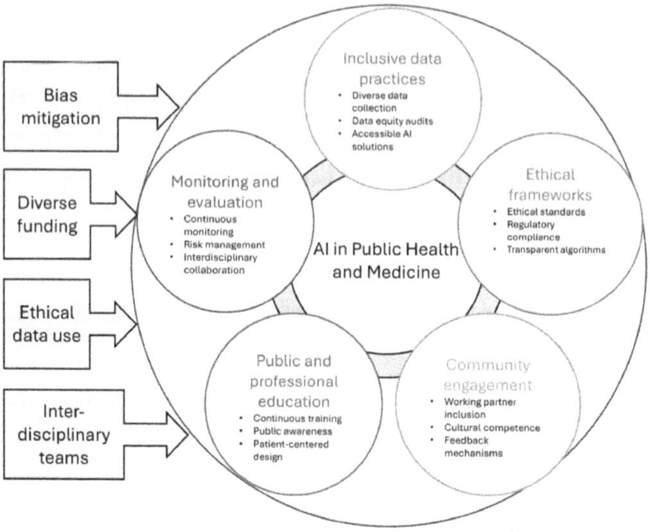

Fig. 6 Ethical Considerations in Using Artificial Intelligence in Public Health

There is a growing need to ensure that AI tools are fair, unbiased, and do not discriminate against specific populations. Furthermore, human oversight is crucial to prevent over-reliance on technology and to ensure clinical judgment remains central in healthcare decisions. Ethical frameworks must also define accountability—clarifying who is responsible when AI systems fail or cause harm. Regulatory standards, continuous auditing, and inclusive AI training practices are necessary to build systems that are both accurate and ethically sound. Ultimately, the goal is to integrate AI into health monitoring in a way that respects patient rights, promotes equity, and supports safe, human-centered healthcare.

6.5.1 Patient Privacy and Data Security

AI systems in health monitoring rely on large volumes of sensitive personal data. Ensuring patient privacy and securing health data is a top ethical concern. Data must be protected using encryption, access controls, and secure storage practices. Informed consent must be obtained before collecting or using patient data. Ethical AI use requires that data sharing complies with regulations like HIPAA or GDPR. Patients should be aware of how their data is used and retain control over their personal information.

6.5.2 Transparency and Explainability

AI decisions in health monitoring must be transparent and explainable, especially when they influence diagnosis, treatment, or health recommendations. Patients and healthcare providers should understand how the AI system works and the reasoning behind its outputs. Black-box AI models may raise ethical concerns if decisions cannot be interpreted. Explainable AI (XAI) helps build trust and supports informed medical decisions. Transparency also facilitates accountability in the case of errors or bias.

6.5.3 Bias and Fairness

AI systems may inherit biases from training data, leading to unfair or inaccurate predictions across different populations. Ethical AI in health monitoring must be trained on diverse, representative datasets to avoid disparities in care. Algorithms should be tested for bias and regularly audited to ensure fair treatment for all demographic groups. Mitigating bias promotes equitable healthcare and prevents discrimination based on race, gender, age, or socioeconomic status.

6.5.4 Accountability and Responsibility

Clearly defined accountability is essential when AI tools are used in health decisions. Healthcare professionals, developers, and institutions must share responsibility for the outcomes of AI-supported interventions. Ethical practice involves documenting decision-making processes and identifying who is responsible if harm occurs. Legal frameworks may need to evolve to address liability issues arising from AI-driven healthcare.

6.5.5 Informed Consent and Patient Autonomy

Patients must be informed when AI is involved in their care and must consent to its use. Ethical use of AI respects patient autonomy by allowing individuals to opt in or out of AI-driven monitoring. Healthcare providers must explain how the AI system works, what data it uses, and the potential risks and benefits. Ensuring meaningful consent enhances trust and empowers patients in their care journey.

6.5.6 Human Oversight and Clinical Judgment

AI should support, not replace, human clinicians. Ethical guidelines emphasize the need for human oversight in AI-assisted healthcare decisions. Clinicians must retain final authority and use their judgment in interpreting AI outputs. This human-in-the-loop approach ensures that AI tools are used responsibly and that patient well-being remains the top priority.

6.6 ADDRESSING DIGITAL HEALTH INEQUITIES

The rapid advancement of digital health technologies has transformed the healthcare landscape, offering new opportunities for remote care, continuous monitoring, and improved patient engagement. However, as digital tools become more integrated into healthcare delivery, they also risk deepening existing health disparities if not implemented equitably. Digital health inequities refer to the uneven access to, usage of, and benefits from digital health solutions among various population groups. These disparities are shaped by multiple intersecting factors, including socioeconomic status, geography, education, age, language proficiency, ethnicity, disability, and technological literacy. For example, individuals in rural or low-income communities may lack access to reliable internet, digital devices, or the knowledge needed to navigate online health platforms. Elderly populations may struggle with new technology due to physical limitations or unfamiliarity, while non-native speakers may find it difficult to use health apps that are not available in their language. These challenges create significant barriers to accessing care through telemedicine, patient portals, health apps, and other digital health services. If left unaddressed, digital health inequities can exacerbate gaps in care, widen health outcome disparities, and reduce trust in healthcare systems. Moreover, systemic issues such as lack of infrastructure, underfunded health systems, and poorly designed digital tools often ignore the unique needs of marginalized communities (Fig. 7).

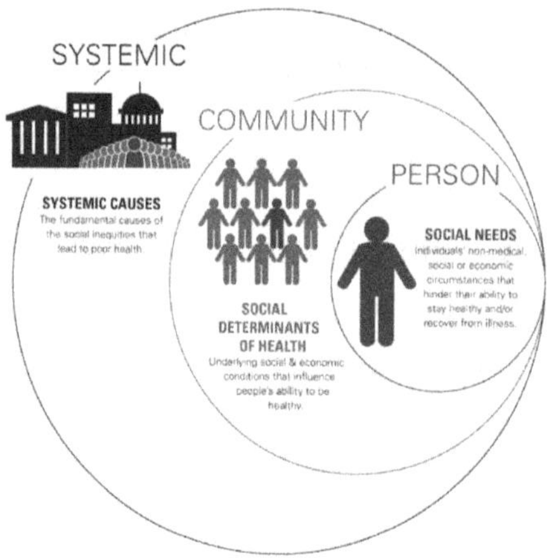

Fig.7 Digital Health Equity

Addressing digital health inequities requires a multi-faceted approach that combines inclusive design, culturally competent solutions, community engagement, education, and strong policy support. It involves creating technologies that are accessible and intuitive for all users, regardless of background, and implementing supportive infrastructure that ensures internet and device access for underserved populations. Efforts must also focus on improving digital literacy, fostering trust, and involving communities in the development and deployment of digital health initiatives. Equitable digital health systems must reflect the diversity of the populations they serve and actively work to remove barriers that limit participation. By centering equity in digital health strategy, we can ensure that technological innovation enhances care for everyone—not just those already privileged by access and resources. Bridging the digital divide is not only a technological challenge but also a moral imperative in the pursuit of universal, inclusive healthcare.

6.6.1 Understanding Digital Health Inequities

Digital health inequities refer to the imbalanced access to and use of digital health technologies across different populations, often leaving marginalized groups behind in the digital health revolution. While innovations like telemedicine, mobile health apps, and remote patient monitoring hold promise for improving healthcare outcomes, not all individuals or communities are equally positioned to benefit. These inequities are shaped by intersecting factors such as socioeconomic status, education level, age, gender, geographic location (especially rural vs. urban), race, and language proficiency. For instance, individuals in low-income or rural areas may lack internet connectivity or digital devices, and older adults may struggle with using new technologies due to limited digital literacy or physical impairments. Additionally, language barriers and culturally irrelevant content can alienate non-native speakers or minority populations. Understanding these disparities is critical for healthcare providers, technology developers, and policymakers who aim to deliver equitable care. Without intentional efforts to close these gaps, digital health tools could exacerbate existing health disparities rather than alleviate them. Therefore, recognizing digital health inequities is the foundational step toward designing inclusive systems, creating fair policies, and ultimately ensuring that all individuals—regardless of background—can benefit from technological advances in healthcare.

6.6.2 Barriers to Access and Use

Numerous barriers hinder equitable access and effective use of digital health technologies, especially for underrepresented or underserved populations. A primary obstacle is the digital divide, where individuals lack consistent internet access due to living in rural areas or belonging to low-income households. Without high-speed internet or smart devices, patients cannot use telehealth platforms or mobile apps designed for monitoring and managing their health. Additionally, the cost of digital tools and services can be prohibitive, limiting their reach among economically disadvantaged communities. Another key barrier is digital literacy—many individuals do not possess the basic skills needed to navigate apps, websites, or patient portals. Physical or cognitive disabilities can further complicate access, especially when technology is not designed to accommodate users with impairments. Language barriers and culturally irrelevant content can alienate non-native speakers or members of ethnic minorities. Some communities may also experience distrust in technology or the healthcare system, often due to historical discrimination or negative past experiences. Fear of data misuse or privacy violations can discourage people from engaging with digital platforms. Addressing these barriers requires not just technology upgrades but also a commitment to equitable infrastructure, education, culturally competent care, and community engagement tailored to the specific needs of different populations.

6.6.3 Inclusive Design and Development

Inclusive design is essential for ensuring that digital health technologies are usable and beneficial for everyone, regardless of their background or abilities. Many digital tools are created with a one-size-fits-all approach, which can unintentionally exclude users who face physical, cognitive, linguistic, or technological challenges. For example, a mobile health app that lacks screen reader compatibility excludes users who are visually impaired, while platforms available only in English may be inaccessible to non-English speakers. To promote equity, designers must prioritize universal accessibility from the beginning of the development process. This involves using clear, simple language, intuitive layouts, support for multiple languages, and compatibility with assistive technologies. Equally important is involving the target users—especially those from marginalized or underrepresented communities—through co-design and feedback processes. Their input ensures that the tools developed are relevant, effective, and aligned with their needs and contexts. Inclusive design is not just about accessibility; it's about fairness, respect, and responsiveness to the diverse realities of users. It enhances engagement, increases adoption rates, and helps digital health tools achieve their intended outcomes across the entire population. By embedding inclusivity into the design philosophy, developers can create health solutions that truly serve all.

6.6.4 Culturally Competent Solutions

Culturally competent digital health solutions are essential to ensuring that all individuals feel seen, respected, and understood within healthcare systems. Cultural competence means acknowledging the varied beliefs, traditions, languages, health practices, and social contexts that influence how people view health and illness. In digital health, this includes designing tools that are sensitive to these differences, such as offering content in multiple languages, using culturally appropriate imagery, and avoiding medical jargon that may be unfamiliar to certain populations. For example, health advice presented in a format that aligns with community norms or faith practices is more likely to be trusted and followed. Involving local stakeholders, community health workers, and cultural leaders in the creation and dissemination of digital health tools can improve trust and adoption. These individuals can serve as bridges between healthcare providers and diverse communities, ensuring that technology is both respectful and relevant. Cultural competence also extends to the user experience—how intuitive, relatable, and welcoming the digital tool feels to someone from a specific background. When health technologies are culturally tailored, they help break down barriers to access and foster more meaningful patient engagement. Ultimately, cultural competence is key to reducing disparities and promoting health equity in the digital age.

6.6.5 Education and Digital Literacy

Digital literacy is a critical enabler of equitable participation in digital health systems. Without the skills and confidence to use technology effectively, individuals may be unable to access vital health information, communicate with healthcare providers, or monitor their own health. Educational efforts must go beyond simply providing devices—they must empower users with practical knowledge on how to operate them. Training should include how to schedule virtual appointments, use patient portals, interpret digital health data, and navigate mobile apps. Tailored learning approaches are important—older adults, for instance, may benefit from hands-on, slower-paced training, while younger users may prefer interactive, mobile-friendly resources. Community centers, libraries, schools, and local health departments can serve as hubs for delivering digital literacy programs. Healthcare providers also play a key role by guiding patients in the use of digital tools and offering support during in-person visits. Materials should be available in multiple languages and formats to reach diverse populations. Boosting digital literacy not only reduces health inequities but also increases individuals' sense of autonomy and engagement in their own care. Ultimately, educating the public and building digital confidence is a long-term investment in both individual and community health outcomes.

6.6.6 Policy and Infrastructure Support

Addressing digital health inequities requires strong policy frameworks and investments in infrastructure that support inclusive and accessible healthcare for all. Governments and institutions must prioritize equitable access to broadband internet, especially in rural and underserved areas where connectivity remains a major challenge. Public funding can support the development and distribution of affordable or subsidized digital devices, ensuring that cost is not a barrier to participation. Policy should also enforce digital accessibility standards for all health technologies, mandating features that accommodate people with disabilities and linguistic diversity. Legal protections around data privacy, consent, and security are vital to building trust among users who may be hesitant to engage with digital health systems. Furthermore, governments should support local innovation through grants, incentives, and partnerships that encourage the development of culturally responsive, community-driven digital health solutions. Policies should be informed by real-world data on usage disparities and shaped in consultation with affected communities. Infrastructure support extends to training programs for healthcare providers, helping them integrate digital tools into their practice effectively and ethically. Overall, a coordinated policy and infrastructure strategy is essential to bridge the digital divide and ensure that digital health advancements benefit everyone, not just the digitally privileged.

7 Chapter

MARKET TRENDS AND INDUSTRY LANDSCAPE

7.0 INTRODUCTION: AN OVERVIEW

The rapid advancement of digital health technologies has transformed the healthcare landscape, offering new opportunities for remote care, continuous monitoring, and improved patient engagement. However, as digital tools become more integrated into healthcare delivery, they also risk deepening existing health disparities if not implemented equitably. Digital health inequities refer to the uneven access to, usage of, and benefits from digital health solutions among various population groups. These disparities are shaped by multiple intersecting factors, including socioeconomic status, geography, education, age, language proficiency, ethnicity, disability, and technological literacy. For example, individuals in rural or low-income communities may lack access to reliable internet, digital devices, or the knowledge needed to navigate online health platforms. Elderly populations may struggle with new technology due to physical limitations or unfamiliarity, while non-native speakers may find it difficult to use health apps that are not available in their language.

These challenges create significant barriers to accessing care through telemedicine, patient portals, health apps, and other digital health services. If left unaddressed, digital health inequities can exacerbate gaps in care, widen health outcome disparities, and reduce trust in healthcare systems. Moreover, systemic issues such as lack of infrastructure, underfunded health systems, and poorly designed digital tools often ignore the unique needs of marginalized communities. Addressing digital health inequities requires a multi-faceted approach that combines inclusive design, culturally competent solutions, community engagement, education, and strong policy support. It involves creating technologies that are accessible and intuitive for all users, regardless of background, and implementing supportive infrastructure that ensures internet and device access for underserved populations. Efforts must also focus on improving digital literacy, fostering trust, and involving communities in the development and deployment of digital health initiatives. Equitable digital health systems must reflect the diversity of the populations they serve and actively work to remove barriers that limit participation. By centering equity in digital health strategy, we can ensure that technological innovation enhances care for everyone—not just those already privileged by access and resources. Bridging the digital divide is not only a technological challenge but also a moral imperative in the pursuit of universal, inclusive healthcare.

7.1 MAJOR PLAYERS IN THE WEARABLE AND DIGITAL HEALTH INDUSTRY

The wearable and digital health industry has witnessed explosive growth over the past decade, transforming how individuals engage with their health and how care is delivered. Driven by advances in sensor technology, mobile computing, data analytics, and artificial intelligence (AI), digital health tools have evolved from basic fitness trackers into sophisticated health monitoring systems capable of detecting early signs of illness, managing chronic diseases, and enabling continuous patient engagement. The shift toward value-based care, increased demand for remote health monitoring, and greater health awareness among consumers—particularly after the COVID-19 pandemic—have accelerated this trend globally. Wearables now go beyond counting steps or tracking calories. They provide real-time insights into heart rate variability, blood oxygen saturation, respiratory patterns, stress levels, sleep cycles, and even ECG readings. These metrics, once only available in clinical settings, are now being tracked passively and continuously in everyday life, giving users and healthcare providers a more complete view of individual health trajectories. As healthcare systems increasingly adopt virtual care models, the ability of wearables to collect, transmit, and analyze health data is becoming essential for early intervention and personalized treatment (Fig. 1).

The market is led by major consumer electronics companies, medical device giants, and innovative startups—all contributing unique capabilities. Companies like Apple, Google, and Samsung have leveraged their consumer tech ecosystems to deliver health-centric devices that combine sleek design with powerful analytics. Devices like the Apple Watch, Fitbit, and Galaxy Watch are not just accessories but integral tools for wellness, fitness, and preventive care. Their integration with mobile apps and cloud platforms has empowered millions of users to take control of their health data and share it securely with caregivers and clinicians. On the other hand, performance-focused wearables from Garmin, Whoop, and Oura cater to athletes and wellness enthusiasts seeking in-depth insights into recovery, strain, and sleep quality.

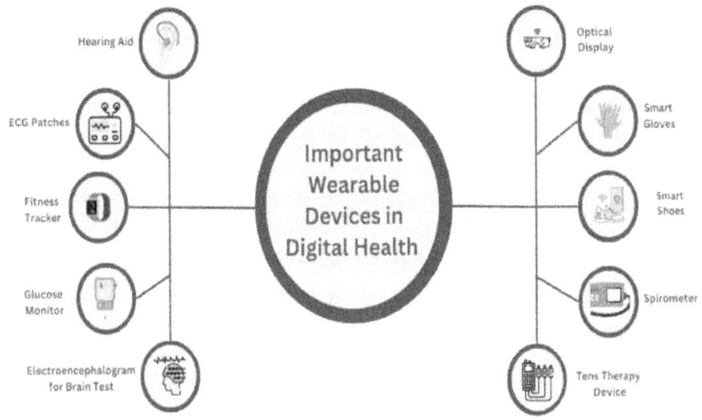

Fig. 1 Integration of wearable technology and artificial intelligence in digital health

These companies are expanding their appeal to broader consumer and research markets by offering validated, high-accuracy metrics that contribute to behavioral change and early illness detection. The Oura Ring, for instance, has gained popularity not only among users but also in scientific studies for monitoring early symptoms of viral infections and tracking recovery patterns. Alongside consumer-oriented players, traditional MedTech companies such as Philips, GE Healthcare, and Siemens Healthineers are bringing clinical-grade monitoring devices into the digital age. They are integrating remote patient monitoring into hospital workflows and chronic care management, leveraging AI and IoT to enable smarter diagnostics, post-discharge care, and hospital-at-home models. Their deep clinical expertise and regulatory compliance make them key partners in healthcare transformation. Meanwhile, a wave of startups and digital health innovators is reshaping the landscape through highly targeted, often FDA-approved wearables designed for specific conditions or populations. Companies like AliveCor, Empatica, BioBeat, and Zio by iRhythm are producing medical-grade devices capable of remote ECG monitoring, seizure detection, respiratory health tracking, and more. These tools are particularly valuable in managing chronic diseases, supporting clinical trials, and expanding access to underserved or rural communities through telehealth solutions.

The future of the wearable and digital health industry is characterized by interoperability, personalization, and integration with healthcare systems. As these technologies continue to mature, the focus is shifting toward building ecosystems that can deliver holistic health experiences—from prevention to diagnosis to treatment and recovery. Collaboration between tech companies, healthcare providers, insurers, and regulators will be critical in ensuring that these innovations are safe, effective, and equitably accessible. The major players in this space are not only redefining consumer health but also driving a systemic shift in how health information is collected, interpreted, and acted upon. Their innovations are at the heart of a more connected, proactive, and patient-centered model of care that holds great promise for the future of global health.

7.1.1 Apple Inc.

Apple is a dominant force in the wearable and digital health landscape, primarily through its Apple Watch and HealthKit platform. The Apple Watch offers advanced features such as ECG recording, irregular heart rhythm notifications, blood oxygen level monitoring, and sleep tracking—all presented in a user-friendly format. Integrated with the iPhone and the Health app, it allows users to view and manage their wellness data securely and in real time. HealthKit enables seamless data sharing between apps and healthcare providers, supporting a growing ecosystem of health-focused apps. Apple's commitment to privacy ensures user data is encrypted and only shared with permission. The company also partners with academic institutions and health organizations for large-scale research, such as studies on heart health and women's health. Apple's recent focus on detecting chronic conditions and falls further positions the brand at the intersection of preventive care and personal health management. With ongoing software updates and hardware improvements, Apple continues to push the boundaries of consumer digital health innovation.

7.1.2 Google (Alphabet Inc.)

Google, through its parent company Alphabet, is deeply involved in shaping the future of digital health. Its acquisition of Fitbit brought an established line of consumer wearables into its portfolio, offering heart rate monitoring, stress tracking, sleep analytics, and active zone minutes to millions of users worldwide. Fitbit devices now integrate closely with the Google ecosystem, including Google Fit and Android Health APIs, offering users a seamless wellness experience. Beyond hardware, Google is investing heavily in artificial intelligence applications in healthcare via DeepMind and Google Health, developing tools for medical imaging diagnostics, predictive modeling, and personalized health insights. Google Cloud is also a major player in storing and analyzing healthcare data securely for institutions. The company is experimenting with AI for diabetic retinopathy screening, cancer detection, and clinical documentation. Through these efforts, Google aims not only to serve consumers but also to provide tools for clinicians and researchers to transform care delivery. It is becoming a full-spectrum digital health provider, from wearables to medical-grade solutions.

7.1.3 Samsung

Samsung has carved a strong presence in the digital health market with its Galaxy Watch series and Samsung Health platform. The Galaxy Watch features robust health tracking tools, including real-time heart rate monitoring, ECG recording, blood pressure tracking (in select markets), oxygen saturation, and advanced sleep analysis. The watches are designed to integrate seamlessly with Android devices and work in tandem with Samsung Health—a comprehensive app that helps users track their fitness, nutrition, stress levels, and menstrual health. Samsung is actively expanding its ecosystem by collaborating with hospitals, academic institutions, and research partners to validate the accuracy of its health sensors and explore clinical use cases. The company's innovation extends to sensors like bioelectrical impedance analysis (BIA) for body composition and SpO2 tracking. Samsung's hardware reliability, coupled with its focus on user-friendly design and health insights, makes it a key competitor in both consumer wellness and emerging clinical applications. Its investments in AI, 5G, and remote health monitoring suggest long-term commitment to connected healthcare.

7.1.4 Garmin

Garmin has built a reputation for producing highly reliable, fitness-focused wearable devices that appeal especially to athletes, outdoor enthusiasts, and health-conscious users. Its product lines, including Forerunner, Fenix, and Vivosmart, offer in-depth health and performance metrics like VO2 max, respiration rate, stress levels, sleep stages, pulse oximetry (SpO2), and heart rate variability. Many devices include built-in GPS for precise tracking of outdoor activities and multisport performance, making them favorites among runners, cyclists, and triathletes. Garmin Connect, the companion app, allows users to visualize their health trends and set goals. With long battery life and rugged design, Garmin's wearables are built for continuous use in demanding conditions. The brand is increasingly being integrated into digital wellness programs, workplace health platforms, and academic health studies. Garmin also offers Enterprise Health solutions for organizations looking to encourage employee wellness. As wearables move into healthcare and research domains, Garmin's accuracy and data depth make it a trusted partner in digital health analytics.

7.1.5 Whoop

Whoop has established itself as a premium health and performance optimization platform aimed at athletes, professionals, and wellness enthusiasts. Its wrist-worn, screenless wearable continuously tracks key physiological metrics, including heart rate variability (HRV), resting heart rate, respiratory rate, and sleep efficiency. The system calculates "strain" and "recovery" scores to guide users in balancing activity and rest for optimal performance. What sets Whoop apart is its subscription-based business model, which gives users access to personalized insights, performance coaching, and community challenges. The platform's data-driven approach has been adopted by professional sports teams, military personnel, and corporate wellness programs. Whoop has also contributed to health research, such as identifying early signs of illness, including COVID-19, through respiratory metrics. The brand emphasizes user education and habit formation, providing detailed feedback and coaching tips. With a focus on continual improvement and a commitment to scientific validation, Whoop is influencing how health data is personalized and applied in real-world scenarios.

7.1.6 Oura Health

Oura Health is the company behind the Oura Ring, a sleek and discreet smart ring that focuses on sleep tracking, recovery, and holistic wellness. Worn on the finger, the device captures detailed biometric data including heart rate, heart rate variability, body temperature, respiratory rate, and sleep cycles. The Oura app provides users with a daily "Readiness Score" to guide activity decisions based on sleep and recovery. Oura is especially popular among biohackers, wellness influencers, and those looking for a minimalistic alternative to wrist-based wearables. Its unobtrusive form factor makes it suitable for 24/7 wear, including sleep tracking without discomfort. The ring has gained traction in health research and was used in studies during the COVID-19 pandemic to identify early symptoms. Oura has also partnered with organizations for corporate wellness and mental health tracking. The company's focus on privacy, personalized insights, and long battery life makes it a standout in the wellness-tech market. As Oura continues to innovate, it remains a leader in passive, continuous health monitoring.

7.1.7 MedTech Companies (Philips, GE Healthcare, Siemens Healthineers)

eading medical technology companies like Philips, GE Healthcare, and Siemens Healthineers are bringing clinical-grade digital solutions into the wearable and remote health space. These companies have long histories in diagnostic imaging, patient monitoring, and hospital equipment, and are now applying their expertise to connected health technologies. Their solutions include wearable biosensors, remote patient monitoring platforms, and AI-assisted diagnostic tools that support chronic disease management and post-discharge care. For instance, Philips' wearable biosensors can track respiratory rate, heart rate, and mobility in real time to alert clinicians about patient deterioration. These MedTech giants integrate wearables with cloud platforms, electronic health records (EHR), and AI analytics, enabling clinicians to monitor patients remotely and intervene early. These solutions support population health management, reduce hospital readmissions, and improve care coordination. Their regulatory experience and global scale give them a competitive advantage in deploying clinical-grade technology, making them indispensable in bridging the gap between hospital care and home-based digital health.

7.1.8 Startups and Innovators

Startups and health-tech innovators play a vital role in pushing the boundaries of wearable technology and personalized health. Companies such as BioBeat, Empatica, AliveCor, and Zio by iRhythm are bringing FDA-cleared, clinical-grade wearables to the market. These devices offer real-time tracking of vitals like ECG, oxygen saturation, blood pressure, and arrhythmia detection, making them valuable in both research and clinical environments. Empatica's wearable can detect seizures and stress, while AliveCor's Kardia device enables consumers to perform ECGs at home. Startups are also targeting niche areas—Bloomlife focuses on maternal health, Spire works on respiratory tracking, and others address mental wellness, diabetes management, and remote rehabilitation. Many of these innovators collaborate with hospitals, research institutions, and pharmaceutical companies to validate and deploy their solutions. Their agility allows them to innovate faster than larger corporations, offering personalized, data-rich, and often AI-powered solutions. As the demand for remote care grows, startups are positioned to revolutionize how healthcare is accessed and delivered.

7.2 MARKET SIZE, GROWTH, AND FORECASTS:

The wearable and digital health market has experienced remarkable growth over the past decade, transforming how healthcare is delivered, monitored, and managed globally. Driven by rapid technological advancements, increasing consumer health awareness, and shifting healthcare paradigms, this market is poised for continued expansion in the coming years. Wearable devices, such as smartwatches and fitness trackers, have become ubiquitous, offering users the ability to continuously monitor vital signs, physical activity, sleep patterns, and more. This real-time data collection empowers individuals to take proactive steps toward managing their health while providing healthcare professionals with valuable insights for personalized care. Simultaneously, the integration of artificial intelligence (AI), machine learning, and big data analytics has significantly enhanced the capabilities of digital health platforms, enabling predictive health insights, early diagnosis, and tailored treatment plans. The global rise in chronic diseases like diabetes, cardiovascular conditions, and respiratory illnesses is further accelerating demand for remote patient monitoring solutions, which facilitate continuous health management beyond traditional clinical settings. Furthermore, the COVID-19 pandemic acted as a catalyst for digital health adoption by highlighting the importance of remote care, telemedicine, and contactless monitoring technologies, prompting healthcare systems worldwide to embrace innovation at an unprecedented pace.

Geographically, North America maintains a dominant position due to its advanced healthcare infrastructure, high digital literacy, and substantial investment in health technology innovation. Europe follows closely, with aging populations and government-led digital health initiatives driving adoption. Meanwhile, the Asia-Pacific region is witnessing the fastest growth, fueled by large populations, increasing smartphone penetration, and a burgeoning middle class eager to adopt health technologies. Emerging markets in Latin America, Africa, and the Middle East are also beginning to embrace digital health solutions, supported by expanding mobile connectivity and targeted government policies. Market forecasts indicate a compound annual growth rate (CAGR) of 12–15% from 2025 to 2030, with the global wearable and digital health market expected to reach an estimated value between USD 300 billion and USD 350 billion by 2030. This impressive growth is underpinned by several factors, including ongoing innovations in wearable sensor technology, the proliferation of digital therapeutics, and the integration of connected health platforms within clinical workflows. Wearables are evolving beyond passive fitness trackers to become comprehensive health management companions that offer real-time diagnostics, medication adherence reminders, and behavioral coaching to promote healthier lifestyles.

In addition to consumer-driven growth, business-to-business (B2B) partnerships are emerging as key growth drivers. Collaborations between wearable manufacturers, health insurers, pharmaceutical companies, and healthcare providers are enabling the development of integrated digital health ecosystems that improve patient outcomes while reducing costs. Moreover, regulatory bodies worldwide are beginning to establish clearer guidelines and approval pathways for clinical-grade digital health solutions, which is expected to accelerate market adoption and innovation. Despite the optimistic outlook, the market faces challenges such as data privacy concerns, cybersecurity risks, high costs of advanced devices in developing regions, and a lack of standardized interoperability across platforms. Addressing these obstacles is critical to unlocking the full potential of wearable and digital health technologies on a global scale. Ongoing efforts to enhance digital literacy, expand broadband access, and harmonize regulations will play a vital role in overcoming these barriers.

The wearable and digital health market represents a dynamic and rapidly evolving landscape shaped by technological innovation, changing consumer behaviours, and the global imperative to improve healthcare delivery. With continued advancements and strategic collaborations, this market is well-positioned to revolutionize healthcare, making it more personalized, accessible, and effective for populations worldwide. As digital health becomes increasingly mainstream, stakeholders must remain agile to capitalize on emerging opportunities and navigate challenges in this transformative era.

7.2.1 Current Market Size

As of 2025, the global wearable and digital health market is valued at approximately USD 150 to 160 billion, reflecting a significant expansion fueled by widespread adoption of innovative health technologies. This broad market encompasses a diverse range of products and services, including fitness wearables, smartwatches equipped with advanced health tracking capabilities, remote patient monitoring (RPM) devices, mobile health (mHealth) applications, and emerging digital therapeutics that deliver software-based treatment solutions. The rapid growth in this sector is a testament to increasing consumer health awareness, the rising prevalence of chronic diseases, and a shift towards proactive health management. Among these, smartwatches with features such as heart rate monitoring, ECG, blood oxygen saturation, sleep analysis, and activity tracking have become mainstream tools for personal health and wellness. The United States dominates the market, holding the largest share due to its mature healthcare infrastructure, high technology adoption rates, and substantial investment in research and development. North America benefits from a tech-savvy population that embraces new digital health innovations and robust regulatory frameworks that support market growth. Europe follows as the second-largest market, driven by government initiatives aimed at digitizing healthcare, an aging population that requires continuous health monitoring, and increased funding for telehealth services. Countries in the Asia-Pacific region, such as China, India, Japan, and South Korea, are experiencing the fastest market expansion, thanks to rapid smartphone penetration, an expanding middle class, and vibrant startup ecosystems focused on digital health innovation.

The surge in consumer demand is further amplified by advancements in wearable sensor technology and artificial intelligence, which have enabled more accurate, real-time health monitoring and personalized data-driven insights. Remote patient monitoring devices have become crucial in managing chronic conditions, reducing hospital visits, and enabling continuous care outside traditional healthcare settings. Meanwhile, mobile health applications are increasingly popular, offering digital coaching, symptom tracking, virtual consultations, and medication management, thus empowering users to take control of their health. Additionally, digital therapeutics—a relatively new but rapidly growing segment—leverages software interventions to treat or manage specific medical conditions such as anxiety, diabetes, and insomnia, offering non-invasive alternatives or complements to traditional therapies. The integration of these digital tools into clinical workflows is accelerating, supported by telehealth infrastructure improvements, cloud computing, and interoperability standards. Furthermore, partnerships between wearable manufacturers, healthcare providers, insurers, and pharmaceutical companies are creating comprehensive digital health ecosystems that enhance patient outcomes and reduce overall healthcare costs. Investment in telehealth infrastructure has surged globally, driven by both private and public sectors, further facilitating market growth. The COVID-19 pandemic acted as a catalyst, highlighting the need for remote monitoring and virtual care solutions, which are now being adopted as standard components of healthcare delivery. However, the market also faces challenges such as ensuring data privacy and security, managing regulatory compliance across different regions, and addressing disparities in digital literacy and access. Overcoming these hurdles will be vital to sustaining growth and expanding the reach of wearable and digital health technologies. The 2025 wearable and digital health market is a dynamic and rapidly evolving space, marked by robust consumer interest, technological innovation, and strategic investments. With continuous advancements in device capabilities, AI-powered analytics, and integrated care models, the market is set to grow significantly, transforming healthcare by making it more personalized, accessible, and preventive worldwide.

7.2.2 Market Growth Drivers

The growth of the wearable and digital health market is propelled by several key drivers that shape consumer demand and industry innovation. Increasing health awareness and the rising prevalence of chronic diseases are pushing individuals to adopt health monitoring technologies. Advances in sensor technology, artificial intelligence, and data analytics are enabling more accurate and personalized health insights. The expansion of smartphone use and improved internet connectivity further facilitate access to digital health tools. Additionally, supportive government policies, rising healthcare costs, and the shift toward remote care and preventive medicine are fueling market expansion. Together, these factors create a dynamic environment for rapid growth and evolving healthcare delivery models.

Several key factors are fueling the expansion of the wearable and digital health market:

- Rising prevalence of chronic diseases (e.g., diabetes, hypertension).
- Aging population with increasing healthcare needs.
- Demand for remote monitoring and home-based care.
- Surge in health-conscious consumers post-COVID-19.
- Integration of AI, cloud computing, and real-time analytics.
- Government initiatives supporting digital transformation in healthcare.

These drivers are pushing both consumers and healthcare providers to adopt wearable health technologies more widely.

7.2.3 Regional Insights

Regional insights provide a critical understanding of how geographic, economic, and cultural factors influence the adoption and growth of wearable and digital health technologies worldwide. Different regions exhibit unique market dynamics shaped by healthcare infrastructure, regulatory environments, technology readiness, and population demographics. North America leads with its advanced digital ecosystem and high healthcare expenditure, while Europe follows with strong government support for health digitization and aging populations. The Asia-Pacific region is experiencing rapid expansion driven by large populations, smartphone penetration, and innovation hubs. Emerging markets in Latin America and Africa face infrastructure and affordability challenges but show promising adoption through mobile health solutions. Analyzing these regional variations helps stakeholders tailor strategies and solutions to meet diverse market needs and unlock growth opportunities globally.

- **North America:** North America continues to lead the wearable and digital health market, driven by high levels of technology adoption and a robust digital infrastructure. The region benefits from significant healthcare spending, strong consumer demand, and advanced research and development ecosystems. The presence of major industry players and startups fosters continuous innovation, particularly in AI integration and personalized health monitoring. Additionally, widespread smartphone usage and high internet penetration support seamless connectivity for digital health platforms. Government initiatives and regulatory frameworks also encourage the adoption of telehealth and remote monitoring technologies. The region's mature healthcare system increasingly embraces digital solutions to improve patient outcomes, manage chronic diseases, and reduce costs. North America's leadership position is likely to remain strong as investments in health IT infrastructure and data security continue to grow.
- **Europe:** Europe ranks as the second-largest market for wearable and digital health technologies, driven by substantial investments in telemedicine and health digitization programs backed by governments. The region faces demographic shifts, including aging populations, which increase demand for remote care and chronic disease management solutions. European countries benefit from strong healthcare infrastructure and progressive policies promoting interoperability and data privacy, enhancing user trust in digital health. The growing emphasis on value-based care further encourages the integration of wearables and mobile health apps in clinical workflows. Additionally, increased funding for health innovation hubs and startups accelerates the development of region-specific solutions. Language diversity and varying healthcare systems across countries pose challenges, but ongoing collaboration aims to standardize and harmonize digital health adoption across the continent.

- **Asia-Pacific:** Asia-Pacific is currently the fastest-growing market for wearable and digital health technologies, fueled by rapid smartphone penetration, expanding middle-class populations, and a surge of innovation from startups. Countries like China, India, Japan, South Korea, and Australia are leading this growth by investing heavily in healthcare digitization and infrastructure development. The region's large population base creates a vast market for affordable and accessible health monitoring solutions. Increasing awareness of preventive healthcare and rising chronic disease prevalence are driving demand for digital health tools. Governments in the region are actively promoting policies to support telehealth and remote monitoring. Despite some challenges related to infrastructure and digital literacy, the region's dynamic economies and technological advancements position it as a key driver of future industry expansion.
- **Latin America and Africa:** Latin America and Africa represent emerging markets with significant potential for growth in digital health, despite facing persistent infrastructure challenges such as limited broadband access and healthcare disparities. In these regions, mobile health adoption is rapidly gaining traction as smartphones become more widespread, providing critical access points for health information and services. Governments and non-governmental organizations are increasingly supporting initiatives to expand digital health through funding, policy reforms, and public-private partnerships. There is growing interest in telemedicine and remote patient monitoring as ways to overcome geographical and resource limitations in healthcare delivery. While digital literacy and affordability remain barriers, innovative, low-cost solutions tailored to local needs are helping to bridge the gap. As infrastructure improves, these regions are expected to become important growth markets in the wearable and digital health ecosystem..

7.2.4 Segment-wise Breakdown

he wearable and digital health industry is a diverse ecosystem composed of several distinct segments, each contributing uniquely to the overall market growth and innovation. Understanding the segment-wise breakdown is essential for grasping how different technologies and applications serve various user needs and healthcare goals. The largest segment, wearable devices, dominates the market by offering continuous health and fitness tracking to millions of consumers worldwide. Meanwhile, remote patient monitoring (RPM) is rapidly gaining momentum as it addresses the growing demand for chronic disease management and elderly care outside traditional healthcare settings. Mobile health apps form another vital segment, providing users with accessible tools for digital coaching, symptom assessment, and virtual healthcare consultations.

Emerging areas such as digital therapeutics focus on software-driven treatments for specific medical conditions, offering new avenues for non-pharmacological intervention. Additionally, the enterprise and clinical use segment is expanding as hospitals, clinics, and corporations adopt these technologies to enhance patient care and employee wellness programs. Together, these segments reflect a dynamic and evolving market landscape, driven by technological innovation, changing healthcare paradigms, and increasing consumer demand for personalized, convenient health solutions. A detailed examination of each segment reveals the unique opportunities, challenges, and growth trajectories shaping the future of digital health.

- **Wearable Devices:** Wearable devices, such as smartwatches and fitness bands, represent the largest and most established segment within the digital health market, accounting for over 50% of the total market share. These devices have gained widespread popularity due to their ability to continuously track vital signs like heart rate, activity levels, sleep patterns, and blood oxygen saturation. Their seamless integration with smartphones and health apps allows users to monitor their wellness in real time. Beyond fitness enthusiasts, wearables are increasingly being used by individuals managing chronic conditions and those interested in preventive health. Manufacturers continue to innovate with improved sensors, longer battery life, and new features like ECG monitoring, expanding the functionality of these devices. As consumer demand grows, wearables remain a cornerstone of the digital health ecosystem.
- **Remote Patient Monitoring (RPM):** Remote Patient Monitoring (RPM) is one of the fastest-growing segments in digital health, driven largely by the rising need to manage chronic diseases and provide care for aging populations outside traditional clinical settings. RPM technologies enable healthcare providers to track patient health data such as blood pressure, glucose levels, and respiratory function remotely, reducing hospital visits and enabling timely interventions. This approach improves patient outcomes by facilitating continuous monitoring, early detection of complications, and personalized treatment adjustments. The COVID-19 pandemic further accelerated RPM adoption as healthcare systems sought to limit in-person contact. With advancements in wireless connectivity and wearable sensors, RPM is poised to become a vital component of home-based healthcare and chronic disease management worldwide.
- **Mobile Health Apps:** Mobile health applications have experienced rapid expansion as users increasingly seek convenient, on-demand health services. These apps offer a broad range of functionalities, including

digital coaching, symptom checkers, medication reminders, and virtual consultations with healthcare professionals. They empower individuals to take charge of their health by providing personalized insights and easy access to medical advice. The rise of smartphones globally has been a significant catalyst for mobile health app adoption, enabling real-time data collection and interaction. Moreover, the integration of AI and machine learning enhances app capabilities by offering tailored recommendations and predictive health analytics. As digital health literacy improves, mobile apps will play an essential role in expanding healthcare access and engagement.

- **Digital Therapeutics (DTx):** Digital Therapeutics (DTx) is an emerging and rapidly growing segment focused on delivering evidence-based therapeutic interventions through software applications. These tools are designed to prevent, manage, or treat medical conditions such as anxiety, diabetes, insomnia, and substance use disorders. Unlike general wellness apps, DTx products undergo rigorous clinical validation and regulatory approval processes, positioning them as complementary or alternative treatments alongside traditional therapies. By leveraging behavioral science, cognitive therapy, and real-time data, digital therapeutics provide scalable, personalized treatment options that can be accessed remotely. This niche market is gaining recognition for its potential to reduce healthcare costs, improve patient adherence, and enhance outcomes, particularly in mental health and chronic disease management.
- **Enterprise and Clinical Use:** The adoption of wearable devices and digital health tools in enterprise and clinical settings is steadily increasing, driven by the need to enhance patient care, improve clinical workflows, and promote employee wellness. Hospitals and clinics are integrating wearables for real-time monitoring of patients' vital signs, supporting telehealth consultations, and facilitating remote diagnostics. This integration improves care coordination and allows for more proactive health management, especially for patients with chronic or complex conditions. In the corporate sector, wellness programs increasingly use wearables and health apps to encourage healthy behaviors, reduce absenteeism, and lower healthcare costs. As digital health solutions prove their value in improving outcomes and operational efficiency, their use within institutional and enterprise environments is expected to continue growing rapidly.

7.2.5 Market Challenges

Despite the impressive growth and promising future of the wearable and digital health industry, there remain significant challenges that could impede widespread adoption and limit the full realization of its potential. One of the foremost concerns is data privacy and cybersecurity. Wearable devices collect vast amounts of sensitive personal health information, making them prime targets for cyberattacks. Ensuring robust data protection and maintaining user trust is critical, especially as regulations around data privacy become more stringent worldwide. In addition, the industry faces regulatory hurdles, particularly for clinical-grade wearables that require stringent approval processes to ensure safety, accuracy, and efficacy. These regulatory challenges can delay product launches and increase development costs. Another major obstacle is the lack of standardization across platforms and devices, which complicates data interoperability and integration with existing healthcare systems. This fragmentation limits the ability of healthcare providers to leverage wearable data fully and can confuse consumers faced with multiple incompatible solutions. Moreover, the high cost of advanced wearable devices poses a significant barrier in emerging economies and among underserved populations, where affordability remains a primary concern. Without addressing pricing and accessibility, these regions risk being left behind in the digital health revolution. Digital literacy is also a critical issue. Many users, especially older adults or those in rural areas, may lack the skills or confidence to effectively use wearable technologies, limiting the impact of these tools on health outcomes. Education and user-friendly designs are essential to overcome this gap. Addressing these multifaceted challenges through technological innovation, policy development, and inclusive design will be key to ensuring that wearable health technologies can achieve their transformative promise on a global scale.

Despite growth, several challenges must be addressed:

- Data privacy and cybersecurity concerns.
- Regulatory hurdles for clinical-grade wearables.
- Lack of standardization across platforms.
- High cost of advanced wearables in emerging economies.
- Limited digital literacy among some user groups.

Overcoming these challenges is key to scaling adoption and unlocking the full potential of digital health solutions.

7.2.6 Market Forecast (2025–2030)

Between 2025 and 2030, the wearable and digital health industry is anticipated to experience robust growth, with projections indicating a compound annual growth rate (CAGR) of 12–15%. This surge is expected to push the global market size from its current valuation of approximately USD 160 billion to between USD 300 and 350 billion by 2030. Several converging factors are driving this expansion.

One of the most significant is the increasing personalization of healthcare, with wearables becoming more attuned to individual health profiles, behaviors, and risk factors. Devices are transitioning from simple fitness trackers to intelligent health management tools capable of real-time diagnostics, chronic condition monitoring, and early illness detection. Artificial Intelligence (AI) and machine learning will play a transformative role during this period, enabling wearables to provide predictive insights, adaptive health recommendations, and anomaly detection with unprecedented accuracy. Health data collected via sensors will be continuously analyzed and interpreted in real time, offering users proactive alerts, medication reminders, and personalized coaching for lifestyle improvement. Integration into electronic health records (EHRs) and clinical workflows will further embed wearables into formal healthcare systems, making them essential tools for physicians and care teams. Another major growth catalyst will be the expansion of business-to-business (B2B) partnerships, particularly with health insurers, pharmaceutical companies, and enterprise wellness providers. Insurers will leverage wearable data to tailor health plans, encourage preventive care, and reduce long-term costs through data-driven decision-making. Pharmaceutical firms will increasingly integrate wearables into clinical trials for real-world evidence and patient monitoring. Moreover, corporate wellness programs will continue to adopt wearables as tools for enhancing employee well-being, productivity, and health engagement. Additionally, aging populations and rising chronic disease burdens globally will create a sustained demand for remote health monitoring, particularly in home settings. Digital health platforms will become more inclusive, accessible, and multilingual, further expanding their reach into emerging markets. Governments and healthcare institutions will likely introduce policy incentives and infrastructure investments to support digital health adoption. By 2030, the wearable and digital health industry will no longer be viewed as supplementary to traditional care, but rather as a core component of a connected, patient-centered, and data-informed healthcare ecosystem. This evolution marks a fundamental shift toward proactive, continuous, and personalized care delivery on a global scale.

7.3 ROLE OF STARTUPS AND INNOVATION HUBS

Startups and innovation hubs play a pivotal role in shaping the wearable and digital health industry by driving rapid technological advancement and fostering a culture of creativity and agility. Unlike large established corporations, startups possess the flexibility to experiment with disruptive ideas and cutting-edge technologies, which often leads to breakthrough innovations in health monitoring, diagnostics, and personalized care. These young companies are instrumental in developing novel sensor technologies, artificial intelligence algorithms, and data analytics platforms that enhance the accuracy, usability, and accessibility of wearable devices. Their contributions are vital in pushing the boundaries of what digital health tools can achieve, enabling the industry to transition from simple fitness tracking toward more sophisticated health management and disease prevention solutions. In addition to their innovative capacity, startups often focus on niche markets or underserved populations that may be overlooked by larger players. This includes specialized areas such as mental health, women's health, chronic disease management, and pediatric care, where tailored solutions can significantly improve patient outcomes. By addressing these unmet needs, startups contribute to making digital health more inclusive and responsive to diverse healthcare challenges. Furthermore, startups tend to adopt a user-centered design philosophy, continuously incorporating feedback from patients, healthcare providers, and caregivers. This iterative development process results in more intuitive and effective health technologies that are better aligned with real-world use cases.

Innovation hubs and incubators provide essential support systems that nurture startups, offering mentorship, access to funding, technical resources, and industry connections. These environments create fertile ground for collaboration between startups, established healthcare organizations, academic institutions, and investors. Such partnerships are crucial for validating new technologies through clinical trials, ensuring compliance with regulatory standards, and facilitating market entry. Innovation hubs also promote knowledge exchange and cross-disciplinary teamwork, which are key drivers of breakthrough discoveries in wearable health tech. By fostering ecosystems that bring together diverse stakeholders, innovation hubs accelerate the pace of product development and commercialization. Startups also play a critical role in expanding the digital health ecosystem by developing interoperable solutions that integrate seamlessly with electronic health records (EHR), telemedicine platforms, and other healthcare infrastructure. This connectivity enhances continuity of care and enables more holistic health management. Moreover, many startups adopt subscription or software-as-a-service (SaaS) business models, offering scalable solutions that can adapt to evolving healthcare needs and regulatory requirements. This agility helps bridge gaps between technology innovation and healthcare delivery.

Globally, innovation hubs in regions such as Silicon Valley, Boston, Berlin, and Bangalore act as vibrant centers of entrepreneurial activity, attracting talent, capital, and expertise. These hubs facilitate cross-border collaborations and knowledge sharing, allowing promising technologies to reach international markets. Additionally, startups and innovation hubs actively engage with policymakers and regulatory bodies to shape frameworks that promote innovation while safeguarding patient safety and data privacy. Their involvement ensures that emerging wearable and digital health technologies are developed and deployed within responsible and compliant guidelines. Overall, startups and innovation hubs are indispensable engines of growth and transformation within the wearable and digital health sector. Their dynamic contributions not only foster technological progress but also help democratize healthcare access and improve patient outcomes worldwide. As the digital health landscape continues to evolve rapidly, the role of startups and innovation hubs will only become more crucial in driving sustainable innovation and creating a future where technology and healthcare converge seamlessly.

7.3.1 Driving Technological Innovation

Startups occupy a unique position at the cutting edge of technological advancement within the wearable and digital health landscape. Freed from the bureaucratic inertia often found in large corporations, they can take bold leaps in sensor design, device form factor, and AI-driven analytics. Many startups are responsible for launching novel biosensors capable of detecting subtle physiological signals—such as continuous glucose monitoring, skin hydration levels, or early indicators of atrial fibrillation—that exceed the capabilities of traditional wearables. These companies typically rely on agile development methodologies, enabling rapid iteration of prototypes, quick validation cycles, and early market feedback loops. This fast-paced innovation pipeline accelerates time to market and shortens development timelines from years to just months. Combined with partnerships for cloud-based AI platforms, startups are also advancing real-time disease prediction algorithms and personalized risk scoring tools that adapt to individual health profiles. By integrating emerging technologies like flexible electronics, voice-activated health prompts, and multimodal sensor fusion, startups are redefining what wearable devices can measure and predict. Their research-and-development models often blend cross-disciplinary teams—engineers, clinicians, UX designers, and data scientists—to create solutions that are not only functional but also user-friendly. These innovations enrich the sector with fresh ideas that larger players adopt or build upon, raising the bar for health-technology advancement across the ecosystem.

7.3.2 Addressing Niche and Unmet Needs

While tech giants often target broadly defined health markets, startups dive into highly specific use cases that remain underserved. For instance, some focus on women's health solutions like fertility awareness, pregnancy tracking, or endometriosis monitoring—areas traditionally overlooked due to their complexity or perceived limited scale. Others specialize in mental wellness, building wearables that detect early signs of anxiety or chronic stress using HRV and sleep pattern analytics. Pediatric wearables that monitor vital signs in neonates and infants are another example of tailored products responding to critical needs in sensitive populations. Startups also target rare disease tracking or remote monitoring for immunocompromised patients, enabling continuous data-driven insights that facilitate early intervention. By tailoring devices and software interfaces around distinct demographic needs, language preferences, or cultural sensitivities, these companies improve adherence and outcomes. They frequently employ human-centered design strategies, conducting immersive user research with specific groups to align features and user flows to lived experiences. In doing so, they create holistic solutions—combining wearable hardware, companion apps, coaching content, and community support networks—that are hyper-contextualized and clinically relevant. Much of their growth relies on measurable user impact, such as improved medication adherence, reduced hospital visits, or elevated quality-of-life scores for underrepresented health populations.

7.3.3 Collaboration with Healthcare Providers and Academia

Partnerships between startups and academic or clinical institutions are foundational for validating the clinical performance and safety of new wearable technologies. These collaborations often involve multi-site clinical trials, user studies, and pilot deployments within hospital systems, giving startups access to real-world environments for device testing. Academic medical centers provide regulatory guidance, IRB support, and clinical expertise that help startups evaluate efficacy, accuracy, and patient usability. Clinical validation processes ensure startups meet standards required for regulatory approval—from FDA clearance to CE marking—and build trust with healthcare providers. These collaborations also enable data collection for peer-reviewed publications, reinforcing the scientific credibility of the technology. Feedback from clinicians helps refine device interfaces, alert thresholds, and data reporting formats to improve workflow integration. By participating in collaborative research consortia, innovation hubs facilitate knowledge exchange across sectors, ensuring that pioneering technologies are grounded in evidence-based medicine. These efforts pave the way for adoption in telehealth protocols, inclusion in care pathways for chronic disease, and use in remote patient monitoring programs. Moreover, successful pilot studies often lead to procurement deals or pilot-scale implementations within hospital systems, providing startup funding and real-world validation.

7.3.4 Access to Funding and Accelerators

Innovation hubs—typically located in tech-centric cities or affiliated with universities—provide early-stage startups with vital access to capital, mentorship, infrastructure, and go-to-market support. Through accelerator programs, startups receive seed funding, workspace, legal and regulatory counsel, and introductions to investors and health system stakeholders. Many hubs specialize in health-tech verticals and can connect startups with medical advisors, clinicians, and venture capital firms with a health focus. These resources enable startups to refine their business model, validate product-market fit, and accelerate paths toward pilot programs and commercialization. Mentorship from serial entrepreneurs and industry veterans helps startups avoid common pitfalls around regulatory compliance, reimbursement strategy, and clinical adoption barriers. Capital deployment often follows milestone-based tranches linked to trial success, user acquisition, or regulatory progress, ensuring startups remain disciplined while scaling. Participation in pitch showcases and demo days amplifies visibility, attracting media attention and strategic partnerships. Infrastructure support, such as lab space, clinical simulation facilities, and biometric testing labs, can significantly reduce development costs. As a result, startups incubated in these ecosystems often advance from concept to prototype, clinical validation, and initial market deployments much faster than those outside support networks.

7.3.5 Promoting Digital Health Ecosystems

Startups contribute not only individual products but also to the broader digital health ecosystem by building interoperable platforms and integrations. Many startups design their wearables and companion apps to communicate seamlessly with electronic health record (EHR) systems, telehealth platforms, or analytics dashboards. They leverage standards like FHIR and HL7 to ensure their data can be shared securely and meaningfully within clinical workflows. Such interoperability enhances continuity of care—providers can access real-time patient data and integrate it into treatment decisions. Some startups offer APIs or SDKs that allow third-party apps to access data streams, enabling partnerships with chronic care management platforms, telemedicine providers, or corporate wellness programs. By embedding their solution into multi-partner ecosystems, these startups amplify user value and generate network effects. Many develop modular solutions—sensor + analytics + coaching content—that can be combined with other health services for bundled offerings. In doing so, they help scale infrastructure for broader adoption: insurers can leverage aggregated anonymized data for population health insights, clinics can deploy remote monitoring programs, and employers can integrate wellness data into HR systems. This ecosystem-oriented approach encourages collaboration rather than siloed development, fueling overall digital health maturation.

7.3.6 Fostering a Culture of Agility and User-Centered Design

Startups often place user experience at the center of their design philosophy, combining rapid prototyping with regular user feedback loops. Through iterative design cycles, they gather input from end users—patients, caregivers, clinicians—to continuously refine hardware ergonomics, app usability, notification design, and interpretability of health insights. This human-centered approach ensures that products are intuitive, accessible, and supportive of user lifestyle and emotional needs. Startups prioritize onboarding flows that reduce friction, such as simple sensor pairing, calibration routines, and clear visualizations of biological data. They frequently employ A/B testing and data-driven UX optimization to improve engagement and long-term adherence. A culture of agility enables teams to pivot quickly based on user feedback or regulatory shifts—adapting features, redesigning dashboards, or altering privacy policies with speed. Compared to traditional health technology firms, startups are more responsive to diverse user requirements—including accessibility features for users with disabilities, novice-friendly mode, and culturally adaptable interfaces. This adaptability fosters inclusivity and greater adoption across user groups otherwise excluded by one-size-fits-all designs.

7.3.7 Expanding Market Reach Through Global Innovation Hubs

Global innovation hubs located in cities such as Silicon Valley, Boston, London, Berlin, Tel Aviv, Bangalore, and Singapore serve as magnets for health-tech entrepreneurs. These clusters offer access to engineering talent, regulatory expertise, clinical networks, and international investors. Many hubs host biotech incubators, NIH-funded research initiatives, and corporate innovation labs—creating dense ecosystems of innovation. Startups benefit from frequent cross-disciplinary events, pitch forums, clinician meetups, and hackathons that spark collaboration. Innovation hubs also facilitate regulatory navigation in multiple regions by helping connect startups with legal and policy experts familiar with FDA, CE, and regional certifications. This access accelerates global commercialization strategies. Regional specialization within hubs (e.g., Berlin's focus on wearables privacy, Bangalore's cost-effective sensor development) helps nurture diverse solutions fitted to different markets. With global networks fostered by these hubs, startups can scale from local pilots to international deployments, adapting products for local regulations, languages, and health system needs.

7.3.8 Driving Policy and Regulatory Advancements

Startups and innovation hubs are increasingly engaging with policymakers, regulatory agencies, and industry groups to contribute to the evolving regulatory landscape for wearable and digital health technologies. Through participation in working groups, standards committees, and pilot policy labs, they help shape guidelines that balance innovation with patient safety. For example, startups may collaborate on shaping the criteria for AI-driven device certifications or real-world evidence standards for remote monitoring. This advocacy helps establish clearer pathways for FDA, EU MDR, and other regulatory approvals. By sharing performance data and human factors insights from real-world use, startups contribute to forming evidence-based policy frameworks. Innovation hubs often host regulatory hackathons, training sessions, and workshops to educate startups about compliance requirements, data governance best practices, and cybersecurity standards. This proactive engagement helps create an enabling environment for new product categories—such as software-as-a-medical-device or digital therapeutics—and reduces uncertainty for future entrants. In turn, policymakers gain practical, technology-grounded perspectives, helping evolve regulations that accommodate innovation while protecting users.

7.4 VENTURE CAPITAL AND INVESTMENT IN DIGITAL HEALTH

Venture capital (VC) has become a critical driving force in the evolution of the digital health and wearable technology sector. As healthcare shifts from reactive treatment to proactive, data-driven care, investors are increasingly recognizing the immense growth potential in digital health innovations. From telemedicine platforms and AI diagnostics to wearable devices and digital therapeutics, a wide array of technologies are being funded to address both longstanding and emerging healthcare challenges. The post-pandemic era has significantly accelerated investor interest, highlighting the value of remote care and virtual health tools during crises. Digital health solutions that once seemed supplementary are now considered essential components of modern care delivery, especially for chronic disease management, mental health support, and population health analytics. This shift has created fertile ground for startups and mid-sized health-tech companies, which are agile enough to respond to gaps in the system with innovation and speed. Emerging sector for investors in India is summarised in Fig. 2.

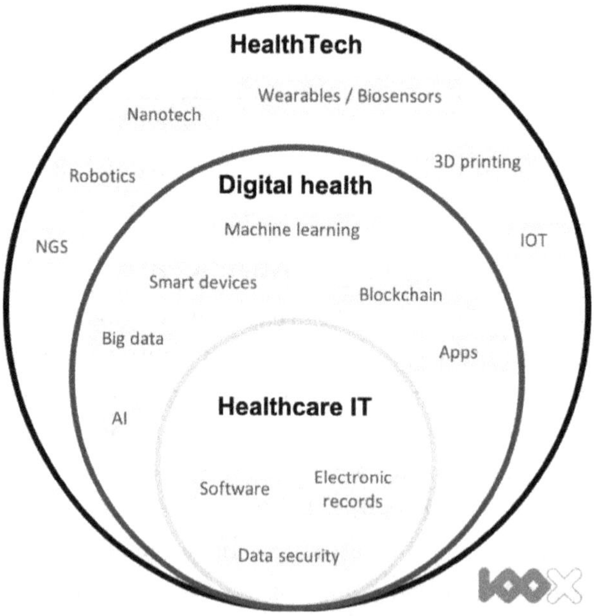

Fig. 2 Emerging sector for investors in India

Venture funding not only provides capital but also helps startups validate their products through clinical trials, refine go-to-market strategies, and scale globally. Early-stage funding enables product development and prototype testing, while later-stage funding supports regulatory approval, international expansion, and strategic hiring. These capital inflows have fostered a dynamic innovation ecosystem where startups, corporates, and research institutions work collaboratively to bring impactful solutions to market. Additionally, corporate venture arms from tech and healthcare giants like Google, Philips, and Johnson & Johnson are actively investing in health-tech startups, offering strategic partnerships, infrastructure support, and access to their global networks. Meanwhile, traditional VCs and private equity firms are targeting areas such as AI-powered diagnostics, wearable sensors, digital mental health, and women's health—segments that show strong growth potential and social impact. Despite the enthusiasm, the space also presents challenges for investors. Regulatory hurdles, data privacy concerns, clinical validation timelines, and reimbursement complexities can slow the path to profitability. However, experienced investors are increasingly adopting longer-term views, betting on companies that demonstrate strong clinical outcomes, user engagement, and interoperability. Overall, venture capital plays a pivotal role in shaping the future of digital health. It fuels the next generation of healthcare technologies, fosters global expansion, and enables scalable solutions that can reduce healthcare disparities. With growing demand, favourable market dynamics, and continuous technological innovation, venture capital investment in digital health is poised to remain a strong pillar of transformation in the global healthcare landscape.

7.4.1 Growing Investor Interest

Investor interest in the digital health sector has surged in recent years, catalyzed by the convergence of healthcare and emerging technologies. The COVID-19 pandemic acted as a tipping point, proving the value of remote care, telehealth, and health monitoring devices. As a result, venture capitalists now view digital health not just as a niche but as a core pillar of future healthcare delivery. The appeal lies in the sector's ability to offer scalable, tech-driven solutions to age-old problems like care access, cost containment, and chronic disease management. Startups that bring AI-enabled diagnostics, virtual care platforms, or real-time monitoring devices to market are especially appealing due to their high growth potential and broad applicability. Additionally, as global healthcare systems strain under increasing patient loads and workforce shortages, investors are betting that digital health will be instrumental in closing these gaps. The promise of high ROI, along with tangible social impact, has made this sector a magnet for both impact-focused and profit-driven investors.

7.4.2 Funding Stages and Trends

The investment lifecycle in digital health spans multiple phases, from early-stage seeding to late-stage IPOs or acquisitions. Seed and Series A rounds often fund product development, initial clinical validation, and market testing. Series B and C help scale operations, expand into new markets, and build regulatory and commercial capabilities. In recent years, the industry has seen a rise in mega-rounds—investments of over $100 million—especially in companies that offer remote patient monitoring, digital therapeutics, or AI-powered clinical tools. Another emerging trend is "crossover" funding, where private equity or hedge funds invest in startups nearing public offering, blurring lines between venture capital and public market strategies. Furthermore, non-traditional investors like sovereign wealth funds and pension funds are entering the space due to its long-term growth potential. Crowdfunding and health-focused accelerators have also contributed to democratizing early-stage capital access. This multi-tiered funding ecosystem is critical in sustaining innovation and market traction across different startup maturities.

7.4.3 Focus Areas for Investment

Investor focus within digital health has shifted from general wellness tools to clinically validated, outcomes-driven solutions. Remote patient monitoring (RPM) technologies have gained significant traction, especially for managing chronic conditions like diabetes, hypertension, and heart disease. AI-based diagnostics are another key area, with applications in radiology, pathology, and predictive analytics. Digital therapeutics (DTx) that deliver evidence-based behavioral interventions for mental health, addiction, or metabolic disorders are also attracting funding due to their scalability and regulatory traction. Women's health—traditionally underfunded—is receiving increased attention, with startups offering fertility trackers, maternal care apps, and hormone health tools. Mental health platforms are booming post-pandemic, offering therapy-on-demand, mood tracking, and cognitive behavioral therapy through digital mediums. Investors are also backing companies that integrate wearables with EHR systems and support data interoperability. Startups that enable compliance with healthcare regulations like HIPAA, GDPR, and FDA's SaMD framework are increasingly favored, as investors seek risk-mitigated opportunities.

7.4.4 Role of Corporate Venture Arms

Corporate venture capital (CVC) has emerged as a powerful force in the digital health investment landscape. Major healthcare and technology firms have established CVC arms—such as Google Ventures (GV), Philips Ventures, and J&J Innovation—to strategically invest in startups aligned with their long-term goals. These CVCs offer more than capital—they provide access to clinical trial sites, regulatory guidance, commercialization channels, and in some cases, early customer bases. Their involvement accelerates product-market fit and credibility, giving startups an edge in competitive fundraising environments. CVCs also use these partnerships to stay ahead of industry trends, explore adjacent markets, and acquire promising companies. Their investments are typically more strategic than traditional VCs, focusing on synergy and integration rather than short-term financial returns. The result is a dynamic where startups benefit from ecosystem access while corporations get early exposure to disruptive technologies—creating mutual growth opportunities.

7.4.5 Regional Investment Hotspots

Digital health investment is concentrated in a few key regions but is rapidly expanding worldwide. The United States continues to dominate, with Silicon Valley, Boston, and New York serving as innovation strongholds. These regions benefit from strong healthcare networks, venture ecosystems, academic institutions, and early adopter populations. Europe is rapidly catching up, driven by robust public health systems, supportive regulation (like the European Health Data Space), and rising healthtech investment in countries like Germany, the UK, France, and the Nordics. The Asia-Pacific region—especially China, India, Singapore, and Japan—is witnessing a digital health boom due to mobile penetration, population size, and tech-savvy younger generations. Investment in Latin America and Africa is still emerging but shows promise, especially in mobile-first solutions and public-private partnerships. Cross-border investments are on the rise, with global funds participating in international rounds to tap into diverse demographics and regulatory frameworks.

7.4.6 Impact on Innovation and Market Growth

Venture funding has a transformative effect on innovation and scalability in digital health. With the right capital, startups can rapidly prototype, test, and validate solutions, bringing products to market in record time. Funding enables access to talent, partnerships with research institutions, and the ability to meet stringent clinical and regulatory standards. It also facilitates international expansion, multilingual product development, and large-scale marketing campaigns. Moreover, with robust backing, startups can invest in building interoperable platforms, user-friendly interfaces, and real-world data capture tools. The cumulative effect is an accelerated pace of digital transformation across the healthcare sector. These innovations improve patient outcomes, reduce operational costs, and support clinicians with actionable insights. Venture funding thus doesn't just fuel business growth—it contributes directly to systemic healthcare improvement, which is particularly critical in the face of aging populations and chronic disease burdens worldwide.

7.4.7 Risks and Investment Challenges

While the digital health space presents immense potential, it is not without significant challenges. Regulatory approval processes can be long, costly, and inconsistent across jurisdictions, posing barriers to scale. Data privacy and security remain top concerns, especially as wearables and health apps handle sensitive personal health data. Ensuring HIPAA, GDPR, or FDA compliance adds operational complexity. The reimbursement landscape is also fragmented, with unclear or delayed payment models for digital interventions. Startups often face difficulty integrating their technologies into existing healthcare systems due to legacy software and clinician resistance. Furthermore, some digital health ventures struggle to prove clinical efficacy, leading to skepticism from both users and providers. Market saturation and a lack of standardization can lead to app fatigue among consumers. For investors, these factors translate into risks around scalability, adoption, and return on investment. Careful due diligence and strategic oversight are necessary to mitigate these risks and maximize impact.

7.4.8 Future Outlook for Digital Health Funding

The outlook for digital health investment remains optimistic. Over the next five years, funding is expected to stay strong, especially in areas that align with global healthcare priorities such as preventive care, aging populations, mental health, and AI ethics. Investors will increasingly seek startups that demonstrate measurable clinical outcomes and economic value, such as reduced hospital readmissions or improved medication adherence. ESG (Environmental, Social, and Governance) considerations will also influence funding decisions, especially in publicly accountable investment portfolios. As markets mature, we may see more mergers and acquisitions, IPOs, and consolidations within the sector. Additionally, public-private partnerships and outcome-based reimbursement models could unlock new funding channels. Emerging technologies like digital twins, personalized genomics, and VR-based therapies may attract a fresh wave of venture capital. Ultimately, digital health will continue to evolve from a disruptive niche into an essential infrastructure, with funding playing a pivotal role in this transformation.

7.5 EMERGING BUSINESS MODELS: SUBSCRIPTION, FREEMIUM, PAAS

Emerging business models are reshaping the landscape of wearable and digital health services, with subscription, freemium, and platform-as-a-service (PaaS) models forming the core of strategic innovation and revenue generation. The subscription-based model has become widely adopted among device manufacturers and health app providers, offering consumers ongoing access to premium features in exchange for monthly or annual fees. With outfits like Whoop, Fitbit Premium, and various mental wellness platforms, subscribers receive personalized insights, advanced analytics, sleep coaching, recovery scores, and guided workout routines. This model ensures steady, predictable revenue streams and supports continuous product improvements and new feature rollouts. It also fosters user engagement and loyalty over longer time horizons as subscribers grow accustomed to the value delivered on an ongoing basis. In contrast, the freemium model lowers barriers to adoption by offering essential features for free—such as basic heart rate tracking, step counting, or stress monitoring—while gating premium or advanced capabilities behind a paid tier. This allows startups and app developers to rapidly build large user bases, test product market fit, and gain visibility without upfront cost to users. Core functionalities provide immediate value, while upsell mechanisms expose high-value features like AI-driven coaching, detailed health reports, or access to expert sessions. They rely on data-driven personalization to entice free users gradually into subscription conversion. When leveraged effectively, the freemium approach creates a natural funnel from broad adoption to monetization, without compromising user trust or engagement.

Meanwhile, the Platform-as-a-Service (PaaS) model is becoming increasingly relevant to healthcare providers, enterprises, and third-party developers. Companies offering PaaS in digital health provide reusable frameworks—APIs, SDKs, or back-end infrastructure—for integrating wearable data, remote monitoring, and analytics into custom applications. Through platforms such as Apple HealthKit, Google Fit APIs, or niche healthcare stack providers, innovation hubs deliver scalable tech foundations that others can build on. This shifts the business model away from selling end-user devices or apps to licensing underlying platforms for health system integration, telehealth augmentation, or clinical decision support tools. PaaS enables healthcare organizations and developers to innovate faster, without having to build complex data pipelines or sensor integrations from scratch. Each business model—subscription, freemium, and PaaS—offers unique advantages. Subscription ensures recurring revenue and predictable cash flow; freemium facilitates rapid user acquisition and low friction product adoption; PaaS offers enterprise-scale flexibility and broader ecosystem reach through licensing and APIs. Many digital health firms now leverage hybrid strategies, combining freemium entry points with subscription upgrades and optional platform integrations for hospitals or insurers. For example, a wearable maker may offer a free wellness app, upsell a subscription for personalized coaching, and separately license a PaaS solution to clinics integrating wearable data into their EHR systems. The premium based business model is depicted in Fig.

3.

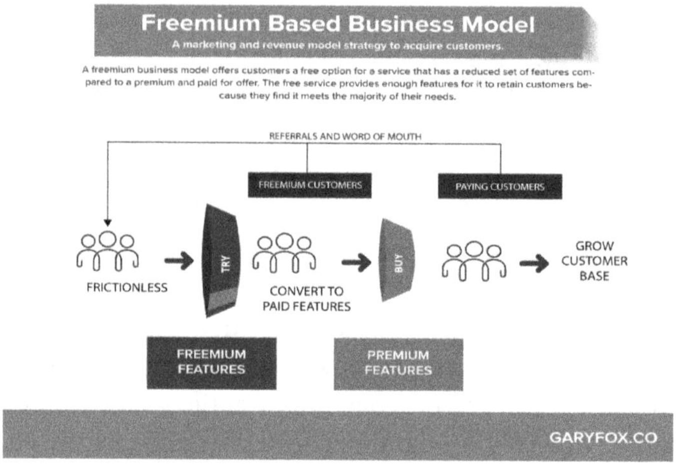

Fig.3 Premium Based Business Model

The success of these models depends on several factors- clarity of value proposition, user retention capabilities, and scalability. Subscriptions work best where users perceive continuous, evolving benefit—such as adaptive sleep coaching, recovery tracking, or chronic condition management. Freemium works when basic features delight users and build trust over time. PaaS demands strong interoperability, data security, compliance with healthcare standards, and ease of integration to gain traction in enterprise settings. Furthermore, monetization strategies depend on maintaining high standards around data privacy, regulatory compliance, and user engagement. Subscription models often invest in customer support and retention features. Freemium models must balance free content with enough premium incentive to convert users. PaaS platforms must establish trust with enterprise partners by offering SaaS-level reliability and healthcare-grade data governance.

Looking ahead, as digital health adoption grows, these business models are poised to evolve further. We may see more bundled offerings—subscription plus enterprise integration service or freemium upsells combined with clinical licensing. Value-based reimbursement and insurance partnerships may drive new hybrid models, with wearables and apps bundled into healthcare plans. Emerging innovations like digital therapeutics (DTx), AI-driven diagnostics, and behavioral health platforms could be monetized through subscriptions or licensing arrangements. Healthcare systems might license PaaS platforms for population health analytics or remote monitoring across patient cohorts. Startups may adopt freemium to attract physician practices, then sell premium analytics or EHR integration as add-ons. Subscription, freemium, and PaaS business models are central to the success and scalability of digital health ventures. They enable diverse revenue streams—from individual consumers to large healthcare enterprises—and catalyze widespread adoption of wearable technology. Companies that master these models while delivering clinical value, regulatory compliance, and seamless user experience will likely emerge as leaders in the evolving digital health ecosystem.

7.5.1 Subscription-Based Model

The subscription model has become a dominant business strategy in the digital health and wearables market. Under this model, users pay a recurring fee (monthly or annually) to access advanced features, analytics, or personalized health insights. Many fitness apps, mental wellness platforms, and wearable device ecosystems (like Whoop or Fitbit Premium) utilize this approach to deliver continuous value through AI-powered recommendations, sleep scoring, or recovery coaching. This model provides companies with a stable revenue stream and encourages long-term user engagement. It also allows for ongoing product updates, seamless integration with other digital health tools, and better customer retention. For users, subscriptions can offer more tailored experiences and evolving content, while companies benefit from improved forecasting and customer lifetime value.

7.5.2 Freemium Model

The freemium model offers users free basic features while charging for premium functionalities. This approach is widely adopted in health apps and wearable software ecosystems, where core capabilities—such as step tracking or heart rate monitoring—are available at no cost, but advanced features like detailed analytics, guided workouts, or expert consultations are gated behind a paywall. The freemium strategy helps companies rapidly grow their user base and attract potential paying customers by offering immediate value without barriers to entry. Over time, companies use engagement data to convert free users into paying subscribers. It also allows startups to validate their product-market fit and build brand awareness before scaling monetization efforts. However, success depends on striking the right balance between free offerings and paid incentives (Fig. 4).

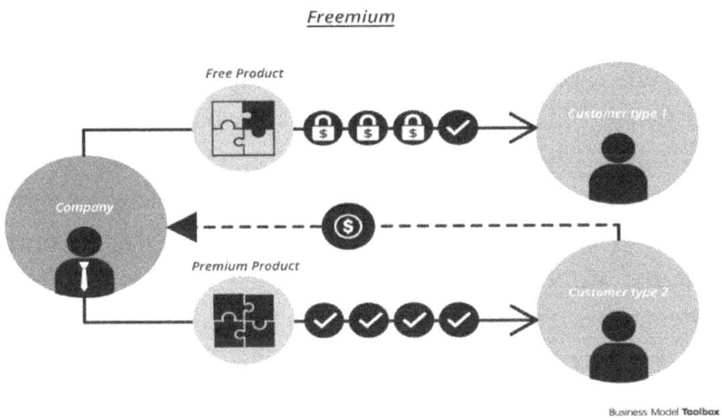

Fig. 4 Freemium Business Model Toolbox

7.5.3 Platform-as-a-Service (PaaS) Model

The Platform-as-a-Service (PaaS) model is becoming an increasingly vital component of the digital health ecosystem, enabling health-tech companies to offer robust, scalable technological infrastructures that others—such as hospitals, researchers, developers, and healthcare solution providers—can build upon. Unlike traditional software delivery models that target individual end-users directly, PaaS operates at an infrastructural level. It provides the building blocks necessary for innovation in digital healthcare, such as application programming interfaces (APIs), software development kits (SDKs), cloud storage, compliance frameworks, and data processing pipelines (Fig.5).

In the context of wearable health technologies and remote patient monitoring, PaaS platforms allow developers to integrate real-time data streams from devices into clinical dashboards, electronic health records (EHRs), or consumer health apps. Health-tech giants like Apple (HealthKit) and Google (Fit APIs) are prominent examples, offering standardized frameworks that ensure compatibility and seamless communication between apps and devices. These platforms facilitate everything from activity tracking and heart rate analysis to chronic disease monitoring and medication adherence management. Moreover, PaaS enables smaller startups or healthcare organizations to reduce development time and costs by avoiding the need to build core infrastructure from the ground up. Instead, they can leverage these ready-made platforms to focus on innovation, UI/UX design, and specialized features. This accelerates time-to-market and increases the likelihood of adoption, especially in time-sensitive medical environments. One of the key strengths of the PaaS model lies in its ability to support interoperability. By adhering to healthcare data standards like FHIR (Fast Healthcare Interoperability Resources) and HL7, PaaS platforms help bridge the gap between various systems, ensuring smoother data exchange and communication across different healthcare providers and technologies. This is critical for building integrated care ecosystems where patient data can travel securely across platforms, devices, and clinical environments. From a business perspective, PaaS models open up B2B revenue opportunities through enterprise licensing, usage-based pricing, and white-label solutions. Health systems, pharmaceutical companies, and digital therapeutics providers are increasingly partnering with PaaS vendors to power their backend infrastructure. These collaborations often result in long-term contracts, enabling vendors to maintain a stable and recurring income stream while offering continuous platform enhancements and technical support. Additionally, PaaS supports data aggregation and analytics, helping healthcare providers derive actionable insights from vast datasets generated by wearable devices. These insights are crucial for predictive modeling, population health management, and clinical decision support systems. With growing demand for personalized and preventive care, the ability to collect, process, and analyze patient data in real time becomes a strategic advantage. The flexibility of PaaS also allows it to serve as the backbone for AI-driven diagnostics, telehealth platforms, and clinical trial management systems. By offering modular, plug-and-play solutions, it enables rapid deployment and customization, catering to diverse user needs across regions, institutions, and medical specialties. Some platforms even include compliance modules that help organizations meet regulatory standards like HIPAA, GDPR, or local data protection laws. The PaaS model is playing a transformative role in digital health by democratizing access to advanced health-tech infrastructure. It empowers innovators, supports clinical excellence, and drives digital transformation across the healthcare continuum. As the demand for scalable, interoperable, and regulation-ready digital health solutions grows, the adoption of PaaS is expected to accelerate, further cementing its position as a foundational pillar in the future of connected healthcare.

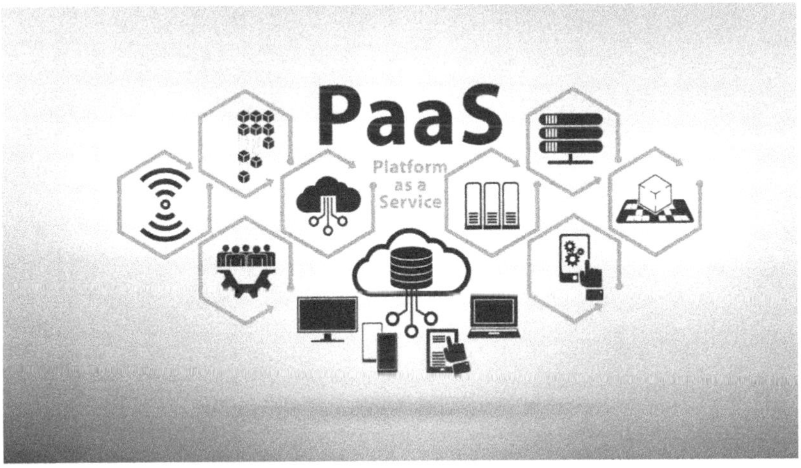

Fig. 5 Platform as a Service

8 Chapter

POLICY, REGULATION, AND STANDARDS

8.0 INTRODUCTION: AN OVERVIEW

The integration of digital technologies in healthcare has created a pressing need for strong policies, regulations, and standards to ensure safety, privacy, and effectiveness. As tools like wearables, mobile apps, and AI diagnostics become more common, global regulators are adapting existing frameworks to address their unique challenges. Key focus areas include data privacy, cybersecurity, ethical use, and clinical validation. Standards such as GDPR, HIPAA, ISO, and HL7/FHIR help establish consistency and interoperability. Regulators are also embracing agile models like sandboxes to support innovation. Ethical concerns around AI bias, consent, and data ownership are increasingly prioritized. International collaboration is crucial to managing cross-border care and data flows. Emerging economies are building digital health policies to match global trends. In all, policy and regulation play a foundational role in building trust and enabling scalable, secure digital health ecosystems.

The rapid evolution of digital health technologies—ranging from wearable devices and mobile health apps to AI-powered diagnostics and digital therapeutics—has transformed how healthcare is delivered, monitored, and experienced. However, this transformation also brings complex challenges that necessitate well-defined policy frameworks, robust regulations, and internationally recognized standards. These elements are essential for ensuring that innovation in healthcare remains safe, secure, equitable, and effective across various contexts and geographies. As healthcare shifts from traditional, episodic care toward continuous, data-driven, and patient-centered models, regulatory bodies worldwide are under pressure to adapt legacy frameworks to accommodate the unique nature of digital technologies. The growing convergence of consumer electronics with medical functionality—like ECGs on smartwatches or AI-powered symptom checkers—blurs the lines between wellness tools and regulated medical devices. In response, regulators such as the U.S. Food and Drug Administration (FDA), the European Medicines Agency (EMA), and the Central Drugs Standard Control Organization (CDSCO) in India are establishing clearer classifications and approval pathways for software as a medical device (SaMD) and connected health tools. Globally, policies related to data privacy, cybersecurity, interoperability, and user consent are central to ensuring ethical and lawful use of digital health tools. Frameworks like the General Data Protection Regulation (GDPR) in the European Union and HIPAA in the United States set high standards for the protection of personal health information. These regulations require healthcare technology providers to incorporate privacy-by-design principles, conduct data protection impact assessments (DPIAs), and ensure transparency and accountability in data processing (Fig. 1).

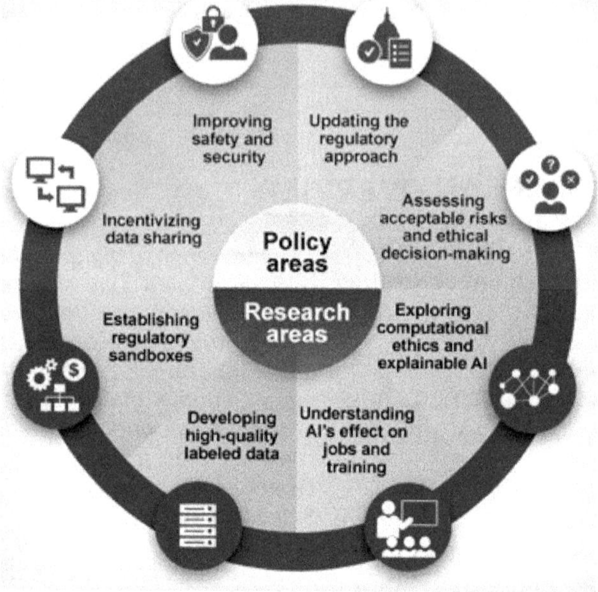
Improving safety and security
Updating the regulatory approach
Assessing acceptable risks and ethical decision-making
Exploring computational ethics and explainable AI
Understanding AI's effect on jobs and training
Developing high-quality labeled data
Establishing regulatory sandboxes
Incentivizing data sharing
Policy areas
Research areas

Fig. 1 Policy and research areas

Another critical dimension of digital health policy involves standardization. Internationally accepted standards such as ISO 13485 for quality management of medical devices, ISO 14971 for risk management, and HL7/FHIR for data exchange promote consistency, safety, and interoperability. These standards are foundational to enabling cross-platform compatibility, secure integration with electronic health records (EHRs), and global scalability of digital health solutions.

Regulatory bodies are also prioritizing real-world evidence and post-market surveillance to ensure that digital health products remain safe and effective over time. Regulatory sandboxes, pilot programs, and adaptive pathways are being introduced in several regions to allow for testing innovation in controlled settings while collecting clinical and user feedback. This agile approach helps regulators stay current with technological advances while minimizing patient risk. Meanwhile, ethical considerations are becoming increasingly embedded in health technology governance. Issues related to algorithmic bias, informed consent in AI systems, data ownership, and equitable access are prompting regulators and policymakers to involve multidisciplinary stakeholders—including ethicists, patients, and clinicians—in the development of regulatory guidelines. The goal is not only compliance but also public trust, patient safety, and long-term sustainability of digital health ecosystems.

The rise of cross-border data flows and telemedicine has further complicated the regulatory landscape, creating a need for international cooperation and harmonized legal frameworks. Organizations such as the World Health Organization (WHO), International Medical Device Regulators Forum (IMDRF), and OECD are working to align national policies and facilitate safe international adoption of digital health technologies. Emerging markets are also shaping the global regulatory narrative. Countries like India, Brazil, and South Africa are creating new digital health missions and public platforms to standardize care delivery, digitize patient records, and promote local innovation. However, regulatory maturity in these regions varies, and international collaboration is critical to avoid fragmentation and duplication. In sum, the intersection of policy, regulation, and standards forms the foundation for a responsible, secure, and innovation-friendly digital health ecosystem. Clear regulatory frameworks not only protect patients and users but also provide clarity to innovators, investors, and healthcare providers. As technologies advance—from wearable sensors and biosignal analytics to AI diagnostics and remote patient monitoring—the importance of agile, forward-looking governance will only grow. The future of digital health depends not just on technological capability but on the robustness and adaptability of the legal, ethical, and regulatory scaffolding that supports it. This chapter explores how policymakers, regulators, standards organizations, and industry stakeholders are shaping the rules that will govern the next era of connected, intelligent, and inclusive healthcare.

8.1 NATIONAL DIGITAL HEALTH MISSIONS AND STRATEGIES

The transformation of healthcare through digital technology is one of the most significant developments in the modern medical landscape. Governments, healthcare providers, and technology companies are increasingly focusing on leveraging digital tools to improve healthcare delivery, accessibility, and efficiency. Digital health initiatives aim to bridge gaps in traditional healthcare systems by introducing innovative technologies such as electronic health records (EHRs), telemedicine, mobile health applications, and data analytics. These initiatives seek to make healthcare more patient-centric, enabling individuals to have better control over their health information and facilitating seamless communication between patients and healthcare providers. One of the key drivers of digital health transformation is the widespread adoption of electronic health records, which replace paper-based systems and enable the secure storage and sharing of patient data. This not only enhances the accuracy and availability of medical information but also reduces redundancies and errors in diagnosis and treatment. Telemedicine, another critical component, has gained prominence by allowing remote consultations and care delivery, especially in rural and underserved areas. This reduces the need for physical travel and enables timely medical intervention, improving outcomes for patients who might otherwise face barriers to accessing healthcare. Moreover, health data analytics and artificial intelligence (AI) are revolutionizing how diseases are detected, monitored, and managed. By analyzing vast amounts of health data, AI-powered tools can identify patterns, predict outbreaks, and assist in personalized treatment plans. Mobile health applications empower individuals to monitor vital signs, track medication adherence, and receive health reminders, promoting preventive care and healthy lifestyles. These technologies also facilitate real-time health monitoring, enabling early detection of potential health issues and reducing hospital admissions.

Governments worldwide are increasingly recognizing the potential of digital health and launching national missions and strategies to promote its adoption. These include frameworks for data privacy and security, standardization of digital health infrastructure, and incentives for technology integration within healthcare systems. The National Digital Health Mission (NDHM) in India, for example, aims to create a digital health ecosystem that provides accessible, affordable, and quality healthcare to all citizens. It focuses on creating a unique health ID for every individual, enabling the integration of health records across providers and fostering interoperability. However, the journey towards digital healthcare transformation is not without challenges. Issues such as data privacy, cybersecurity, and digital literacy need to be addressed to ensure trust and widespread adoption. Infrastructure gaps in rural and remote areas, including internet connectivity and technological access, can limit the reach of digital health services. Additionally, healthcare professionals require training to effectively use digital tools and incorporate them into clinical practice. Despite these challenges, the benefits of digital health initiatives are profound. They have the potential to reduce healthcare costs by minimizing unnecessary tests and hospital visits, streamline workflows for healthcare providers, and enhance patient satisfaction through personalized care. Furthermore, digital health supports public health efforts by enabling better surveillance, reporting, and management of health crises such as pandemics. Initiatives to transform healthcare through digital technology represent a paradigm shift towards more efficient, equitable, and patient-focused healthcare delivery. By harnessing the power of digital tools, healthcare systems can improve outcomes, expand access, and empower individuals to take charge of their health. Continued investment, innovation, and collaboration across sectors will be essential to realize the full potential of digital health and ensure it benefits people globally.

8.1.1 Improve accessibility, affordability, and quality of health services

The primary objectives of digital health initiatives revolve around improving the accessibility, affordability, and quality of health services for all individuals, regardless of their geographic location or socio-economic status. Accessibility is enhanced by leveraging digital technologies such as telemedicine, mobile health applications, and electronic health records, which help overcome traditional barriers like distance, limited healthcare infrastructure, and shortage of healthcare professionals in rural or underserved areas. Through digital platforms, patients can consult doctors remotely, receive timely advice, and access their health information anytime, making healthcare more inclusive and convenient. Affordability is addressed by reducing the costs associated with healthcare delivery—digital tools help minimize unnecessary hospital visits, streamline administrative processes, and enable early diagnosis and preventive care, which in turn lower the overall financial burden on both patients and healthcare systems. Moreover, digital health encourages the use of cost-effective technologies, such as AI-driven diagnostics and remote monitoring devices, which reduce reliance on expensive in-person procedures. Improving the quality of healthcare is another key objective, achieved by enabling more accurate and comprehensive patient data management, enhancing clinical decision-making through AI and data analytics, and fostering personalized treatment plans. Digital records reduce medical errors, facilitate coordinated care among multiple providers, and ensure continuity of care. Collectively, these objectives aim to create a patient-centric health ecosystem that is efficient, equitable, and sustainable, ensuring that high-quality healthcare services are accessible and affordable for all sections of society.

8.1.2 Electronic Health Records (EHR), Telemedicine, Health Data Analytics:

Digital health technologies like Electronic Health Records (EHR), Telemedicine, and Health Data Analytics are revolutionizing the way healthcare is delivered, accessed, and managed globally. EHRs are centralized digital repositories of patient information that include medical histories, diagnoses, prescriptions, lab reports, and treatment plans. They eliminate the limitations of paper-based systems by ensuring real-time access to accurate, up-to-date patient data for healthcare providers. This enhances coordination among multiple specialists, reduces errors, and improves treatment outcomes. EHRs also empower patients by enabling them to track their medical history, appointments, and prescriptions online. Telemedicine complements EHRs by offering remote healthcare services through video calls, mobile apps, and virtual platforms. It significantly improves healthcare accessibility, especially in remote or underserved regions where hospitals and specialists may be unavailable. Patients can consult doctors, receive prescriptions, and even access mental health services from the comfort of their homes. This reduces travel time, healthcare costs, and hospital congestion while ensuring continuous care, particularly for chronic diseases and elderly patients. Health Data Analytics ties these systems together by analyzing vast amounts of health data generated through EHRs, telemedicine platforms, wearable devices, and diagnostic tools. Using technologies like artificial intelligence (AI) and machine learning (ML), analytics can detect disease trends, predict health risks, and optimize clinical decisions. It helps healthcare providers personalize treatment, monitor patient outcomes, and identify areas for public health improvement. Governments and institutions use analytics for pandemic tracking, vaccination planning, and policy-making. However, successful implementation depends on robust data privacy laws, skilled professionals, and equitable access to technology. Together, EHRs, telemedicine, and health analytics form the backbone of modern digital healthcare ecosystems, enabling faster, smarter, and more inclusive healthcare delivery. These tools not only improve efficiency but also promote patient-centered care and long-term public health benefits.

1. Electronic Health Records (EHR): Electronic Health Records (EHRs) are a foundational component of digital health, designed to store and manage patients' medical information in a digital format. EHRs contain comprehensive data such as patient history, diagnoses, medications, treatment plans, immunization records, laboratory results, and radiology images. Unlike paper records, EHRs are easily accessible, secure, and can be updated in real-time by authorized healthcare providers. This ensures continuity of care, especially when patients visit multiple facilities or are referred to specialists. EHRs improve clinical efficiency by reducing documentation errors, duplication of tests, and delays in accessing information. Through interoperability frameworks, EHR systems can share data across different hospitals and health networks, creating a seamless patient experience. Patients benefit from greater involvement in their own care, as many systems offer portals that allow individuals to view their records, schedule appointments, and receive health alerts. Healthcare professionals, in turn, can use EHR data to make more informed decisions, track patient progress, and coordinate care across teams. Government initiatives such as India's Ayushman Bharat Digital Mission aim to assign a unique Health ID to citizens, linking their health data across the digital ecosystem. While the benefits are significant, challenges include ensuring data privacy, standardization across platforms, and training healthcare workers in digital literacy. Despite these issues, EHRs represent a transformative shift toward more accurate, efficient, and personalized healthcare services that can adapt to the dynamic needs of populations (Fig. 2).

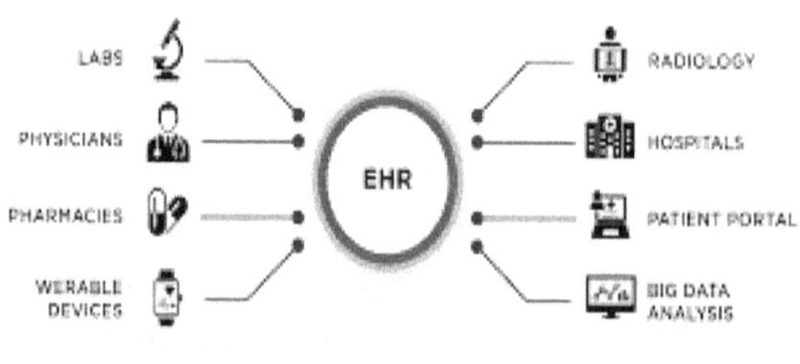

Fig. 2 Electronic Health Records (EHRs)

2. Telemedicine: Telemedicine refers to the delivery of healthcare services remotely using telecommunications technology such as video calls, mobile apps, and online platforms. It plays a vital role in increasing access to healthcare, especially in rural or underserved areas where medical professionals and facilities are limited. With telemedicine, patients can consult with doctors, receive prescriptions, follow-up care, and even access mental health services without the need for physical travel. This not only reduces transportation costs and waiting times but also ensures timely intervention and continuity of care. Telemedicine became a lifeline during the COVID-19 pandemic, helping healthcare systems manage high patient loads while minimizing exposure risks. It supports real-time consultations as well as store-and-forward systems, where data such as X-rays or reports can be sent to specialists for review. Telemedicine is particularly beneficial for chronic disease management, elderly care, and post-surgery follow-ups. Governments and private players are promoting telehealth platforms through regulatory support and public-private partnerships. In India, platforms like eSanjeevani provide free teleconsultation services across states. However, the success of telemedicine depends on reliable internet access, digital literacy among users, and clear legal guidelines on data security and medical liability. When implemented effectively, telemedicine democratizes healthcare access, empowers patients, and reduces the burden on urban hospitals. As technology evolves, telemedicine will continue to play a pivotal role in shaping patient-centered, efficient, and equitable healthcare delivery across the globe. Benefits of HER telehealth integration is given in Fig. 3.

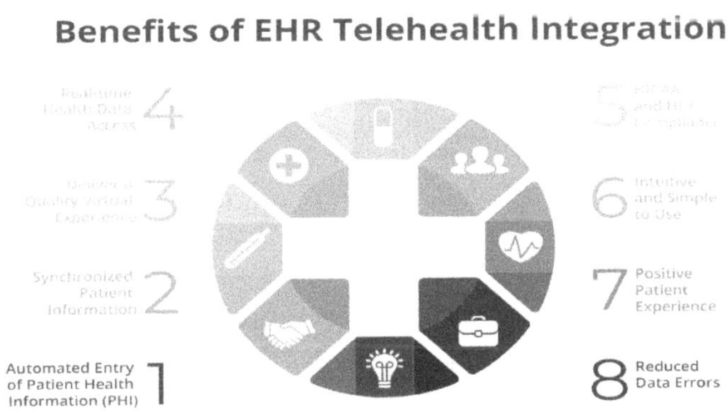

Fig.3 Benefits of HER Telehealth Integration

3. Health Data Analytics: Health data analytics is the process of collecting, analyzing, and interpreting vast amounts of health-related data to improve decision-making and healthcare outcomes. In the digital health ecosystem, data is continuously generated from sources like EHRs, wearable devices, teleconsultations, diagnostic labs, and insurance claims. Health analytics turns this raw data into actionable insights that can help detect disease patterns, predict outbreaks, assess treatment effectiveness, and personalize patient care. For example, predictive analytics can identify high-risk patients for diabetes or heart disease and alert healthcare providers for early intervention. AI and machine learning tools enhance these capabilities by uncovering hidden trends and automating data interpretation. Public health agencies use analytics to monitor disease trends, optimize resource allocation, and plan vaccination campaigns. Hospitals and clinics apply data-driven strategies to reduce readmission rates, improve operational efficiency, and enhance patient satisfaction. On a national level, health analytics supports policy decisions, such as identifying gaps in healthcare delivery or evaluating the impact of health programs. Despite its advantages, challenges like data privacy concerns, lack of standard data formats, and limited skilled professionals remain. Ensuring ethical use and maintaining trust is crucial when handling sensitive personal health data. When implemented with the right safeguards, health data analytics becomes a powerful tool to create evidence-based healthcare, reduce costs, and foster innovation in both preventive and curative services. Its growing relevance underscores the shift from reactive to proactive healthcare models (Fig. 4).

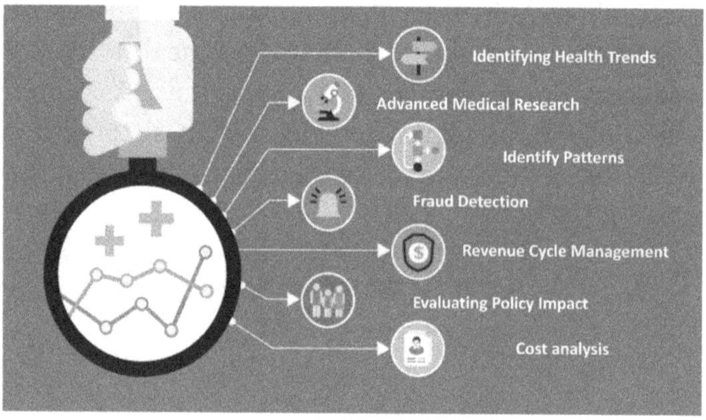

Fig. 4 Health data analytics

8.1.3 Government Programs- National Digital Health Mission (NDHM), Ayushman Bharat Digital Mission (ABDM):

1. National Digital Health Mission (NDHM)

The National Digital Health Mission (NDHM) was launched by the Government of India on 15th August 2020 with the vision of creating a comprehensive digital health infrastructure for the country. It aimed to digitize the entire healthcare ecosystem by introducing key components such as Health ID, DigiDoctor, Health Facility Registry, Personal Health Records (PHR), and Electronic Medical Records (EMR). The central goal of NDHM was to ensure that every citizen has access to a digital health ID that links all their health information in a secure and interoperable system. This ID enables individuals to share their medical records with healthcare providers across India seamlessly, ensuring continuity of care even when visiting different doctors or hospitals.

Important Facts about the National Digital Health Mission	
Launch Date	15th August 2020 – 74th Independence Day
Comes under which Ministry	It is implemented by the National Health Authority (NHA) under the Ministry of Health and Family Welfare
Objective	To create a national digital health ecosystem that supports universal health coverage
Official Website	https://ndhm.gov.in/

NDHM was designed to address long-standing challenges in the Indian healthcare system, such as fragmented patient records, poor communication between providers, and lack of standardization in data sharing. With digital platforms, NDHM sought to bridge the rural-urban healthcare gap by promoting telemedicine and making healthcare services accessible to even the remotest areas. It also aimed to empower patients by giving them control over their own health data while maintaining strict data privacy and consent protocols. NDHM promoted interoperability between systems to avoid duplication of tests, streamline insurance processes, and enhance clinical efficiency.

The mission also emphasized the importance of digital literacy among healthcare workers and encouraged hospitals, labs, and pharmacies to integrate their systems with the NDHM ecosystem. By creating a unified digital backbone for health services, NDHM was expected to enable better planning, resource allocation, and policy-making at both national and state levels. The mission marked a foundational step in building a "Digital Health for All" environment, enabling a shift from reactive healthcare to a preventive, personalized, and predictive model. It laid the groundwork for what later evolved into the more comprehensive Ayushman Bharat Digital Mission (ABDM).

Background of National Digital Health Mission

1. **National Health Policy 2017 Envisions:**
   - Highest level of health and wellbeing for all at all ages
   - Preventive and promotive health care orientation in all development policies
   - Universal healthcare access
2. MoH&FM set up a committee under J. Satyanarayana to develop an implementation framework for the National Health Stack
3. The Satyanarayana committee recommended drafting a National Digital Health Blueprint to lay down the building blocks and action plan for a digital health mission.

4. National Digital Mission Blueprint recommended the establishment of an entity called National Digital Health Mission to provide for a digital healthcare ecosystem for healthcare services across the country.

National Health Authority that is the apex authority to implement the National Digital Health Mission is also the implementing authority of Ayushman Bharat.

Objectives of National Digital Health Mission

1. **Establishment of Digital Health Systems**
   - Core digital health data managed by these systems
   - To manage the Infrastructure requirements for seamless exchange of services.
2. **Creation of Registries**
   - It will have all credible data of clinical establishments, healthcare professionals, health workers, drugs, and pharmacies
3. Enforcement of adoption of open standards by all national digital health stakeholders
4. **Establishment of Standardized personal health records**
   - It will take inspiration from international standards
   - Based on an individual's informed consent, the records can be easily shared between individuals and healthcare professionals, and services providers.
5. Enterprise-class health application systems
   - The aim will be to achieve health-related Sustainable Development Goals (SDGs).
6. Adoption of cooperative federalism while coordinating with states and union territories.
7. Promotion of private players' participation along with the public health authorities
8. Making healthcare services portable nationally.
9. Promotion of Clinical Decision Support (CDS) Systems by healthcare professionals.
10. **Digitally manage:**
    - Identifying people, doctors, and health facilities,
    - Facilitating electronic signatures
    - Ensuring non-repudiable contracts
    - Making paperless payments
    - Securely storing digital records, and
    - Contacting people

The National Digital Health Mission is set to be built alongside the existing public digital infrastructure like PM Jan-Dhan Yojana.

Components of National Digital Health Mission

There are four components:

1. National Health Electronic Registries
2. A Federated Personal Health Records (PHR) Framework – It will fight twin challenges of:
    - Access to healthcare reports/data by the patients and the healthcare provider for treatment
    - Making the data available for medical research
3. A National Health Analytics Platform
4. Other Horizontal Components like:
    - Unique Digital Health ID,
    - Health Data Dictionaries
    - Supply Chain Management for Drugs,
    - Payment gateways

2. Ayushman Bharat Digital Mission (ABDM)

The Ayushman Bharat Digital Mission (ABDM), officially launched on 27th September 2021, is the expanded and upgraded version of the earlier NDHM. Building on the foundations laid by NDHM, ABDM aims to create a nationwide digital health ecosystem that connects patients, healthcare providers, health facilities, insurers, and digital health applications. One of its core components is the Ayushman Bharat Health Account (ABHA) – a unique 14-digit health ID provided to every citizen, which stores and manages their personal health records digitally and securely.

ABDM's vision is to enable universal health coverage by leveraging digital technologies to provide accessible, affordable, and high-quality healthcare to all. It aims to improve efficiency, transparency, and accountability in healthcare service delivery. The mission supports the integration of EHRs, telemedicine platforms, e-pharmacies, and digital health applications under a common framework that ensures interoperability and data protection. It also includes registries for healthcare professionals and health facilities to build a trustworthy and verified digital network across India.

What sets ABDM apart is its citizen-centric approach, where individuals have full control over their health data—right from consent management to the ability to share records with a chosen provider. ABDM promotes the use of open standards and APIs to ensure that all stakeholders—from startups to large hospitals—can build and connect services to the platform. It has also introduced the ABDM Sandbox, which allows developers and service providers to test their digital health solutions in a controlled environment.

ABDM plays a key role in supporting the Ayushman Bharat Pradhan Mantri Jan Arogya Yojana (PM-JAY) by improving the tracking of beneficiaries, claim processing, and fraud detection. It promotes the use of AI, blockchain, and analytics to improve population health management and resource utilization. Despite challenges like digital infrastructure gaps, privacy concerns, and the need for capacity building, ABDM represents a transformative leap toward building an equitable, inclusive, and efficient health system in India. By integrating technology into every level of healthcare, ABDM is turning the vision of "Digital Health for All" into a reality.

National Digital Health Eco-system

It is a National Digital Health Eco-system that supports Universal Health Coverage in an efficient, accessible, inclusive, affordable, timely, and safe manner, through provision of a wide-range of data, information and infrastructure services, duly leveraging open, interoperable, standards-based digital systems, and ensuring the security, confidentiality and privacy of health-related personal information (Fig. 5).

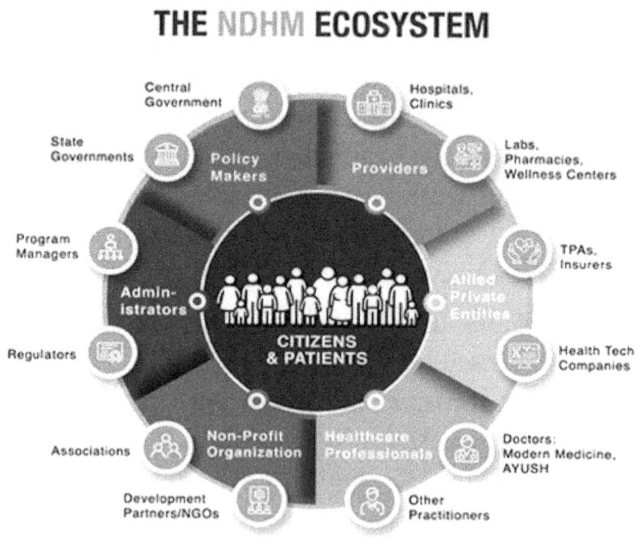

Fig. 5 The NDHM Ecosystem

8.1.4 Strategic Goals

Integration of healthcare data, patient-centric services, secure data sharing: The integration of healthcare data, patient-centric services, and secure data sharing forms the foundation of a modern, efficient, and responsive healthcare system. As healthcare becomes increasingly digital, strategic goals are shifting toward unifying fragmented data sources, enhancing patient engagement, and protecting sensitive information. Seamless integration of healthcare data across providers and systems allows for more accurate diagnoses, continuity of care, and personalized treatment plans. At the same time, prioritizing patient-centric services ensures that individuals are not just passive recipients of care, but active participants in managing their health.

Technologies such as Electronic Health Records (EHRs), Internet of Things (IoT) devices, and mobile health applications are driving this transformation. However, with the rapid digitization of health information, ensuring secure data sharing becomes paramount. Blockchain, encryption protocols, and strict access controls are being adopted to protect patient privacy while enabling authorized sharing. These strategic goals not only enhance care delivery but also improve efficiency, reduce duplication, and empower patients with greater control over their health data (Fig. 6).

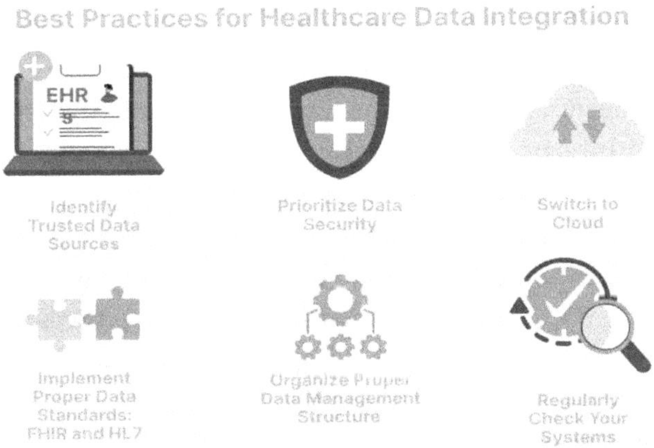

Fig. 6 Practices for Healthcare Data Integration

A well-integrated and secure healthcare ecosystem supports real-time decision-making, predictive analytics, and better outcomes across the care continuum. Ultimately, achieving these goals requires strong leadership, regulatory support, cross-industry collaboration, and ongoing technological innovation.

- **Integration of Healthcare Data:** The integration of healthcare data refers to the unification of patient records, diagnostics, treatment history, lab results, prescriptions, and imaging into a single, interoperable ecosystem. By standardizing data formats and ensuring compatibility across systems, healthcare providers can access comprehensive patient profiles in real-time. This approach improves clinical decision-making, reduces medical errors, and avoids repetitive diagnostic tests. Integrated healthcare systems also promote continuity of care, especially for patients transitioning between general physicians, specialists, and hospitals. In emergency settings, immediate access to critical data such as allergies, medications, and previous diagnoses can save lives. Integration fosters better population health management by enabling large-scale analytics, disease surveillance, and early detection. Through centralized health information exchanges (HIEs), data becomes accessible yet securely compartmentalized. Artificial Intelligence (AI) and Machine Learning (ML) technologies thrive in such environments, offering predictive analytics based on integrated data. Chronic disease management is also enhanced, as physicians can monitor long-term health patterns. Integration also supports remote monitoring and telemedicine by feeding consistent data into virtual care platforms. Public health officials can aggregate anonymous data for policy planning and outbreak responses. Insurance providers benefit from fewer disputes when all records are unified. The challenges to integration include diverse legacy systems, lack of standard protocols, and resistance from institutions. National policies on interoperability must be enforced to overcome such barriers. Privacy considerations must be baked into design to avoid compromising patient trust. APIs and FHIR (Fast Healthcare Interoperability Resources) standards are central to making this integration scalable. In rural or under-resourced settings, cloud-based integration offers a cost-effective model. A digital health ID system linked to patient data can further simplify access. Data silos must be broken down through collaboration and shared infrastructure investments. Eventually, integration can serve as the backbone for a national digital health mission, where every citizen's health journey is traceable and optimizable. It also accelerates clinical research, as structured and interoperable data can be anonymized and mined. Integration is not a one-time event but a continuous effort requiring governance, compliance, and adaptive technologies. Success demands participation from government, private sector, and civil society. Ultimately, integrated data systems can revolutionize healthcare delivery and public health monitoring at scale.

- **Patient-Centric Services:** Patient-centric services place the individual at the heart of healthcare design, delivery, and decision-making. The focus shifts from provider convenience to patient empowerment, creating an experience tailored to individual needs, preferences, and lifestyles. Personalized care plans, developed collaboratively between clinicians and patients, form the cornerstone of this model. These services encompass easy access to medical records, remote consultations, health education, and chronic disease management. Digital platforms play a pivotal role by offering mobile apps, online appointment booking, and secure messaging with doctors. Emotional and psychological support is also integral, acknowledging the full spectrum of patient well-being. The design of hospital environments, waiting times, and communication clarity all influence patient satisfaction. Accessibility is key: services must be inclusive of differently-abled individuals and linguistically diverse populations. Feedback mechanisms allow patients to express concerns and rate services, ensuring continuous improvement. Wearable technology and home monitoring devices empower patients to track vital signs and lifestyle factors in real time. These insights promote proactive engagement in their own health journey. Transparency in billing, treatment options, and medication effects builds trust. Patient advocacy groups can collaborate with health providers to bridge care gaps and improve outcomes. Family involvement, especially for geriatric and pediatric cases, enhances care coordination. Culturally competent care, which respects beliefs and values, ensures dignity and compliance. Health literacy programs help patients make informed decisions. Patient portals should be intuitive, secure, and multilingual. Mental health, often overlooked, must be integrated into patient-centric models. Social determinants of health such as income, education, and housing should be addressed holistically. Regular satisfaction surveys and personalized follow-ups contribute to loyalty and trust. Artificial intelligence can analyze user behavior to offer smart nudges and reminders. In rural areas, mobile health units and telehealth bridge accessibility gaps. The elderly population especially benefits from home-based care plans. Ultimately, patient-centric services lead to better adherence, fewer hospital readmissions, and enhanced quality of life. Policy frameworks and funding must support innovation in this space. Healthcare workers must be trained in empathy, communication, and shared decision-making. Successful patient-centric models require a balance of technology, human touch, and systemic support.

- **Secure Data Sharing:** Secure data sharing is a foundational pillar for modern, digital healthcare systems where trust, privacy, and integrity are non-negotiable. With the proliferation of electronic health records (EHRs), genomic data, imaging, and wearable device outputs, the need for secure yet efficient data exchange has become paramount. Secure sharing allows different stakeholders—clinicians, labs, insurers, pharmacies—to collaborate seamlessly without compromising patient confidentiality. Encryption, multi-factor authentication, and access control protocols are critical technologies used to safeguard data at rest and in transit. Blockchain technology is emerging as a promising solution for tamper-proof health data transactions. Data anonymization techniques ensure that personal identifiers are removed when data is used for research or analytics. National regulations like HIPAA (in the US) and GDPR (in the EU) set the legal framework for privacy and breach accountability. Role-based access ensures that only authorized personnel can view or modify data. Patients themselves must have control over who accesses their health records, fostering transparency. Secure sharing enables second opinions, cross-border care, and seamless referrals. Cybersecurity training for hospital staff is essential to prevent phishing and social engineering attacks. Audit trails help trace data usage and ensure compliance. Cloud platforms must adhere to industry certifications such as ISO 27001 or HITRUST. Regular vulnerability assessments and penetration testing reduce risk exposure. Consent management systems allow patients to approve or deny specific data uses. Secure APIs are necessary for integrating third-party tools like health apps. Health Information Exchanges (HIEs) must implement standardized protocols for data exchange. During pandemics, secure sharing allows rapid but responsible data dissemination. Breaches can lead to identity theft, loss of trust, and legal consequences, emphasizing the importance of proactive security. Data backup and disaster recovery systems ensure business continuity. International collaboration on cyber norms for healthcare is growing in importance. Machine learning can detect anomalies in access patterns, flagging suspicious activities. Vendors and partners must also be held to strict data handling agreements. Public awareness campaigns should inform citizens about their data rights. Innovation in this space must prioritize privacy by design. Ultimately, secure data sharing builds a resilient, interconnected healthcare ecosystem that prioritizes both progress and protection.

8.1.5 Technology Focus- AI, IoT, Blockchain for healthcare security and efficiency:

In the rapidly evolving landscape of modern healthcare, the integration of emerging technologies has become essential for enhancing both operational efficiency and patient safety. Among the most transformative technologies making a profound impact are Artificial Intelligence (AI), the Internet of Things (IoT), and Blockchain. These technologies are not only redefining how healthcare services are delivered but also playing a critical role in addressing the growing challenges of data security, privacy, interoperability, and real-time decision-making. AI has brought significant advancements to healthcare by enabling intelligent systems that support clinical decisions, automate administrative tasks, and improve diagnostic accuracy. Through machine learning algorithms and data analytics, AI helps predict disease patterns, detect abnormalities in medical images, and recommend personalized treatment plans. It reduces the workload on healthcare professionals while ensuring timely and precise interventions. The Internet of Things has revolutionized patient care by connecting a wide array of medical devices and sensors that monitor patient health in real-time. From wearable fitness trackers to remote monitoring tools for chronic disease management, IoT enhances patient engagement, promotes preventive care, and facilitates immediate medical responses. The real-time data collected through IoT devices is instrumental in improving hospital efficiency and enabling home-based healthcare. However, as healthcare becomes more digitized and interconnected, it also becomes increasingly vulnerable to cyber threats (Fig. 7).

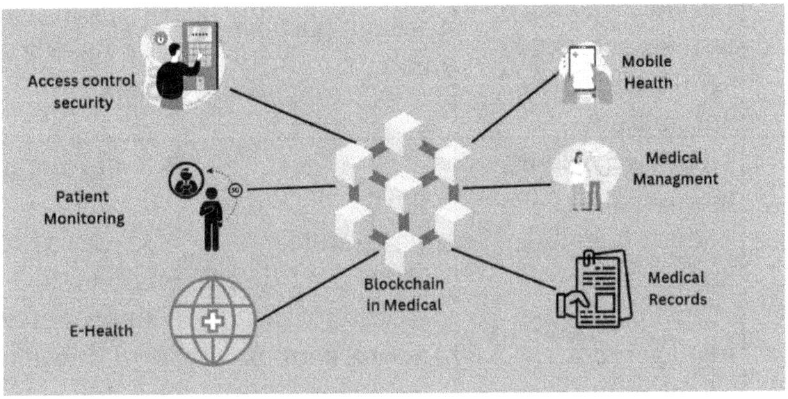

Fig. 7 Generative AI, IoT, and blockchain in healthcare: application, issues, and solutions

The sensitive nature of patient health information demands robust security mechanisms. This is where Blockchain plays a pivotal role. By providing decentralized, tamper-proof ledgers, Blockchain ensures that patient records remain secure, accurate, and accessible only to authorized parties. It also enhances trust among stakeholders by providing transparency in data sharing, patient consent management, and drug traceability. The convergence of AI, IoT, and Blockchain in healthcare creates a powerful synergy. Together, they facilitate smarter, safer, and more efficient healthcare delivery systems. For instance, AI can analyze vast volumes of IoT-generated health data to detect health risks in real-time, while Blockchain secures this data against tampering. This integrated approach helps healthcare providers streamline operations, reduce costs, improve diagnostics, and protect sensitive patient data. In essence, these three technologies are not standalone innovations but interconnected components of a next-generation digital healthcare ecosystem. Their combined application offers the potential to transform healthcare into a more patient-centric, responsive, and secure system. From hospitals to home care, from clinical research to patient outreach, AI, IoT, and Blockchain are reshaping the way healthcare is conceptualized and delivered. As we look toward the future, embracing these technologies is no longer optional—it is a necessity for healthcare systems that aspire to be resilient, efficient, and secure in the face of evolving patient needs and technological advancements (Table-1).

Table 1: Summary of the Technology Focus: AI, IoT, and Blockchain for Healthcare Security and Efficiency

Technology	Key Applications	Security Contributions	Efficiency Improvements
AI	- Clinical decision support - Medical imaging & diagnostics - Predictive analytics - Administrative automation	- Detects anomalies & cyber threats - Prevents fraud through pattern analysis	- Automates routine tasks - Enhances diagnostic speed & accuracy - Reduces readmissions
IoT	- Remote patient monitoring - Smart hospital infrastructure - Chronic disease management - Real-time alerts	- Device-level data encryption - AI-assisted threat detection - Access control	- Real-time data sharing - Reduces hospital visits - Improves asset & workflow management
Blockchain	- Secure EHR storage - Patient consent via smart contracts - Supply chain tracking - Decentralized data sharing	- Immutability of records - Decentralized access logs - Identity management	- Enables interoperability - Reduces fraud - Speeds up claims & consent processes
Integration	- AI + IoT: Predictive monitoring - Blockchain + IoT: Trusted device data - AI + Blockchain: Secure data insights	- End-to-end traceability - Verified data inputs - Tamper-proof analytics	- Coordinated care delivery - Smart workflows - Streamlined operations

1. **Artificial Intelligence (AI) in Healthcare:** Artificial Intelligence (AI) in healthcare is revolutionizing the way medical services are delivered by enabling smarter, faster, and more personalized care. By analyzing vast amounts of data—from electronic health records to imaging scans—AI supports accurate diagnoses, treatment planning, and patient monitoring. It reduces the burden on healthcare professionals by automating routine tasks and streamlining workflows. AI-driven tools enhance clinical decision-making, predict health trends, and detect anomalies in real-time. This leads to improved patient outcomes, lower operational costs, and

more efficient use of resources. As healthcare becomes increasingly data-driven, AI is emerging as a cornerstone of modern medical innovation (Fig 8).

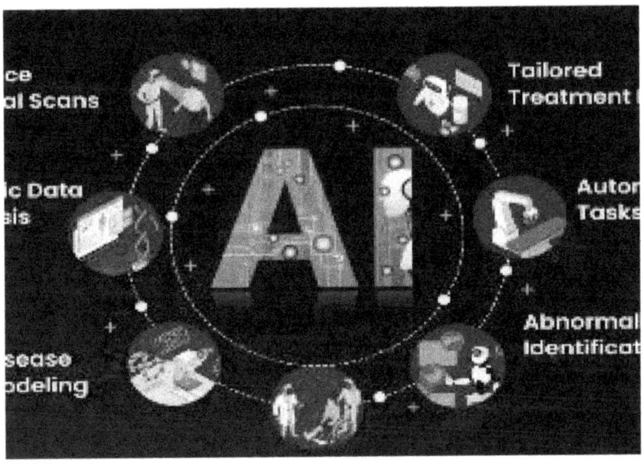

Fig. 8 Applications of Generative AI in Healthcare

- **Clinical Decision Support:** AI-powered Clinical Decision Support Systems (CDSS) are revolutionizing the way healthcare providers make clinical judgments. These systems analyze vast datasets—ranging from electronic health records (EHRs) to genetic information and clinical guidelines—to offer evidence-based recommendations. By processing this data in real-time, AI can identify patterns and correlations that may not be immediately visible to clinicians. This supports more accurate diagnoses, tailored treatment plans, and faster medical interventions. It reduces cognitive load on physicians, especially in complex cases involving multiple comorbidities. AI can also flag potential drug interactions or contraindications based on the patient's history. Importantly, CDSS platforms improve the consistency of care by standardizing decision-making. They contribute to better patient outcomes and fewer medical errors. Additionally, integrating AI with natural language processing allows it to interpret physician notes and unstructured data. This enriches clinical context and improves recommendations. As healthcare systems move towards precision medicine, AI-driven support is becoming an essential partner at the point of care.
- **Medical Imaging & Diagnostics:** AI, especially deep learning, is bringing a paradigm shift to medical imaging and diagnostics. Sophisticated neural networks are trained on millions of annotated images, enabling them to detect anomalies with a level of accuracy often comparable to—or even surpassing—human radiologists. These models can recognize early signs of diseases such as cancer, pneumonia, or brain disorders by examining X-rays, MRIs, CT scans, and ultrasounds. They help in reducing diagnostic delays and minimizing oversight due to human fatigue. AI accelerates image analysis, allowing faster turnaround times for reports, which is crucial in

emergency settings. Furthermore, it can quantify lesion sizes, monitor changes over time, and suggest potential diagnoses. It ensures consistent interpretations across different institutions and imaging professionals. AI also facilitates image enhancement, noise reduction, and segmentation, improving visualization. Integration with cloud platforms allows remote analysis, aiding underserved or rural regions. Ultimately, AI enhances diagnostic precision, speeds up workflows, and supports better-informed clinical decisions.

- **Predictive Analytics:** AI-driven predictive analytics is transforming healthcare from a reactive to a proactive system. By leveraging historical patient records, environmental data, wearable device inputs, and real-time clinical metrics, AI models can anticipate health events before they occur. For example, it can forecast the likelihood of patient deterioration in ICUs, enabling timely interventions. It helps in identifying individuals at high risk for chronic diseases, such as diabetes or cardiovascular conditions, facilitating early prevention strategies. In public health, predictive analytics models forecast disease outbreaks and track infection spread patterns, aiding policy responses and resource allocation. Hospitals use AI to predict bed occupancy, staff needs, and medication demands, optimizing operational efficiency. Insurers and providers use it to identify at-risk populations and improve care management. It can also predict hospital readmissions, reducing costs and improving outcomes. Personalized risk scores enhance patient engagement and adherence to care plans. Overall, predictive analytics is enabling a shift toward smarter, more anticipatory healthcare delivery.
- **Administrative Efficiency:** AI significantly boosts administrative efficiency in healthcare by automating repetitive and time-consuming tasks. It streamlines medical billing, insurance coding, and claims processing with high accuracy, reducing administrative burden and human error. AI chatbots and virtual assistants manage appointment scheduling, patient reminders, and basic triage, freeing up staff for more critical duties. Document management systems powered by natural language processing extract relevant data from forms, lab results, and notes, minimizing manual data entry. Revenue cycle management becomes more efficient as AI flags billing inconsistencies or coding mismatches. In human resources, AI assists in workforce planning and shift optimization, improving productivity. Hospital supply chains also benefit from AI, which predicts inventory needs and automates procurement. AI can also analyze patient satisfaction data to identify service gaps. These optimizations lead to shorter wait times, lower administrative costs, and improved patient experiences. By relieving

administrative stress, healthcare workers can focus more on patient-centered care.

- **Security Role:** AI plays a critical role in enhancing the cybersecurity posture of healthcare organizations. With the growing volume of digital health data, protecting patient privacy and securing infrastructure is more vital than ever. AI-based systems monitor network traffic, user behaviors, and access logs to detect anomalies that might indicate cyber threats. These systems can identify unusual login patterns, unauthorized access attempts, or suspicious file transfers in real time. Machine learning models adapt to evolving threats and reduce reliance on static rule-based systems. AI can also classify sensitive data and enforce access controls automatically based on context. In the case of ransomware attacks or breaches, AI aids in faster detection and response, limiting damage. It ensures compliance with regulations like HIPAA by monitoring audit trails and data integrity. Furthermore, AI supports intrusion detection systems and firewalls in filtering malicious traffic. By integrating AI into security operations, healthcare organizations can proactively safeguard patient data and maintain trust in digital systems.

2. Internet of Things (IoT) in Healthcare: Internet of Things (IoT) in healthcare is transforming the medical field by connecting devices, sensors, and systems to enable real-time monitoring and data sharing. IoT allows healthcare providers to remotely track patients' vital signs, manage chronic conditions, and respond to emergencies faster. Wearable devices, smart beds, and connected diagnostic tools improve both hospital operations and patient engagement. This technology enhances early detection of health issues and supports personalized, proactive care(Table-2). Additionally, IoT helps optimize resource usage and reduce hospital readmissions. As connectivity grows, IoT is paving the way for a smarter, more responsive healthcare ecosystem (Fig. 9).

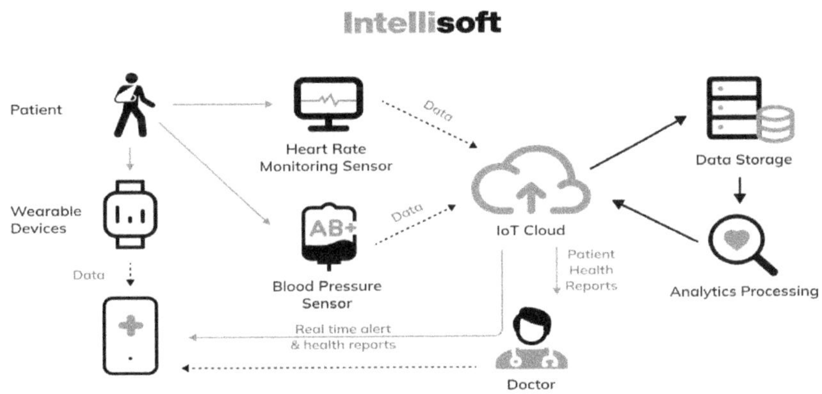

Fig.9 Internet of Things (IoT) in healthcare

Table -2 : Summary of the Internet of Things (IoT) in Healthcare

Aspect	Description
Definition	Integration of IoT devices and technologies to monitor and manage healthcare.
Key Components	Wearable devices, sensors, mobile apps, cloud computing, and medical devices.
Applications	Remote patient monitoring, chronic disease management, telemedicine, smart hospitals, fitness tracking.
Benefits	Real-time data collection, improved patient care, reduced hospital visits, cost efficiency, personalized treatment.
Examples	Smartwatches for ECG monitoring, insulin pumps, smart beds, connected inhalers.
Challenges	Data privacy, cybersecurity, device interoperability, high costs, regulatory compliance.
Future Trends	AI integration, blockchain for data security, predictive analytics, 5G adoption, robotics in care.

- **Remote Patient Monitoring:** Remote Patient Monitoring (RPM) leverages IoT-enabled wearables and smart devices to continuously track vital signs such as heart rate, blood pressure, oxygen saturation, and glucose levels. These devices transmit real-time health data directly to healthcare providers, allowing for timely interventions and adjustments in treatment plans. RPM is especially beneficial for elderly patients, post-surgical care, and those with mobility limitations. It reduces the need for frequent hospital visits, enabling patients to receive quality care from the comfort of their homes. With AI integration, RPM systems can detect trends or anomalies, prompting early medical action. This not only improves outcomes but also empowers patients to be more involved in managing their health. RPM also assists healthcare systems in prioritizing high-risk cases and reducing readmission rates. Physicians can make data-informed decisions without needing physical consultations. Insurance companies and providers also benefit from reduced costs. Ultimately, RPM increases convenience, improves disease management, and enhances patient satisfaction.

- **Connected Infrastructure:** IoT creates a connected healthcare infrastructure where devices like smart beds, infusion pumps, and asset tracking systems communicate seamlessly to optimize hospital workflows. Smart beds can monitor patient movement, adjust automatically for comfort, and alert staff in case of falls or emergencies. Infusion pumps can be remotely monitored and adjusted, ensuring precise medication delivery without manual oversight. Real-time tracking systems for medical equipment reduce search times, prevent loss, and improve resource allocation. Integration of IoT with hospital management systems enhances staff coordination, bed occupancy tracking, and emergency preparedness. Connected infrastructure improves patient flow and reduces wait times in emergency departments. It also minimizes operational inefficiencies and ensures faster responses to critical situations. By creating a smart environment, hospitals can improve service quality while lowering administrative overhead. Additionally, analytics derived from infrastructure data support continuous improvement initiatives. This interconnectedness makes hospitals safer, more responsive, and more efficient.

- **Chronic Disease Management:** IoT plays a crucial role in managing chronic diseases like diabetes, hypertension, COPD, and heart conditions through continuous monitoring and data-driven interventions. Devices such as smart glucometers, digital blood pressure cuffs, and connected inhalers collect daily health metrics and send them to caregivers in real time. This constant stream of data enables physicians to detect early warning signs, adjust medications promptly, and personalize care plans based on individual health trends. Patients can receive real-time feedback, leading to better self-management and adherence to treatment protocols. The proactive nature of IoT reduces emergency room visits and hospital admissions for chronic patients. Moreover, caregivers and family members can stay informed about patient status, creating a support network that promotes better outcomes. AI algorithms analyze collected data for predictive insights and tailored alerts. This continuous loop of feedback fosters a more preventive and patient-centric care approach. Overall, IoT enhances the quality of life for patients with long term conditions.
- **Data-Driven Alerts:** IoT devices generate data-driven alerts by continuously monitoring patients and detecting anomalies in vital signs or activity patterns. When abnormalities such as arrhythmias, oxygen drops, or sudden falls are detected, the system immediately sends notifications to healthcare providers, caregivers, or emergency services. These real-time alerts enable rapid medical intervention, potentially saving lives in critical situations. In hospital settings, such alerts can indicate equipment malfunctions, medication errors, or breaches in safety protocols. AI-enhanced analytics further improve alert accuracy by reducing false positives and prioritizing the most urgent cases. Alerts can also be customized based on patient history and care protocols. For patients at home, wearable devices can send alerts to family members or call for emergency services autonomously. Data-driven alerting ensures proactive care, minimizes human error, and bridges the gap between patient and provider in real-time. This continuous monitoring builds a safety net that empowers both clinicians and patients.

- **Security Concerns:** While IoT significantly enhances healthcare delivery, it also introduces critical security vulnerabilities. IoT devices are often deployed with limited computing power and minimal security features, making them attractive targets for cyberattacks. Breaches in IoT endpoints can lead to unauthorized access to sensitive patient data or manipulation of medical devices. Therefore, robust security measures—such as end-to-end encryption, secure boot processes, and multi-factor authentication—are essential. Network segmentation and device-level firewalls can help contain threats. AI can assist in threat detection by identifying unusual patterns in device behavior, flagging potential attacks in real time. Regular software updates and device patching are crucial to maintaining defenses against evolving threats. Compliance with healthcare regulations like HIPAA and GDPR is also necessary to ensure legal protection of patient data. Manufacturers and healthcare providers must work collaboratively to establish secure standards. In a connected environment, cybersecurity is not optional—it's a fundamental requirement for patient safety and system reliability.

3. Blockchain in Healthcare: Blockchain in healthcare offers a transformative approach to managing data security, transparency, and interoperability. By using a decentralized and tamper-proof ledger, blockchain ensures that medical records are securely stored and only accessible to authorized users. It enhances trust between patients, providers, and institutions by enabling verifiable data sharing without compromising privacy. Smart contracts can automate processes like consent management and insurance claims. From securing patient identities to tracking pharmaceutical supply chains, blockchain strengthens every layer of the healthcare system (Table-3). As digital health expands, blockchain provides a resilient foundation for secure, transparent, and efficient operations (Fig. 10).

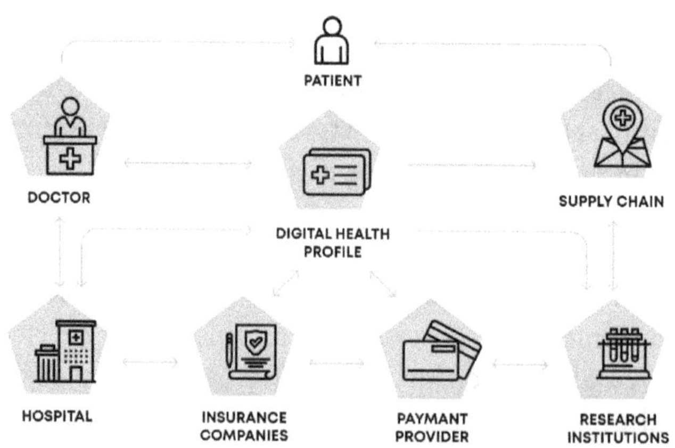

Fig.10 Blockchain in healthcare

Table 3: Summary of Blockchain in Healthcare

Aspect	Description
Definition	A decentralized, secure ledger technology used to store and share healthcare data.
Key Features	Immutability, transparency, decentralization, enhanced security, smart contracts.
Applications	Electronic Health Records (EHR), medical supply chain management, clinical trials, billing & claims processing, patient consent management.
Benefits	Improved data security, enhanced interoperability, fraud prevention, streamlined operations, patient control over data.
Examples	MedRec (MIT), Chronicled, Guardtime, Medicalchain, IBM Blockchain in Healthcare.
Challenges	Regulatory uncertainty, scalability, integration with legacy systems, data privacy concerns, high implementation cost.
Future Trends	Blockchain + AI for predictive healthcare, patient-owned data marketplaces, increased adoption in telehealth, interoperability standards.

- **Data Integrity:** Blockchain ensures the integrity of healthcare data by creating an immutable and tamper-proof ledger for storing medical records. Each transaction or data entry is time-stamped and cryptographically secured, making it impossible to alter without leaving a trace. This guarantees that patient data remains accurate, authentic, and unchanged over time. It is especially vital in clinical trials, diagnostics, and legal contexts where data accuracy is paramount. Immutable records also reduce the risk of medical errors stemming from altered or missing information. Audit trails are automatically maintained, enabling quick verification of changes and access history. Hospitals and regulators benefit from increased transparency, which boosts compliance and trust. Moreover, in cases of data breaches, blockchain ensures that compromised data can be identified and isolated without affecting the integrity of the entire system. This permanence helps prevent fraud and unauthorized modifications. As healthcare digitization grows, ensuring data integrity becomes a foundational requirement—one that blockchain is uniquely equipped to provide.
- **Patient Consent Management:** Blockchain revolutionizes patient consent management by using smart contracts to provide secure, programmable access to personal health data. Traditionally, consent forms are paper-based or stored in disparate systems, leading to delays, confusion, or misuse. With blockchain, patients can grant, revoke, or modify access to their medical records in real time through a digital identity system. Smart contracts automatically execute these permissions based on predefined rules, ensuring transparency and compliance with patient preferences. This allows patients to take full control of who views or uses their health

data, whether it's a doctor, researcher, or insurer. Such systems support informed decision-making and protect against unauthorized data sharing. It's especially useful in multi-institutional care, where consistent access rights are crucial. The blockchain ledger keeps a record of all consent actions, enabling complete auditability. Consent becomes dynamic rather than static, evolving as the patient's situation changes. In essence, blockchain empowers patients and reinforces trust in digital healthcare systems.

- **Interoperability:** One of the biggest challenges in healthcare is achieving seamless interoperability across different systems and institutions. Blockchain addresses this by serving as a universal, decentralized ledger that allows secure and standardized data exchange. Unlike traditional systems, where information silos hinder communication, blockchain enables the integration of electronic health records (EHRs) across hospitals, clinics, labs, and pharmacies. It ensures that data remains consistent and synchronized across platforms while maintaining patient privacy and security. Providers can access a complete and up-to-date medical history, improving diagnosis accuracy and continuity of care. Patients benefit from not having to repeat tests or explain their history multiple times. Blockchain also supports metadata tagging and indexing, which simplifies record retrieval. Integration with APIs and healthcare information systems enhances its adaptability. In emergencies, access to reliable patient data can be lifesaving. Ultimately, blockchain-powered interoperability reduces redundancy, lowers costs, and facilitates coordinated, patient-centric care delivery.
- **Supply Chain Security:** Blockchain brings end-to-end transparency and traceability to the healthcare supply chain, addressing issues of fraud, counterfeiting, and inefficiency. Each transaction in the supply chain—from manufacturing to distribution to patient delivery—is recorded in a shared, immutable ledger. This creates a verifiable audit trail that ensures the authenticity and origin of medical products, such as pharmaceuticals, vaccines, and medical devices. By scanning a product's QR code or RFID tag linked to a blockchain record, stakeholders can instantly verify its journey and condition. It helps prevent the infiltration of fake or expired medications into the system—a serious concern, especially in developing regions. Smart contracts can automate compliance checks and trigger alerts if anomalies are detected. Blockchain also ensures that cold-chain conditions are met for temperature-sensitive drugs. Regulators, suppliers, and healthcare providers gain full visibility into the supply network. This

transparency not only ensures patient safety but also boosts operational efficiency and trust across the supply chain.

- **Data Access Control:** Blockchain enhances data access control through decentralized identity management and permissioned access systems. Instead of relying on centralized servers that are prone to breaches, blockchain distributes control to individual users—primarily the patients. Each patient is issued a unique cryptographic identity, allowing them to manage who can view or edit their health information. Access is granted via digital keys and tracked on the blockchain ledger, ensuring transparency and accountability. If access is no longer needed, patients can instantly revoke permissions. This model supports fine-grained access, where different roles (e.g., doctors, insurers, researchers) receive only the data relevant to them. It aligns with privacy laws like HIPAA and GDPR by ensuring that data is accessed and processed only with explicit consent. Blockchain can also integrate biometric authentication for added security. This level of granular control significantly reduces data misuse and unauthorized exposure. By placing control back in the hands of patients, blockchain fosters a more secure and ethical healthcare data ecosystem.

4. Integration for Enhanced Security and Efficiency: The combined application of Artificial Intelligence (AI), the Internet of Things (IoT), and Blockchain is creating a powerful, integrated ecosystem that significantly enhances both security and efficiency in healthcare. AI leverages real-time data from IoT devices to detect health anomalies, predict risks, and guide timely interventions, improving diagnostic accuracy and operational responsiveness. Meanwhile, Blockchain secures this data by ensuring its authenticity, immutability, and controlled access across networks. For example, IoT-enabled wearables monitor vital signs, AI interprets the data to detect early warning signs, and Blockchain protects that data from tampering or misuse. This triad also ensures secure, efficient sharing of electronic health records (EHRs) across institutions without compromising privacy. Smart contracts automate patient consent and streamline insurance claims, while predictive analytics optimize resource allocation. Together, these technologies reduce administrative burden, improve patient outcomes, and enhance data transparency (Table-4). Their integration is not just a technological advancement—it is a strategic necessity for building a modern, resilient, and patient-centric healthcare system (Fig. 11).

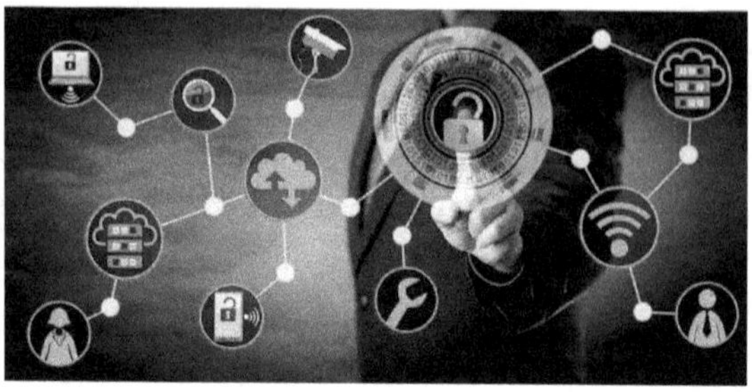

Fig. 11 Smart surveillance is elevating security through IoT integration

Table 4 : Summary of Integration for Enhanced Security and Efficiency in Healthcare

Aspect	Description
Definition	Combining advanced technologies (e.g., IoT, Blockchain, AI) to improve security and operational efficiency in health-care.
Technologies Involved	IoT, Blockchain, Artificial Intelligence (AI), Cloud Comput-ing, Big Data, EHR systems.
Security En-hancements	Encrypted data sharing, secure authentication, decentral-ized records, real-time threat detection.
Efficiency Im-provements	Automated workflows, faster diagnosis, reduced adminis-trative burden, better data access and sharing.
Use Cases	Secure remote monitoring, AI-based diagnostic tools, blockchain-based patient consent, automated billing.
Benefits	Enhanced data protection, improved patient outcomes, lower operational costs, streamlined processes.
Challenges	Integration complexity, high costs, interoperability issues, training requirements, regulatory compliance.
Future Outlook	Fully connected health ecosystems, zero-trust security models, AI-led decision-making, real-time healthcare deliv-ery.

- **AI + IoT: Enhancing Predictive Healthcare:** The integration of Artificial Intelligence (AI) with the Internet of Things (IoT) has opened new frontiers in predictive and personalized healthcare. IoT devices such as smart wearables, remote monitors, and implantable sensors continuously collect real-time patient data like heart rate, glucose levels, and respiratory activity. AI processes this massive stream of data using machine learning models to identify patterns, detect anomalies, and generate actionable insights. This allows healthcare providers to predict health deteriorations or emergencies before they occur, facilitating early interventions. It significantly helps in managing chronic diseases, reducing hospital admissions, and improving patient compliance with treatment plans. For instance, AI can alert a clinician when a patient's vitals deviate from expected norms, even slightly, prompting preemptive care. It also prioritizes cases based on risk levels, helping with better triage and resource use. Combined, AI and IoT support remote monitoring, faster decision-making, and enhanced operational efficiency in both in-hospital and at-home care environments. This synergy strengthens proactive care and reduces dependency on reactive models.

- **Blockchain + IoT: Building Trust and Traceability:** The convergence of Blockchain and IoT in healthcare ensures that the data collected from connected medical devices is not only comprehensive but also secure, traceable, and verifiable. IoT sensors continuously generate sensitive health information, which, if left unprotected, is susceptible to tampering, hacking, or misuse. Blockchain addresses these vulnerabilities by providing a decentralized ledger where all device interactions and data logs are time-stamped and immutable. This creates a transparent, auditable trail of where data originated, how it has been accessed, and by whom. In supply chains, blockchain-integrated IoT devices track pharmaceuticals, vaccines, and surgical tools from manufacturer to patient, minimizing the risk of counterfeit products. Device calibration records, usage logs, and maintenance histories can also be recorded on blockchain, ensuring accountability and performance validation. This integration enhances trust among patients, clinicians, and regulators, as all data transactions are verifiable and resistant to fraud. It supports regulatory compliance and patient safety, especially in critical care and drug delivery scenarios. The fusion of IoT's sensing capabilities with blockchain's security infrastructure forms a robust foundation for trusted, data-driven healthcare operations.
- **AI + Blockchain: Secure Intelligence with Verified Data:** Pairing AI with Blockchain technology in healthcare enables the development of intelligent systems that rely on secure, verified, and traceable data. While AI requires vast amounts of high-quality data to train models and generate predictions, blockchain ensures that this data is authentic, unaltered, and comes from trusted sources. This is particularly important in clinical research, diagnostics, and personalized medicine, where decisions must be based on accurate and ethically sourced data. AI can process blockchain-logged patient histories, genomic data, or imaging records to identify disease risks, recommend treatments, or simulate outcomes. In return, blockchain tracks each AI decision, providing transparency and traceability that supports explainable AI in healthcare. It can also enforce data usage policies through smart contracts, ensuring AI systems use only consented and relevant data.

This integration fosters patient trust while ensuring regulatory compliance. It's especially valuable in decentralized clinical trials, telemedicine, and AI-driven drug discovery. Together, AI and blockchain balance the power of predictive analytics with the necessity of data integrity, security, and transparency.

- **Triad Synergy: AI, IoT, and Blockchain for Intelligent, Secure Healthcare:** The true potential of healthcare innovation emerges when AI, IoT, and Blockchain technologies are integrated into a single, synergistic system. In this triad, IoT devices gather real-time patient data, AI analyzes this information to provide predictive insights or trigger interventions, and Blockchain secures the data, ensuring its integrity and controlled access. This creates a closed-loop healthcare ecosystem that is intelligent, responsive, and trustworthy. For example, a wearable device could detect an irregular heartbeat, AI could assess the risk of cardiac arrest, and blockchain would log the event securely while sharing it with authorized care teams instantly. Such integrated systems enhance care delivery, especially in remote settings and for chronic disease management. They also automate administrative workflows like consent handling, insurance verification, and supply chain tracking. The triad enables holistic digital health transformation by supporting secure data sharing, real-time responsiveness, and informed decision-making. As healthcare systems become more complex and data-centric, this fusion provides a robust infrastructure for patient-centered, efficient, and secure operations. It represents the future of smart healthcare.

8.1.6 Challenges-Data privacy, infrastructure gaps, digital literacy

In the rapidly evolving landscape of digital healthcare, several critical challenges continue to hinder the full realization of its potential. Among the most pressing are data privacy, infrastructure gaps, and digital literacy. As healthcare systems integrate advanced technologies like Electronic Health Records (EHRs), IoT devices, and AI-driven platforms, safeguarding sensitive patient data has become increasingly complex. Data breaches and unauthorized access not only threaten individual privacy but also undermine trust in digital health solutions. Simultaneously, infrastructure gaps remain a major barrier, particularly in rural and under-resourced regions. Inconsistent internet connectivity, outdated hardware, and the lack of standardized systems prevent seamless data exchange and efficient care delivery. These limitations restrict access to real-time health monitoring and telemedicine services, exacerbating healthcare inequalities. Moreover, digital literacy poses another significant challenge. Both healthcare professionals and patients often lack the necessary skills to effectively use digital tools, leading to underutilization, errors, and frustration. Without targeted education and training, the benefits of digital transformation may remain out of reach for many. Addressing these interconnected challenges is crucial to building a secure, inclusive, and efficient digital healthcare ecosystem (Table-5).

Table -5: Summary of the Challenges of Data Privacy, Infrastructure Gaps, Digital Literacy in healthcare

Challenge	Description	Impact	Potential Solutions
Data Privacy	Protection of sensitive patient information like medical history, genetic data, and treatment records.	Risk of breaches, identity theft, loss of patient trust.	Strong encryption, access controls, compliance with regulations, patient consent management.
Infrastructure Gaps	Lack of reliable internet, outdated IT systems, uneven technology distribution, especially in rural areas.	Limited access to digital health services, data silos, inefficiency.	Investment in broadband, modernization of legacy systems, standardized interoperability frameworks.
Digital Literacy	Limited skills and knowledge among healthcare providers and patients to use digital health tools effectively.	Underutilization of technology, increased errors, patient exclusion.	Training programs, user-friendly interfaces, ongoing education for all stakeholders.

1. Data Privacy

- **Sensitive Nature of Health Data:** Healthcare data is among the most sensitive types of personal information, encompassing details such as medical histories, diagnostic reports, genetic profiles, and ongoing treatment records. This data not only reflects an individual's current health status but can also reveal deeply personal aspects such as hereditary risks and mental health conditions. Because of its highly confidential nature, any unauthorized access or breach can lead to severe consequences for patients, including discrimination, stigma, and emotional distress. Moreover, compromised health data can result in identity theft or financial fraud if linked with other personal identifiers. Protecting this data is therefore crucial, not only to uphold patient privacy but also to maintain trust in healthcare providers and digital health technologies. As healthcare systems increasingly rely on electronic records and cloud storage, the risk associated with data exposure grows, emphasizing the need for robust security frameworks. The sensitivity of this information mandates that healthcare organizations adopt stringent data governance policies and invest in advanced encryption and secure storage solutions. Ensuring confidentiality and integrity of health data is fundamental to delivering safe, ethical, and effective care in the digital age.

- **Cybersecurity Threats:** The rapid adoption of digital health platforms has introduced a new array of cybersecurity challenges that healthcare organizations must navigate. Cybercriminals are increasingly targeting hospitals, clinics, and health IT providers because of the valuable and often vulnerable data they hold. Common cyber threats include ransomware attacks that lock healthcare systems until a ransom is paid, phishing scams designed to trick employees into revealing login credentials, and sophisticated hacking attempts to steal patient records. Such breaches can cause widespread disruption of medical services, putting patients' lives at risk by delaying treatments or losing critical health information. Additionally, cyberattacks can result in hefty financial losses and legal penalties for healthcare institutions, alongside significant reputational damage. The healthcare sector's traditional underinvestment in cybersecurity infrastructure makes it a soft target for attackers. As healthcare becomes more interconnected through IoT devices and telemedicine platforms, the attack surface expands, requiring continuous monitoring and advanced threat detection systems. Proactive cybersecurity strategies, staff training, and incident response planning are essential to safeguard digital health ecosystems from evolving threats.
- **Lack of Standard Regulations:** One of the critical obstacles to secure data sharing in healthcare is the absence or inconsistency of standard privacy regulations across different regions and countries. While some areas have established comprehensive laws—such as HIPAA in the United States or GDPR in the European Union—many others operate under outdated frameworks that fail to address the complexities of modern digital health technologies. This regulatory patchwork complicates cross-border data exchange and interoperability, as healthcare providers must navigate varying compliance requirements. The lack of harmonized standards also creates loopholes that can be exploited, putting patient data at risk. Furthermore, regulations often lag behind technological advancements, meaning emerging tools like AI analytics, blockchain, and IoT devices are sometimes left unregulated or ambiguously governed. This uncertainty can deter innovation or result in inconsistent application of privacy principles. Policymakers, industry stakeholders, and healthcare providers must collaborate to develop clear, adaptive, and enforceable regulations that balance innovation with patient protection. Consistent legal frameworks are essential to foster trust, enable secure data sharing, and ensure equitable access to digital health services globally.

- **Patient Consent and Control:** Ensuring patients have meaningful control over their personal health data is a fundamental yet complex challenge in digital healthcare. Informed consent requires that patients fully understand who is accessing their data, for what purposes, and how it will be used or shared. However, this transparency is difficult to achieve when data flows across multiple systems, providers, and third-party applications, each with varying privacy practices. Patients may inadvertently consent to broad data use agreements without clear knowledge of downstream sharing or potential risks. Moreover, the technical mechanisms to enforce consent preferences—such as granular access controls or revocation options—are often limited or non-existent in current health IT infrastructures. Balancing usability with privacy rights necessitates designing user-friendly consent management tools that empower patients to make informed decisions. Without effective consent frameworks, patient trust erodes, which can lead to reduced data sharing and less effective care coordination. Healthcare organizations must prioritize patient autonomy by adopting transparent policies, leveraging technologies like blockchain for auditability, and educating patients about their rights and options. Empowering patients to control their health data is key to ethical, patient-centric digital health ecosystems.

2. Infrastructure Gaps

- **Unequal Technology Distribution:** One of the most significant infrastructure challenges in healthcare is the uneven distribution of technology across regions. Rural and underdeveloped areas often lack access to basic necessities like high-speed internet and reliable electricity, which are essential for deploying digital health solutions. Without these foundational services, implementing telemedicine, remote patient monitoring, or real-time data sharing becomes nearly impossible. This digital divide exacerbates existing health disparities, limiting access to quality care for populations that may already be underserved. Even where basic infrastructure exists, the availability of modern healthcare IT systems is frequently limited, restricting the ability to collect, store, and analyze patient data efficiently. This lack of technological resources stifles innovation and reduces the potential impact of digital health initiatives. Addressing this issue requires coordinated efforts from governments, private sector, and international organizations to invest in infrastructure development and ensure equitable technology access. Closing this gap is vital for creating a healthcare ecosystem where all individuals benefit from digital advances, regardless of their location or socio-economic status.

- **Legacy Systems:** Many healthcare providers, especially longstanding hospitals and clinics, continue to rely on legacy IT systems that were not designed to integrate with modern digital health technologies. These outdated systems often operate on obsolete software and hardware, creating isolated data silos that impede the smooth exchange of health information. The inability of legacy systems to communicate with newer platforms leads to inefficiencies, duplicated efforts, and potential errors in patient care. For example, manual data entry or paper-based records remain common in many facilities, slowing down clinical workflows and limiting data accuracy. Moreover, upgrading or replacing these systems can be complex, costly, and risky, as it may disrupt ongoing operations. This resistance to change can hinder the adoption of advanced solutions like AI-driven diagnostics or real-time remote monitoring. Healthcare organizations must balance maintaining day-to-day operations with the need for modernization, often requiring strategic planning and phased implementation. Finding scalable, interoperable solutions that can bridge the gap between legacy and emerging systems is critical to advancing healthcare digital transformation.
- **Interoperability Issues:** Interoperability remains a major challenge in healthcare, as various providers and systems use different data formats, standards, and technologies. This fragmentation prevents seamless sharing and integration of patient information, which is essential for coordinated care, especially when patients receive treatment from multiple providers. Without interoperability, vital data such as lab results, medication histories, or imaging reports may be unavailable or delayed, increasing the risk of errors and redundant testing. The lack of standardized protocols means healthcare organizations often need to rely on costly custom interfaces or manual data reconciliation. Furthermore, emerging technologies such as IoT devices and AI analytics demand consistent and high-quality data inputs, which are difficult to ensure in non-interoperable environments. Addressing this challenge requires the adoption of universal standards like HL7 FHIR and collaborative efforts across industry stakeholders. Improving interoperability enhances patient outcomes by enabling real-time information exchange, supports better clinical decision-making, and increases operational efficiency.
- **High Implementation Costs:** The financial burden of upgrading healthcare infrastructure to support digital health solutions can be prohibitive for many organizations. Investments are required not only for purchasing new hardware and software but also for hiring skilled personnel capable

of managing and maintaining advanced systems. Smaller clinics and rural hospitals, in particular, may lack the budget to undertake such costly transformations, leading to slower adoption of digital technologies. High implementation costs also include expenses related to staff training, data migration, system customization, and ongoing cybersecurity measures. These financial challenges can discourage healthcare providers from embracing innovation, perpetuating reliance on inefficient manual processes. Additionally, the return on investment may not be immediately apparent, as benefits like improved patient outcomes and operational savings accrue over time. To overcome this barrier, funding models such as government grants, public-private partnerships, and scalable cloud-based solutions can help lower upfront costs. Strategic planning, cost-benefit analysis, and phased rollouts are essential to maximize investment impact and ensure sustainable digital health adoption.

3. Digital Literacy

- **Healthcare Professionals' Readiness:** A major challenge in digital healthcare adoption is the readiness of healthcare professionals to effectively use advanced digital tools. Many doctors, nurses, and administrative staff lack comprehensive training in emerging technologies such as Electronic Health Records (EHRs), telemedicine platforms, and AI-based diagnostic tools. This gap can lead to operational inefficiencies, increased risk of errors, and even resistance to adopting new systems. Without sufficient digital literacy, healthcare workers may struggle to navigate software interfaces, interpret data outputs, or integrate technology into clinical workflows. Furthermore, the stress and workload pressures in healthcare environments can reduce the time available for training. Inadequate preparation not only hampers the benefits of digital transformation but can also compromise patient safety and care quality. To address this, healthcare organizations must invest in structured training programs, hands-on workshops, and ongoing support. Cultivating digital proficiency among professionals is essential for maximizing technology's potential and improving healthcare delivery.
- **Patient Digital Skills:** Digital literacy challenges extend beyond healthcare providers to patients themselves. Many individuals, especially the elderly, less educated, or economically disadvantaged, may find it difficult to use digital health tools such as mobile apps, telemedicine services, or wearable monitoring devices. This limits their ability to access essential healthcare remotely, participate in self-management programs, or share health data securely. The lack of digital skills can lead to frustration, decreased engagement, and lower adherence to treatment plans. Moreover, patients

unfamiliar with technology might be less likely to trust digital platforms, further hindering adoption. Bridging this gap requires targeted patient education initiatives, intuitive app designs, and support services like helplines or community training sessions. Enhancing patient digital literacy empowers individuals to take greater control of their health and helps reduce disparities in healthcare access and outcomes.

- **Language and Accessibility Barriers:** Another critical issue in digital health is the lack of multilingual and accessible platform designs. Many digital health tools are created primarily in dominant languages, with limited consideration for non-native speakers or those with limited language proficiency. This can exclude significant patient populations from benefiting fully from telehealth, health apps, or online portals. Additionally, platforms often lack features to accommodate persons with disabilities, such as screen readers, voice commands, or adjustable text sizes, which are essential for visually impaired or physically challenged users. Without inclusive design, digital health risks widening health inequities by leaving vulnerable groups behind. Addressing these barriers requires deliberate efforts to incorporate multiple languages, culturally sensitive content, and accessibility standards from the outset. Inclusive digital health solutions enhance usability and foster equitable healthcare access for diverse populations.
- **Need for Ongoing Training:** The fast pace of innovation in digital healthcare necessitates continuous education and skill development for both healthcare providers and patients. New technologies, software updates, regulatory changes, and evolving best practices require ongoing training programs to keep users proficient and confident. However, many healthcare organizations underestimate or underfund these efforts, resulting in outdated knowledge and suboptimal use of digital tools. Lack of refresher courses, workshops, and e-learning opportunities can lead to frustration and decreased efficiency. Moreover, as digital health ecosystems grow more complex, specialized training in areas like data privacy, cybersecurity, and AI interpretation becomes increasingly important. Establishing a culture of lifelong learning through regular training sessions, certifications, and user support enhances adaptability and ensures that healthcare professionals and patients can fully leverage technological advancements.

8.1.7 Impact-Enhanced healthcare delivery, better disease management, cost reduction

The integration of advanced technologies in healthcare has significantly transformed the way medical services are delivered, leading to enhanced healthcare delivery, better disease management, and substantial cost reductions. By leveraging digital tools such as remote monitoring devices, telemedicine, and data analytics, healthcare providers can offer more timely, accurate, and personalized care to patients. This shift not only improves patient outcomes but also increases access to care, especially for those in remote or underserved areas. Better disease management is achieved through continuous monitoring and early detection, allowing for proactive interventions that prevent complications and hospitalizations. Additionally, digital health solutions streamline administrative processes, reduce redundancies, and minimize errors, which collectively drive down operational costs. The efficient use of resources and improved coordination among healthcare teams further contribute to lowering healthcare expenses. As a result, both providers and patients benefit from a system that is more effective, patient-centered, and economically sustainable. This impact highlights the critical role of technology in shaping the future of healthcare delivery worldwide.

Enhanced Healthcare Delivery: The integration of digital technologies has revolutionized healthcare delivery, making it more efficient, accessible, and patient-centered. Telemedicine platforms and remote monitoring devices enable healthcare providers to offer consultations and continuous care regardless of patients' geographic locations, breaking down barriers related to distance and mobility. Real-time access to patient data allows for faster diagnosis and more informed clinical decisions, reducing delays in treatment. Digital tools also facilitate better coordination among multidisciplinary teams, improving communication and care planning. Automated administrative systems decrease paperwork and streamline workflows, allowing clinicians to focus more on patient care. Furthermore, personalized medicine powered by data analytics tailors treatments to individual patient needs, enhancing the overall quality of care. These advancements collectively contribute to improved patient satisfaction and health outcomes. Enhanced healthcare delivery not only optimizes resource utilization but also fosters a more responsive and resilient healthcare system capable of adapting to future challenges.

Better Disease Management: Digital health technologies have significantly improved disease management by enabling continuous monitoring, early detection, and timely interventions. Wearable sensors and mobile apps track vital signs and symptoms in real-time, providing patients and clinicians with valuable data to manage chronic conditions such as diabetes, hypertension, and heart disease. This constant flow of information helps detect health deteriorations before they become critical, allowing for preventive care that reduces hospital admissions and complications. Patient engagement tools encourage adherence to medication and lifestyle changes, empowering individuals to take an active role in their health.

Furthermore, data analytics and AI-driven predictive models help identify high-risk patients and optimize treatment plans tailored to their unique profiles. Telehealth services expand access to specialists and support networks, improving management for those with complex conditions. Collectively, these technologies transform reactive care into proactive, continuous disease management, resulting in better patient outcomes and quality of life.

Cost Reduction: The adoption of digital health solutions contributes significantly to reducing healthcare costs by improving efficiency and eliminating waste. Automated administrative processes reduce paperwork and billing errors, cutting down on overhead expenses and freeing up staff resources. Remote patient monitoring and telemedicine reduce the need for costly in-person visits and hospital stays by managing health issues proactively and preventing complications. Early diagnosis and timely intervention minimize expensive emergency treatments and long-term care requirements. Digital tools also streamline supply chain management and optimize resource allocation, further reducing operational costs. Additionally, improved data sharing and interoperability reduce duplicative tests and procedures, saving both time and money. These cost savings benefit healthcare providers, payers, and patients alike, making healthcare more affordable and sustainable. By balancing quality care with cost efficiency, digital health innovations support the development of value-based healthcare models that prioritize outcomes over volume.

8.2 FDA AND REGULATORY APPROVAL FOR DIGITAL DEVICES

The rapid advancement of digital health technologies has dramatically reshaped the landscape of modern healthcare, offering innovative solutions to enhance diagnosis, treatment, and patient engagement. From mobile health (mHealth) applications that track daily wellness metrics to wearable devices that monitor heart rate, glucose levels, or sleep patterns, these tools are becoming essential in promoting preventive care and chronic disease management. More sophisticated innovations such as AI-powered diagnostic tools can now analyze medical images with accuracy comparable to human specialists, while remote patient monitoring (RPM) systems allow clinicians to track patient vitals in real-time, even outside traditional healthcare settings. As these technologies become increasingly integrated into clinical practice, there is a growing imperative to establish robust regulatory frameworks to ensure their safety, effectiveness, accuracy, and reliability. In the United States, the Food and Drug Administration (FDA) serves as the primary authority for regulating medical devices, including those with digital components. The FDA's oversight is critical to maintaining public trust in health technologies, as it ensures that products reaching the market are rigorously tested, scientifically validated, and function safely within their intended use.

The FDA defines a "medical device" broadly under the Federal Food, Drug, and Cosmetic Act, which includes any instrument, apparatus, implement, machine, software, or related article that is used for diagnosing, curing, mitigating, treating, or preventing disease, or that affects the structure or function of the body. As such, many digital health products—especially those that provide clinical decision support or are involved in disease diagnosis or treatment—fall under this definition and are subject to formal regulatory review.

This oversight extends to emerging technologies such as Software as a Medical Device (SaMD), which encompasses software that performs medical functions independently of hardware, such as an AI model that detects diabetic retinopathy from retinal images. Similarly, mobile apps that function as diagnostic tools or dosage calculators must demonstrate safety and efficacy to gain FDA clearance or approval. Devices are typically categorized by risk: Class I (low risk), Class II (moderate risk), and Class III (high risk)—with regulatory pathways like 510(k) clearance, De Novo classification, or Premarket Approval (PMA) required depending on classification. Each pathway involves varying levels of documentation, clinical validation, and post-market surveillance. Beyond national borders, other countries maintain their own regulatory bodies with similar mandates. For example, the European Medicines Agency (EMA) and European Commission oversee digital medical devices in the EU through the Medical Device Regulation (MDR), which recently tightened requirements for safety and transparency. In India, the Central Drugs Standard Control Organization (CDSCO) governs the approval and monitoring of medical devices and has begun establishing guidelines for digital health and software-based products. While objectives across these agencies are aligned—focusing on public health, patient safety, and product integrity—their processes, timelines, and documentation standards often differ, posing challenges for companies seeking global market entry. Moreover, the pace of digital innovation often outstrips existing regulatory frameworks, requiring agencies like the FDA to adapt quickly. Recognizing this, the FDA has introduced several forward-thinking initiatives, including the Digital Health Innovation Action Plan, SaMD regulatory guidance, and the Digital Health Software Precertification Program, aimed at expediting review processes while maintaining safety standards. These efforts reflect a shift toward more agile, transparent, and iterative regulatory models that align with the fast-moving nature of software development and AI evolution. Importantly, regulatory approval is not a one-time event. Post-market surveillance and real-world evidence collection are essential to monitor the ongoing performance of digital health products, detect unforeseen risks, and inform future updates. This is especially crucial for AI-based tools that learn and evolve over time, necessitating adaptive regulatory approaches such as the FDA's proposed framework for AI/ML-based Software as a Medical Device (SaMD), which includes a Predetermined Change Control Plan to manage algorithm updates responsibly. As digital health technologies become more deeply embedded in patient care, the role of regulatory agencies like the FDA and their international counterparts is more important than ever. Their work ensures that innovation does not come at the cost of patient safety and that products introduced into the healthcare system are trustworthy, transparent, and clinically valid. Establishing clear and consistent regulatory pathways is essential for fostering innovation, protecting public health, and building a sustainable digital health ecosystem globally.

8.2.1 "Medical Device" under FDA

The U.S. Food and Drug Administration (FDA) defines a medical device in broad terms under the Federal Food, Drug, and Cosmetic Act (FD&C Act), encompassing not only traditional hardware devices but also modern digital technologies. A digital product is classified as a medical device if it is intended for use in the diagnosis, cure, mitigation, treatment, or prevention of disease, or if it affects the structure or any function of the body. This definition captures a wide range of innovative technologies, including mobile ECG monitors that track cardiac activity, AI-powered imaging tools that assist radiologists in identifying abnormalities, and digital therapeutics that deliver evidence-based behavioral interventions for conditions like depression or insomnia. Also included are insulin dosing calculators and smart inhalers that actively participate in medical decision-making. In contrast, apps focused solely on general wellness—such as fitness trackers, diet logs, or meditation timers—typically fall outside the scope of FDA regulation unless they make explicit medical claims or are used for clinical purposes. The distinction between regulated and unregulated digital tools is crucial, as it determines whether a product must undergo rigorous evaluation for safety, effectiveness, and data integrity before entering the market. As digital health evolves, understanding this classification helps developers, clinicians, and patients make informed decisions about the tools they use in healthcare.

8.2.2 Classification of Digital Devices (Class I, II, III)

To ensure patient safety and appropriate regulatory oversight, the FDA classifies medical devices, including digital health technologies, into three categories: Class I, Class II, and Class III. This classification is based on the level of risk the device poses to patients and users, as well as the degree of regulatory control required. Class I devices are considered low-risk and are subject to the least regulatory burden, often requiring only general controls such as good manufacturing practices and proper labeling. Examples include digital thermometers or wellness tracking apps. Class II devices pose moderate risk and require more stringent controls, including 510(k) premarket notification, where the manufacturer must demonstrate that the new device is substantially equivalent to an already approved device. Devices like smart blood pressure monitors or glucose meters often fall into this category. Class III devices are high-risk and typically sustain or support life, are implanted, or present potential risks of serious harm. These require Premarket Approval (PMA), involving extensive clinical testing and scientific evidence. Examples include AI-driven diagnostic platforms for cancer detection or implantable defibrillators with software components. Understanding these classes helps developers choose the correct regulatory path and ensures safe innovation in digital healthcare.

The FDA categorizes medical devices based on risk to the patient:

- **Class I (Low Risk):** Class I medical devices pose the least amount of risk to patients and users and are typically subject to general regulatory controls. These include standards related to manufacturing practices, proper labeling, and record-keeping. Most Class I devices are non-invasive and do not directly affect the patient's health outcomes, making them suitable for simplified regulatory oversight. Many of these devices are exempt from premarket review, allowing for quicker entry into the market. Examples include fitness trackers, basic health apps that monitor steps or hydration, and digital scales. These tools support general wellness and healthy living but do not provide diagnostic or treatment functionalities. While the regulatory burden is minimal, manufacturers must still ensure their products meet quality standards and do not make medical claims. Class I classification enables innovation while maintaining a baseline of consumer safety and product accountability.
- **Class II (Moderate Risk):** Class II devices involve moderate risk and require both general and special regulatory controls to ensure safety and effectiveness. These devices often perform critical functions like monitoring health conditions or assisting in diagnosis, but they are not life-sustaining. Manufacturers must typically submit a 510(k) premarket notification, demonstrating that their product is substantially equivalent to an existing, legally marketed device. Examples include glucose monitors, smart thermometers, digital blood pressure cuffs, and clinical decision support software. Class II regulations may also require performance standards, post-market surveillance, and labeling requirements. This classification strikes a balance between promoting innovation and ensuring devices are safe, accurate, and effective before being widely used in clinical or home settings. It is the most common category for digital health tools currently on the market.
- **Class III (High Risk):** Class III medical devices carry the highest risk and are used in situations where failure could result in serious injury or death.

These include life-sustaining, life-supporting, or implantable devices, as well as those used in critical diagnostic or therapeutic contexts. Because of the high stakes, Class III devices require a rigorous Premarket Approval (PMA) process, which involves clinical trials, safety and efficacy data, and manufacturing inspections. Examples include AI-based cancer diagnostic platforms, robotic surgical systems, and implantable pacemakers with digital components. The PMA process is time-consuming and resource-intensive but ensures that only the most thoroughly vetted technologies reach the market. Class III devices are subject to intense post-market surveillance to monitor real-world performance. Regulatory rigor in this category is essential to maintaining trust, safety, and clinical effectiveness in advanced digital health innovations. The classification determines the regulatory path a device must take to reach market.

8.2.3 Regulatory Pathways for Approval

As digital health technologies continue to expand across the healthcare landscape, ensuring their safety, efficacy, and reliability becomes a critical responsibility of regulatory bodies. In the United States, the Food and Drug Administration (FDA) provides several defined regulatory pathways through which medical devices—including digital tools—must pass before entering the market. These approval routes are determined by the device's risk classification, novelty, and intended use, and each pathway is designed to match the level of scrutiny with the potential risk posed to patients. Selecting the right pathway is essential for developers and manufacturers, as it affects the timeline, cost, and required documentation for product launch. The most commonly used regulatory route is the 510(k) premarket notification, applicable mainly to Class II (moderate-risk) devices. In this process, manufacturers must demonstrate that their device is "substantially equivalent" to a legally marketed predicate device. This allows for streamlined clearance while maintaining safety standards. For novel devices with no predicate but deemed to pose low to moderate risk, the De Novo pathway offers a viable option. It allows innovative technologies to gain market entry while establishing a new device classification. For Class III (high-risk) devices, such as AI diagnostic platforms or implantable digital systems, the Premarket Approval (PMA) process is mandatory. PMA is the most stringent pathway, requiring extensive clinical trials, laboratory testing, risk analysis, and long-term data to prove the device's safety and effectiveness. This route ensures that life-sustaining or life-supporting technologies meet the highest regulatory standards.

In some cases, especially for low-risk digital health tools, the FDA may exercise enforcement discretion, meaning it does not actively regulate the product as long as it does not make specific medical claims. Additionally, the FDA is adapting to evolving technologies by piloting modern frameworks, such as the Digital Health Software Precertification Program, to streamline oversight of software-based medical tools. Understanding these regulatory pathways is essential not only for compliance but also for promoting trust, transparency, and widespread adoption of digital health innovations. Each pathway serves as a vital checkpoint in ensuring that digital devices entering the healthcare system are safe, effective, and beneficial to patients and providers alike.

The primary FDA pathways for digital medical devices include:

- **510(k) Clearance:** The 510(k) premarket notification is one of the most commonly used regulatory pathways for Class II (moderate-risk) medical devices. To gain clearance, manufacturers must demonstrate that their device is "substantially equivalent" to a previously FDA-cleared device, known as a predicate device. This means the new product must have a similar intended use and technological characteristics, or show no new safety concerns. While this pathway does not typically require full clinical trials, it often demands bench testing, usability studies, and performance data. Digital health products such as glucose monitors, smart thermometers, and diagnostic software frequently use this route. The 510(k) process is generally faster and less costly than other pathways, making it suitable for iterative innovations and minor technological advancements. It strikes a balance between regulatory efficiency and public safety, facilitating the growth of mid-level digital health tools in the market.
- **De Novo Classification:** The De Novo classification pathway is designed for novel medical devices that have no predicate device but are deemed to be of low to moderate risk. It provides an entry point for first-of-its-kind innovations that cannot use the 510(k) route due to their uniqueness. To qualify, a manufacturer must demonstrate that their device does not pose significant risk and that special controls can ensure its safety and effectiveness. Examples include AI-driven software for early disease detection or new digital therapeutic platforms. While it may require more supporting evidence than 510(k), it avoids the clinical trial demands of PMA. Once cleared through the De Novo pathway, the device can serve as a predicate for future 510(k) submissions, opening the door for industry-wide innovation. This route supports emerging technologies while preserving rigorous safety standards.
- **Premarket Approval (PMA):** The Premarket Approval (PMA) process is the most rigorous and comprehensive regulatory pathway, required for Class III (high-risk) devices. These are typically devices that are life-sustaining, life-supporting, or have a high potential for harm if they malfunction.

PMA requires extensive clinical data, including evidence from controlled human trials, as well as documentation on manufacturing processes, design controls, and quality systems. Examples include implantable cardiac devices, robotic surgical systems, and AI-powered diagnostic platforms used in critical care. The PMA review process is time-consuming and resource-intensive, often taking several months to years. Despite its complexity, it ensures that only the most thoroughly evaluated technologies enter the market, safeguarding patients and upholding high clinical standards. It is essential for the safe deployment of groundbreaking, high-impact digital health innovations.

- **Enforcement Discretion:** In specific cases involving low-risk digital health tools, the FDA may exercise enforcement discretion, choosing not to actively regulate the product under existing medical device laws. This typically applies to general wellness apps, fitness trackers, or digital meditation guides that do not make disease-specific claims. While these tools may promote healthy behaviours or offer health insights, they are not used for diagnosis, treatment, or prevention of diseases and thus fall outside strict regulatory oversight. The FDA's discretionary approach supports innovation and market access for startups and developers while still promoting transparency and responsible marketing. However, if these products begin making medical claims, they may fall under regulatory scrutiny. Enforcement discretion enables a lighter-touch framework that encourages consumer health engagement without stifling technological progress.

8.2.4 Software as a Medical Device (SaMD)

Software as a Medical Device (SaMD) refers to software that is intended for medical use independent of any physical hardware. Unlike traditional medical devices embedded in instruments or machines, SaMD functions on general-purpose platforms like smartphones, tablets, or cloud-based systems. These tools can perform a wide range of tasks—from monitoring vital signs and managing chronic diseases to diagnosing conditions using AI algorithms. Regulatory bodies such as the FDA and International Medical Device Regulators Forum (IMDRF) recognize SaMD as a distinct category and have developed specific frameworks for its evaluation. Since SaMD can directly influence clinical decisions, it must meet stringent safety, effectiveness, and performance standards. Risk classification depends on the software's intended use, clinical context, and the severity of conditions it addresses. As digital health expands, SaMD plays a crucial role in making care more accessible, personalized, and data-driven, while posing unique challenges in validation, updates, and cybersecurity.

The FDA and global regulators have adapted to Software as a Medical Device (SaMD)—software intended to be used for medical purposes without being part of a hardware device. This includes:

- AI-based imaging interpretation tools.
- Algorithms for stroke detection.
- Digital mental health therapeutics.

The International Medical Device Regulators Forum (IMDRF) provides guidance to harmonize SaMD regulation globally. The FDA has aligned its framework with these standards to support innovation while ensuring patient safety.

8.2.5 AI and Machine Learning-Based Devices

The integration of Artificial Intelligence (AI) and Machine Learning (ML) into medical devices is transforming modern healthcare by enhancing diagnostic accuracy, automating clinical workflows, and enabling predictive care. These advanced technologies analyze vast amounts of health data—from imaging scans to electronic health records—to identify patterns that might be overlooked by human clinicians. AI/ML-based devices can support early disease detection, personalize treatment plans, and optimize hospital resource management. Examples include AI algorithms for detecting cancer in radiology images, triaging emergency room cases, or predicting patient deterioration in intensive care units. Due to their adaptive nature, many of these systems continuously learn and improve from new data, which presents both opportunities and regulatory challenges. Ensuring transparency, fairness, and safety becomes critical, especially when decisions influence life-saving treatments. The FDA has begun developing tailored regulatory frameworks, including the proposed Predetermined Change Control Plan, to oversee evolving AI systems without stifling innovation. As these tools continue to grow in complexity, they will play an increasingly vital role in delivering efficient, data-driven, and personalized care.

As AI and machine learning enter healthcare, the FDA has introduced specific guidelines for AI/ML-based software:

- Initial approvals follow traditional pathways (510(k), De Novo, or PMA).
- The FDA has proposed a "Predetermined Change Control Plan", allowing developers to update algorithms post-approval within defined boundaries.
- Transparency, reproducibility, and ongoing performance monitoring are required to ensure safety and trust.

These evolving regulations reflect the dynamic nature of AI and its impact on clinical care.

8.2.6 Cybersecurity and Data Privacy Requirements

As healthcare systems adopt digital technologies such as connected devices, cloud-based platforms, and remote monitoring tools, ensuring cybersecurity and data privacy has become a top priority. Medical data is among the most sensitive and valuable information, containing personal identifiers, diagnoses, genetic data, and treatment histories. This makes healthcare a frequent target for cyberattacks, including ransomware, phishing, and unauthorized data access. Regulatory bodies like the FDA, HIPAA (Health Insurance Portability and Accountability Act) in the U.S., and GDPR in Europe set strict guidelines for protecting patient information. Manufacturers of digital health devices must build systems with secure data encryption, access controls, authentication protocols, and update mechanisms to defend against evolving threats. The FDA also requires cybersecurity documentation during the device approval process, especially for connected or cloud-based products. Continuous monitoring, vulnerability testing, and post-market updates are essential to maintaining trust. In AI and software-based devices, data integrity and algorithm security are also critical to preventing manipulation or bias. As healthcare becomes more digitized, robust cybersecurity strategies and compliance with privacy laws are essential to safeguard both patient welfare and system reliability.

Digital devices must also meet cybersecurity standards to protect patient data:

- FDA requires manufacturers to submit cybersecurity documentation during the approval process.
- Devices must include features for secure software updates, access control, and risk management.
- Compliance with broader laws like HIPAA (Health Insurance Portability and Accountability Act) is often required for handling protected health information (PHI).

Ensuring data integrity and system resilience is critical to both safety and user trust.

8.2.7 Post-Market Surveillance and Reporting

Post-market surveillance and reporting are critical components of the regulatory framework that ensure ongoing safety and effectiveness of medical devices after they enter the market. Once a digital health device or software receives regulatory approval, continuous monitoring is necessary to detect any adverse events, malfunctions, or cybersecurity vulnerabilities that may arise during real-world use. Manufacturers are required to collect, analyze, and report data on device performance, including any incidents that could cause harm to patients or users. Regulatory agencies like the FDA mandate periodic safety updates and may request recalls or corrective actions if significant risks are identified. This ongoing vigilance helps to identify rare or long-term issues that clinical trials may not have revealed. Additionally, post-market data can inform future product improvements and updates, ensuring devices remain safe as technology and clinical practices evolve. With the rise of connected devices and software that can be remotely updated, post-market surveillance has become more dynamic and integral to patient safety. Transparency and timely reporting foster trust between manufacturers, regulators, healthcare providers, and patients, supporting a safer and more effective digital healthcare ecosystem.

Even after approval, digital health devices are subject to post-market surveillance:

- Manufacturers must report adverse events or malfunctions to the FDA.
- Ongoing performance data may be required, especially for AI/ML systems.
- The FDA can mandate recalls or additional safety measures if new risks emerge.

Post-market oversight ensures that devices continue to perform safely and effectively as they are adopted in real-world settings.

8.2.8 Challenges in Regulatory Approval

Post-market surveillance and reporting are critical components of the regulatory framework that ensure ongoing safety and effectiveness of medical devices after they enter the market. Once a digital health device or software receives regulatory approval, continuous monitoring is necessary to detect any adverse events, malfunctions, or cybersecurity vulnerabilities that may arise during real-world use. Manufacturers are required to collect, analyze, and report data on device performance, including any incidents that could cause harm to patients or users. Regulatory agencies like the FDA mandate periodic safety updates and may request recalls or corrective actions if significant risks are identified. This ongoing vigilance helps to identify rare or long-term issues that clinical trials may not have revealed. Additionally, post-market data can inform future product improvements and updates, ensuring devices remain safe as technology and clinical practices evolve. With the rise of connected devices and software that can be remotely updated, post-market surveillance has become more dynamic and integral to patient safety. Transparency and timely reporting foster trust between manufacturers, regulators, healthcare providers, and patients, supporting a safer and more effective digital healthcare ecosystem.

Several challenges remain in the regulatory space for digital devices:

- Rapid innovation can outpace existing regulatory frameworks.
- Global discrepancies in regulations complicate market entry for developers.
- Data quality and bias in AI tools require stricter validation.
- Interoperability standards and cybersecurity risks add complexity.

The FDA continues to refine its approaches through public consultation, pilot programs (e.g., the Digital Health Software Precertification Program), and global collaboration.

8.3 HEALTH TECHNOLOGY ASSESSMENT (HTA) OF MONITORING TOOLS

Health Technology Assessment (HTA) is a comprehensive, multidisciplinary evaluation process that systematically examines the medical, economic, social, organizational, and ethical aspects of health technologies. In the context of monitoring tools, HTA plays a vital role in assessing digital and clinical devices designed to continuously or intermittently track patient health indicators—such as blood pressure, glucose levels, heart rate, respiratory rate, or oxygen saturation. These tools are increasingly essential in managing chronic diseases, enabling early detection of complications, personalizing care plans, and supporting remote healthcare delivery models. HTA ensures that healthcare systems make evidence-informed decisions about adopting these technologies by analyzing their clinical effectiveness, safety profile, and real-world usability. It also considers the cost-effectiveness of the monitoring tool, comparing health outcomes and resource use against alternative methods or standard care. This includes evaluating whether the tool reduces hospitalizations, improves medication adherence, or contributes to better disease management outcomes. Furthermore, HTA investigates organizational implications such as staff training, integration with existing IT systems, workflow changes, and interoperability with electronic health records. It also addresses ethical and social dimensions, including data privacy, equitable access, patient autonomy, and the impact on vulnerable populations. The patient's perspective—especially regarding usability, comfort, and trust—is also incorporated to ensure patient-centered care. Overall, HTA equips policymakers, clinicians, insurers, and health authorities with the necessary insights to determine if a monitoring tool adds real value to clinical practice. By balancing innovation with evidence, HTA helps safeguard health system sustainability while promoting effective, safe, and equitable technological integration into patient care.

8.3.1 Components of HTA for Monitoring Tools

Health Technology Assessment (HTA) is a comprehensive, multidisciplinary process used to evaluate the medical, economic, ethical, and societal implications of health technologies. When applied to monitoring tools—such as wearable devices, remote patient monitoring systems, and AI-enabled diagnostic platforms—HTA helps stakeholders determine their value, effectiveness, and feasibility for integration into clinical practice. As digital health tools become increasingly central to modern care delivery, particularly in chronic disease management, post-acute care, and preventive medicine, a structured HTA ensures that these technologies meet standards of safety, efficacy, cost-effectiveness, and user acceptability. Components of HTA for monitoring tools include clinical effectiveness, which assesses whether a tool leads to improved health outcomes compared to existing alternatives. The technological evaluation looks at accuracy, reliability, cybersecurity, and the ability to scale and adapt to different care settings. Economic evaluation examines the cost-effectiveness of the tool, including initial investment, maintenance, and long-term financial impact on health systems. Ethical, legal, and social aspects (ELSA) explore patient autonomy, data privacy, informed consent, and potential health disparities that may arise from unequal access or biased algorithmic decision-making (Fig. 12).

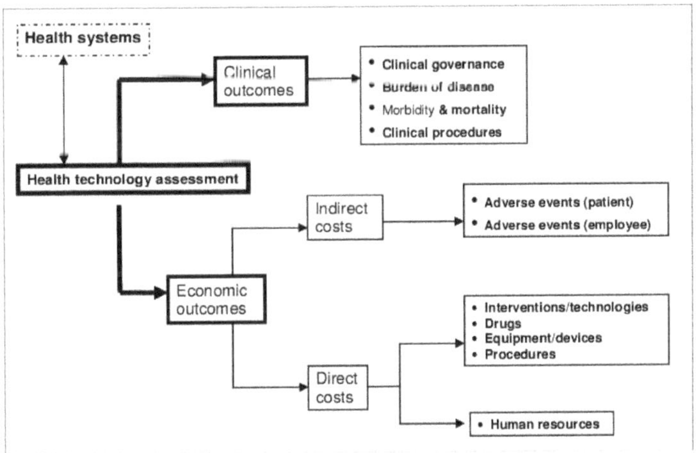

Fig. 12 Various components of health technology assessments

Equally important are patient and caregiver perspectives, which assess usability, satisfaction, and overall experience—factors that directly affect adherence and real-world effectiveness. Furthermore, HTA considers coverage decisions (whether insurance or national health plans will reimburse the tool), clinical guideline inclusion, and adoption and diffusion patterns across healthcare settings. In some cases, HTA may even recommend de-implementation of outdated or ineffective tools to optimize resource use. Together, these components form a holistic framework, guiding policy, practice, and innovation toward safe, equitable, and sustainable healthcare improvements through digital monitoring technologies.

- **Clinical Effectiveness:** Clinical effectiveness is a central component of Health Technology Assessment (HTA) that focuses on evaluating how well a monitoring tool contributes to improved patient outcomes. It examines the tool's ability to provide accurate, timely, and clinically relevant information that supports diagnosis, treatment decisions, and ongoing management. Key metrics assessed include diagnostic accuracy, sensitivity, specificity, and reliability of the device in real-world settings. This evaluation also considers whether the tool can detect early signs of deterioration or complications, allowing for prompt clinical intervention. Tools that demonstrate high precision and consistency across different patient populations and conditions are considered clinically effective. Clinical effectiveness is typically supported by data from randomized controlled trials (RCTs), observational cohort studies, and real-world evidence collected in routine clinical practice. These data help determine if the tool leads to measurable improvements in health indicators, reduced hospital admissions, or enhanced quality of life. Ultimately, assessing clinical effectiveness ensures that monitoring tools deliver tangible health benefits and support evidence-based care.
- **Safety:** Safety is a critical dimension of Health Technology Assessment (HTA) that focuses on identifying and evaluating any potential risks or adverse effects associated with the use of a monitoring tool. This includes analyzing issues such as device malfunction, technical failures, user error, and misinterpretation of data, all of which could lead to incorrect clinical decisions or delayed interventions. The safety assessment ensures that the tool does not introduce new hazards into the care process. Special attention is given to vulnerable populations—such as the elderly, children, pregnant women, and individuals with chronic conditions—who may be more susceptible to harm due to physiological or cognitive limitations. The evaluation also examines whether the tool has undergone rigorous testing for accuracy, durability, and fail-safe mechanisms, and whether users have clear instructions and training to minimize misuse. By identifying and mitigating potential safety risks, HTA helps ensure that monitoring tools contribute positively to patient care without compromising well-being, supporting both clinical reliability and patient trust.
- **Economic Evaluation:** Economic evaluation is a vital component of Health Technology Assessment (HTA) that assesses the financial value of a monitoring tool in relation to its clinical benefits. It helps determine whether a tool provides good value for money and informs reimbursement and investment decisions by healthcare systems and policymakers. One

common method is Cost-Effectiveness Analysis (CEA), which compares the cost of the monitoring tool to its health outcomes, often expressed as cost per Quality Adjusted Life Year (QALY) gained. This helps assess whether the tool delivers meaningful health improvements at a reasonable cost. Cost-utility and cost-benefit analyses go further by considering both direct costs (such as device price and maintenance) and indirect savings, like reduced hospital admissions, fewer emergency visits, or improved disease control over time. In addition, a budget impact analysis may be conducted to evaluate the short- and long-term affordability of implementing the tool across a healthcare system. This analysis helps decision-makers understand the potential financial burden or savings at a population level. Overall, economic evaluation ensures that monitoring tools not only work well but also use healthcare resources efficiently.

- **Organizational Impact:** Organizational impact refers to the evaluation of how the introduction of a monitoring tool affects the structure and operation of healthcare delivery systems. As part of Health Technology Assessment (HTA), this component examines whether the new technology aligns with or disrupts current clinical workflows, and whether it demands changes in staff roles, resource allocation, or process redesign. It assesses the training needs for healthcare providers, patients, or caregivers to use the tool effectively and safely. For instance, some monitoring tools may require specialized staff or technical support, while others may simplify routine tasks or reduce the need for in-person visits. In addition, the assessment looks at how well the tool can interoperate with electronic health records (EHRs) and integrate into existing care pathways without duplicating efforts or creating data silos. A seamless integration enhances care coordination and ensures that data collected through monitoring is accessible and actionable for clinicians. Understanding organizational impact is essential to ensure smooth implementation and long-term sustainability of the monitoring tool within healthcare settings.
- **Ethical, Legal, and Social Aspects (ELSA):** Evaluates issues like data privacy, informed consent, equity of access, and the potential for health The Ethical, Legal, and Social Aspects (ELSA) of digital health technologies are crucial considerations in ensuring their responsible development and use. Key concerns include data privacy and security, as remote monitoring systems, AI-driven diagnostics, and wearable sensors often collect sensitive personal health data. Safeguarding this information against breaches and misuse is essential to maintain trust and comply with regulations such as GDPR or HIPAA. Informed consent must be clearly obtained, ensuring users understand what data is collected, how it is used, and their rights

regarding that data. Equity of access is another critical issue. Digital tools must be designed inclusively to avoid widening existing health disparities, particularly among marginalized populations with limited internet access, digital literacy, or affordability. Technologies should enhance healthcare accessibility, not exacerbate inequalities. AI algorithms must also be transparent and free from bias to prevent discriminatory outcomes based on race, gender, or socioeconomic status. Further, the social implications of increased digital health surveillance must be carefully considered. Continuous monitoring might improve outcomes but could also lead to overmedicalization or anxiety. ELSA evaluation ensures that innovations align with broader societal values, balancing technological advancement with respect for autonomy, fairness, and human dignity.

- **Patient and Caregiver Perspectives:** Patient and Caregiver Perspectives play a vital role in the successful adoption and effectiveness of digital health technologies. Incorporating qualitative data—such as feedback on experiences, preferences, and usability—helps ensure that tools are designed with the end user in mind. This user-centered approach is crucial for building systems that meet real-world needs, especially in chronic disease management or elder care, where caregiver involvement is often significant. Understanding how patients and caregivers perceive a tool's ease of use, accessibility, and relevance can directly influence adherence and engagement. Devices or platforms that are intuitive, non-intrusive, and customizable tend to receive higher satisfaction ratings and lead to better health outcomes. Moreover, involving patients and caregivers early in the design process fosters a sense of ownership and trust, increasing the likelihood of long-term use. Tools that align with user preferences—such as minimal disruption to daily life or offering clear, actionable insights—are more likely to be accepted and integrated into routine care. Therefore, collecting and analyzing lived experiences is essential not just for usability, but also for refining digital solutions that genuinely support health and well-being.
- **Technological Aspects:** Technological Aspects are fundamental in evaluating the effectiveness and sustainability of digital health monitoring tools. This includes a thorough review of the design, ensuring the interface is user-friendly, adaptable, and suited for diverse populations. The accuracy and reliability of data collection are critical—devices must consistently deliver precise measurements to support informed clinical decisions. Maintenance needs, such as battery life, hardware durability, and software support, also impact long-term usability. Scalability is a

key factor, particularly in systems intended for widespread deployment across various settings or population groups. A tool must be capable of maintaining performance and data integrity even as user numbers grow. The lifespan of both hardware and software components should be sufficient to justify investment, while update requirements must be manageable to ensure functionality and security without overburdening users or healthcare providers. Cybersecurity is a growing concern, especially with the integration of cloud-based storage, wireless communication, and AI analytics. Devices must be protected against data breaches, unauthorized access, and malware, requiring ongoing security updates and compliance with data protection regulations. Overall, a robust technological framework underpins the reliability, safety, and scalability of digital health solutions.

Examples of Monitoring Tools Evaluated by HTA

- Continuous Glucose Monitors (CGMs) for diabetes management.
- Wearable ECG monitors for arrhythmia detection.
- Remote patient monitoring (RPM) systems for post-operative care.
- Pulse oximeters used during COVID-19 home monitoring.
- Digital apps for mental health and medication adherence.

8.3.2 Outcomes of HTA in Monitoring Tools

- **Coverage Decisions:** Coverage by national health systems or insurance plans is a critical determinant of a digital health tool's adoption and accessibility. Health Technology Assessment (HTA) plays a key role in evaluating whether a tool offers sufficient clinical and economic value to justify reimbursement. If a device or platform demonstrates cost-effectiveness, improved outcomes, and patient benefit, it is more likely to be funded by public or private payers. Lack of coverage, on the other hand, can severely limit uptake, especially in lower-income populations. Reimbursement decisions often hinge on HTA evidence, making rigorous evaluation essential for market access. In many countries, inclusion in reimbursement lists also enhances the credibility and perceived legitimacy of a health technology.
- **Clinical Guidelines:** The integration of a digital health tool into clinical guidelines significantly boosts its credibility and encourages widespread professional use. Recommendations from authoritative bodies—such as medical societies or specialist associations—are based on comprehensive evidence reviews, often including HTA findings. These guidelines provide a roadmap for clinicians, reinforcing the tool's safety, effectiveness, and

appropriate use cases. Endorsement in clinical protocols helps standardize care and reduces variability in practice. Moreover, clinicians are more likely to adopt technologies that are formally supported within their field, further promoting consistent, evidence-based care delivery across institutions.

- **Adoption & Diffusion:** The rate at which a digital health tool is adopted and diffused across healthcare systems often depends on the strength of HTA findings. Positive assessments can drive procurement decisions in hospitals, clinics, and even community-based or home care settings. Adoption is further accelerated when stakeholders—including clinicians, administrators, and policymakers—are convinced of a technology's benefits through clear, evidence-based reports. Conversely, weak or inconclusive HTA results may delay or restrict uptake. Widespread diffusion also depends on training, infrastructure readiness, and stakeholder engagement. A strong HTA framework can provide the necessary confidence and guidance to scale implementation effectively and equitably.
- **De-implementation:** While HTA often promotes new innovations, it also plays a crucial role in de-implementation—the process of phasing out tools that are ineffective, obsolete, or disproportionately costly. This is essential for maintaining a high-quality, efficient healthcare system. By rigorously assessing outcomes, costs, and comparative performance, HTA can identify technologies that no longer meet clinical or economic standards. De-implementation frees up resources for more beneficial innovations and reduces the risk of patient harm from outdated or unvalidated tools. It also supports a culture of continuous improvement and accountability within health systems, ensuring that care remains evidence-based and value-driven.

8.4 INTEROPERABILITY STANDARDS (FHIR, HL7, ETC.)

In the evolving landscape of digital health, interoperability has become a cornerstone for achieving integrated, efficient, and patient-centered care. It refers to the capacity of various healthcare information systems, medical devices, and applications to access, exchange, interpret, and cooperatively utilize data in a synchronized and meaningful way. This functionality is critical in today's complex healthcare environments, where patients often receive care from multiple providers, using diverse platforms and systems. Interoperability standards—such as FHIR (Fast Healthcare Interoperability Resources) and HL7 (Health Level Seven)—play a vital role in ensuring that digital systems can "speak the same language." These standards provide common frameworks and data structures that allow different technologies to transmit and interpret health information consistently and securely. For example, FHIR uses modern web technologies and

APIs to enable real-time data sharing across electronic health records (EHRs), mobile apps, and remote monitoring devices. HL7, one of the oldest and most widely adopted standards, supports structured messaging and documentation that allows clinical data to flow between systems with minimal friction. By enabling seamless communication between technologies, interoperability standards improve clinical workflows, support decision-making, and facilitate continuity of care. They help eliminate redundant testing, prevent medical errors, and enhance patient safety by ensuring that healthcare professionals have access to complete and up-to-date information at the point of care. For patients, this translates into smoother care transitions, more personalized treatment plans, and a more cohesive healthcare experience overall. Moreover, interoperability underpins many critical public health functions, including population health management, telemedicine, research, and health system analytics. During emergencies—such as pandemics or natural disasters—interoperable systems allow for rapid data aggregation and coordinated response strategies across regions and institutions. They also support advanced use cases such as AI-based diagnostics, clinical decision support tools, and personalized medicine, which rely heavily on real-time, accurate data inputs from multiple sources. Despite its importance, achieving full interoperability remains a challenge due to variations in technology maturity, data governance policies, and vendor-specific barriers. However, international efforts—led by organizations such as HL7 International, ONC (Office of the National Coordinator for Health Information Technology), and ISO—continue to drive standardization and adoption. Compliance with standards like FHIR is increasingly being mandated in national digital health strategies, ensuring that future systems are built with openness, scalability, and data fluidity in mind.

In conclusion, interoperability standards are not just technical protocols—they are enablers of better health outcomes, operational efficiency, and system-wide innovation. Their proper implementation ensures that healthcare becomes more connected, collaborative, and capable of meeting the needs of both patients and providers in the digital age.

Two of the most prominent standards in health information exchange are HL7 and FHIR.

8.4.1 HL7 (Health Level Seven)

HL7 (Health Level Seven) is a globally recognized set of international standards developed by Health Level Seven International. These standards are specifically designed to facilitate the exchange, integration, sharing, and retrieval of electronic health information across different healthcare systems. First introduced in the late 1980s, HL7 has since become a cornerstone in the development of healthcare information technology (IT) infrastructure.

HL7 provides a framework that enables various healthcare providers and systems to communicate effectively. It ensures that medical data—such as patient records, lab results, prescriptions, and billing information—can be shared seamlessly between different software platforms. This interoperability is crucial in today's healthcare environment, where multiple organizations often need to collaborate on a single patient's care. The HL7 standards cover a range of data exchange formats, including HL7 Version 2 (widely used in hospitals), HL7 Version 3 (which includes more structured data), and HL7 FHIR (Fast Healthcare Interoperability Resources), a newer standard designed for web-based applications. Each version has its specific strengths and use cases. HL7 promotes efficiency, reduces errors, and improves patient outcomes by enabling real-time data exchange. Its adoption helps eliminate redundant data entry, minimizes delays in care, and supports decision-making by ensuring that accurate information is readily available. HL7 plays a vital role in modernizing healthcare systems by setting a common language for health data communication, thereby improving the quality, safety, and coordination of care worldwide.

- HL7 is a set of international standards developed by Health Level Seven International for the exchange, integration, sharing, and retrieval of electronic health information.
- It has been in use since the late 1980s and is foundational in healthcare IT systems.

Key Versions:

- **HL7 v2.x:** HL7 Version 2.x is the most widely implemented standard in healthcare organizations, especially in hospital settings. It facilitates communication between systems like laboratory information systems (LIS), admission-discharge-transfer (ADT) systems, billing, and radiology systems. This version uses a message-based format that relies on plain text and delimiters to structure data. While it is highly efficient and lightweight, the messages are not easily human-readable, making interpretation challenging without specialized tools. Despite its simplicity, v2.x is highly flexible and customizable, which has contributed to its long-standing popularity. It supports near real-time messaging, enabling quick updates across different systems. However, this flexibility has also led to inconsistent implementations across vendors. HL7 v2.x is widely regarded for its stability and widespread support. It is still in use today in thousands of healthcare institutions worldwide. For many legacy systems, HL7 v2.x remains the operational backbone of data exchange.
- **HL7 v3:** HL7 Version 3 was developed to address the limitations of HL7 v2.x by providing a more rigorous and consistent data model. It introduced the

Reference Information Model (RIM), aiming for semantic interoperability across diverse healthcare systems. Unlike the text-based v2.x, HL7 v3 uses XML, making the messages more structured and self-descriptive. This allows for more precise and meaningful data exchange, reducing misinterpretation. However, the increased complexity of its data models and XML syntax made implementation more challenging. Adoption has been slower, especially in comparison to v2.x, due to the steep learning curve and the need for specialized tools and expertise. Many healthcare organizations found it resource-intensive to migrate or build systems using v3. Nonetheless, HL7 v3 set the foundation for future standards like CDA and FHIR. It is still used in specific scenarios that require high levels of data structure and interoperability. Overall, HL7 v3 marked an evolution in HL7's design philosophy.

- **CDA (Clinical Document Architecture):** The Clinical Document Architecture (CDA) is a document-based standard developed as part of the HL7 Version 3 framework. It is used to structure clinical documents such as discharge summaries, progress notes, and imaging reports in a machine-readable and human-readable format. CDA uses XML to encode clinical content, ensuring that it is both interoperable and displayable to end users. Each CDA document includes a header (with metadata like patient ID, provider, and document type) and a body (containing the clinical narrative). This dual nature allows for consistent sharing of rich clinical data across healthcare organizations. CDA is widely used in national and regional health information exchanges (HIEs) due to its ability to preserve clinical context. It supports digital signatures and version control, enhancing document integrity. Although creating CDA documents can be complex, the standard has proven valuable for maintaining longitudinal patient records. It has laid the groundwork for future standards such as C-CDA and FHIR documents. CDA continues to play a key role in structuring healthcare documentation globally.

Use Cases:

- **Lab Result Messaging:** Lab result messaging is a critical function in healthcare interoperability, enabling the electronic transmission of laboratory test results from diagnostic laboratories to hospitals, clinics, and physicians. Using standards such as HL7 v2.x, these messages ensure that test outcomes—whether blood work, pathology, or microbiology results—are delivered quickly and accurately to the appropriate healthcare providers. Timely lab result delivery improves clinical decision-making, reduces delays in diagnosis, and enhances patient care. Lab messages often include patient demographics, test identifiers, results, reference ranges, and abnormal flags. Automated messaging minimizes manual data entry errors and facilitates better integration with electronic health record (EHR) systems. This functionality is particularly important in emergency settings, where rapid access to lab data can be life-saving.

- **ADT (Admission, Discharge, Transfer) Notifications:** ADT notifications are foundational messages in healthcare systems that communicate patient movement events within a facility, such as admissions, discharges, and transfers. These real-time notifications help synchronize patient data across various departments, ensuring everyone involved in a patient's care has up-to-date information. ADT messages typically include patient identifiers, admission details, attending physician information, and bed assignments. Hospitals use them to track patient flow, optimize resource use, and improve care coordination. For example, when a patient is admitted to a ward, an ADT message ensures that labs, radiology, and billing systems are immediately updated. These notifications are also key for public health monitoring, case management, and transitions of care between facilities. Their reliable, timely transmission helps reduce errors and streamline operations.
- **Prescription and Pharmacy Information Exchange:** Prescription and pharmacy information exchange supports the secure and standardized transfer of medication-related data between prescribers, pharmacies, and healthcare systems. This process is vital for ensuring patients receive the correct medications without delay. Through HL7 messaging standards or newer approaches like FHIR, electronic prescriptions (eRx) can be sent directly from a clinician's system to a pharmacy, reducing the risk of errors from handwritten scripts. These messages can include drug identifiers, dosages, frequencies, refill information, and instructions. They also support medication reconciliation, allergy checks, and drug interaction alerts within EHR systems. For pharmacists, this improves workflow efficiency and enables better communication with providers. Overall, electronic prescription exchange enhances patient safety, reduces prescription fraud, and facilitates coordinated medication management.

8.4.2 FHIR (Fast Healthcare Interoperability Resources)

FHIR, or Fast Healthcare Interoperability Resources, is a modern health data exchange standard developed by HL7 International. It was created to overcome the complexity and limitations of earlier HL7 standards like v2.x and v3, aiming to provide a more flexible, developer-friendly approach to healthcare interoperability. FHIR leverages widely used web technologies such as RESTful APIs, JSON, XML, and HTTPS, making it faster, more secure, and easier for software developers to implement compared to traditional standards. This shift to web-based architecture aligns healthcare IT more closely with modern software practices and enables real-time access to health information across diverse platforms. FHIR is designed to support a wide range of health information workflows, including clinical, administrative, and research scenarios. One of FHIR's key innovations is its modular design, which is based on discrete components called "resources." Each resource represents a specific type of healthcare data, such as Patient, Observation, Medication, AllergyIntolerance, Encounter, or Condition. These resources are the building blocks of FHIR, and they can be combined, extended, or linked to create complex health data structures. Resources are designed to be standalone, yet composable, allowing systems to retrieve and manipulate only the specific data they need. This modularity enables fine-grained data exchange and avoids the overhead of processing entire documents or massive messages, as seen in older HL7 standards. For example, a mobile app can request just a patient's medication list or vital signs using a simple API call, without downloading an entire record. FHIR also supports strong terminologies and coding systems, such as SNOMED CT, LOINC, and ICD-10, helping ensure semantic consistency and interoperability. Another key advantage of FHIR is its support for mobile apps, cloud-based services, wearable device integration, and patient-facing technologies. Its compatibility with OAuth2.0 and OpenID Connect enables secure authentication and authorization, which is essential for protecting sensitive health data. As a result, FHIR is gaining rapid adoption globally, not just in hospitals but also in public health systems, health information exchanges (HIEs), and third-party app ecosystems. It plays a central role in initiatives such as the U.S. 21st Century Cures Act, which mandates greater patient access to health data through standardized APIs. While FHIR is still evolving, its community-driven development and open standards approach make it highly adaptable to the future of digital health. Ultimately, FHIR represents a major leap forward in creating a connected, patient-centered, and data-driven healthcare system.

Benefits:

- **Easier Integration with Mobile Apps and Cloud-Based Systems:** FHIR is specifically designed with modern development environments in mind, making it highly compatible with mobile apps and cloud-based platforms. Its use of standard web technologies like RESTful APIs and JSON means developers can build healthcare applications using the same tools they use for other modern web and mobile services. This ease of integration accelerates innovation, allowing third-party developers to create secure and responsive apps for both providers and patients. Whether it's a mobile app that tracks chronic conditions or a cloud service that aggregates patient data from multiple hospitals, FHIR facilitates smooth, real-time data exchange without the need for complex middleware or custom connectors.

- **Strong Support for Real-Time Data Exchange:** One of FHIR's most powerful features is its ability to support real-time data exchange between healthcare systems. With its RESTful API architecture, FHIR allows data to be requested and delivered instantly, enabling timely access to critical clinical information. This capability is especially valuable in emergency care, decision support, and coordinated care scenarios where up-to-date information can make a life-saving difference. FHIR's real-time exchange also supports alerts, notifications, and monitoring systems that improve responsiveness and reduce errors. It shifts healthcare from a batch-based model to a dynamic, always-on data environment.
- **Enables Patient Access to Their Own Health Data:** FHIR is transforming patient engagement by enabling individuals to easily access their health data through apps and portals. With FHIR-enabled APIs, patients can view lab results, medication lists, visit summaries, and more—directly from their smartphones or web browsers. This access empowers patients to take a more active role in managing their health, improving transparency and communication with providers. It also supports compliance with healthcare regulations such as the 21st Century Cures Act in the U.S., which mandates that patients must be able to access and share their medical data electronically. FHIR is a key enabler of patient-centered care.
- **High Interoperability Across Different Systems and Vendors:** FHIR was built to address the long-standing challenge of poor interoperability in healthcare IT. By offering a standardized, resource-based data model and using common data formats and protocols, FHIR ensures that data can move fluidly between different EHR systems, labs, pharmacies, insurers, and health information exchanges. It reduces vendor lock-in and facilitates collaboration across organizations and software platforms. This high level of interoperability leads to better data continuity, fewer errors during transitions of care, and more efficient workflows across the entire healthcare ecosystem. FHIR is helping to build a connected healthcare future where systems "speak the same language."

Use Cases:

- **Mobile Health Apps That Retrieve Patient Data from EHRs:** One of the most impactful use cases of FHIR is enabling mobile health apps to securely retrieve patient data directly from Electronic Health Records (EHRs). With standardized APIs, FHIR allows apps to access specific data like allergies, lab results, appointments, or medications in real time. This means patients can use their smartphones to view their health records, track chronic conditions, or even share data with new providers instantly. It empowers patients with greater control over their health while supporting providers in offering personalized, data-driven care.

- **Sharing Immunization Records or Medication History:** FHIR streamlines the exchange of immunization records and medication histories between healthcare systems, pharmacies, and public health registries. This is particularly important for ensuring continuity of care, especially when patients move between providers or regions. Through FHIR resources like Immunization and MedicationStatement, clinicians can view up-to-date vaccination statuses or medication regimens, reducing duplicate prescriptions or missed immunizations. This functionality also supports school requirements, travel documentation, and outbreak tracking in public health initiatives.
- **Population Health Dashboards:** FHIR supports the creation of population health dashboards that aggregate and analyze data from multiple sources to identify trends, gaps in care, and at-risk populations. By pulling structured data from various EHR systems using FHIR APIs, healthcare organizations can monitor metrics like vaccination rates, readmission trends, or chronic disease management across large groups. These dashboards enable data-driven decision-making for health system administrators, public health officials, and care managers, ultimately improving population-level outcomes and resource allocation.
- **Remote Patient Monitoring (RPM):** Remote Patient Monitoring (RPM) solutions leverage FHIR to transmit patient-generated health data from wearable devices, home monitors, or mobile apps back to healthcare providers. Whether it's tracking blood pressure, glucose levels, or heart rate, FHIR allows for secure, real-time data exchange between the patient's device and their care team. This ensures timely interventions, supports chronic disease management, and reduces the need for in-person visits. RPM powered by FHIR improves patient engagement, enhances outcomes, and supports the shift toward proactive, value-based care.

8.4.3 Other Important Standards & Frameworks

In addition to HL7 and FHIR, the healthcare industry relies on a variety of other important standards and frameworks to ensure effective data exchange, consistency, and interoperability. These standards support different aspects of health information management, from medical imaging to clinical terminology and patient records. For example, DICOM is essential for the storage and transmission of medical images like X-rays and MRIs, ensuring they can be viewed and shared across systems. LOINC provides universal codes for lab tests and clinical observations, allowing accurate interpretation of test results across institutions. SNOMED CT offers a standardized vocabulary for clinical terms, enhancing the clarity and consistency of diagnoses and treatment documentation. ICD-10 is a global disease classification system used for coding conditions, symptoms, and causes of death. Frameworks like IHE help different standards—such as HL7 and DICOM—work together seamlessly, improving system integration. OpenEHR, on the other hand, focuses on a vendor-neutral, long-term health data architecture, promoting patient-centric record keeping across a lifetime. Together, these tools form a robust foundation for digital health infrastructure worldwide (Table-6).

Table-6: Standard/Framework and their description

Standard/Framework	Description
DICOM (Digital Imaging and Communications in Medicine)	Standard for storing and transmitting medical images (e.g., X-rays, MRIs).
LOINC (Logical Observation Identifiers Names and Codes)	Standard for identifying lab results and clinical observations.
SNOMED CT	A standardized vocabulary for clinical terms, widely used in EHRs for consistency in diagnosis and treatment documentation.
ICD-10 (International Classification of Diseases)	Coding standard for diseases, signs, symptoms, and conditions.
IHE (Integrating the Healthcare Enterprise)	Framework that helps different systems use standards (like HL7 and DICOM) to work together.
OpenEHR	A standard for health data architecture focused on lifelong, vendor-neutral patient records.

8.4.4 Levels of Interoperability

Interoperability in healthcare refers to the ability of different information systems, devices, and applications to access, exchange, and use health data cohesively. It operates across multiple levels to ensure both technical compatibility and meaningful data exchange. Foundational interoperability is the most basic level, enabling systems to connect and exchange data without ensuring how that data is interpreted. Structural interoperability goes a step further by standardizing data formats and organization, allowing systems to understand the structure and syntax of the information exchanged. Semantic interoperability ensures that both sending and receiving systems interpret the data consistently and accurately, using shared terminologies like SNOMED CT and LOINC. At the highest level, organizational interoperability deals with non-technical aspects such as policies, legal agreements, and governance to support smooth, compliant, and secure data sharing across institutions. Together, these levels create a comprehensive framework for effective and meaningful health information exchange (Table-7).

Table -7 : Interoperability in healthcare and their description

Level	Description
Foundational	Enables basic data exchange between systems.
Structural	Ensures data exchanged between systems is organized and formatted for interpretation.
Semantic	Ensures that both systems interpret the exchanged data meaningfully (using terminologies like SNOMED, LOINC).
Organizational	Aligns policy, legal, and governance standards for seamless exchange.

8.4.5 Challenges in Interoperability

- **Lack of Standard Adoption Across All Vendors and Regions:** One of the biggest hurdles in achieving full interoperability is the inconsistent adoption of data standards across vendors, healthcare organizations, and geographic regions. While standards like HL7, FHIR, and DICOM exist, not all EHR or health IT systems implement them uniformly—or at all. Some vendors use proprietary formats or partial implementations, leading to compatibility issues and fragmented data exchange. This lack of standardization hinders seamless communication between systems, creating barriers to coordinated care and patient data mobility. Smaller vendors or under-resourced regions may lack the technical infrastructure or expertise to adopt emerging standards. The situation is further complicated when multiple healthcare providers serve patients across different networks. Uniform adoption and enforcement of standards are essential for achieving true interoperability at scale.
- **Legacy Systems That Do Not Support Modern APIs or Standards:** Many healthcare organizations continue to rely on legacy systems that were built long before modern interoperability standards like FHIR and RESTful APIs were introduced. These older systems often use outdated protocols, lack integration capabilities, and require manual workarounds to exchange data. Replacing or upgrading them is costly, time-consuming, and sometimes risky to ongoing clinical operations. As a result, these systems become bottlenecks in digital transformation efforts. Even when newer systems are introduced, legacy infrastructure can limit the scope and effectiveness of integration. In some cases, middleware or data converters are used to bridge the gap, but these solutions are often fragile and inefficient. The continued reliance on outdated technology slows innovation and compromises the quality of care.

- **Data Privacy and Security Concerns, Especially with Cloud-Based Tools:** The shift to cloud-based healthcare solutions and patient-facing apps has raised significant concerns about data privacy and security. Sensitive health information must be protected under laws like HIPAA (in the U.S.) or GDPR (in the EU), yet cloud environments pose new risks for unauthorized access, data breaches, and misuse. Healthcare data is a prime target for cyberattacks due to its high value on the black market. Ensuring end-to-end encryption, secure authentication, access controls, and audit trails is essential but often difficult to implement consistently. Additionally, many organizations are wary of storing health data off-premises, fearing loss of control or non-compliance. Balancing innovation with strict security measures remains a persistent challenge in achieving trust and widespread adoption of interoperable solutions.
- **Semantic Inconsistency – Same Data Interpreted Differently Across Systems:** Semantic interoperability ensures that exchanged data retains the same meaning across different systems—but achieving this is complex. Even when systems use similar formats, inconsistent use of medical terminologies, coding systems, or labels can result in misinterpretation. For example, one system might record a blood glucose measurement in mg/dL while another uses mmol/L, or different terms may be used for the same condition. This inconsistency can affect clinical decision-making, reporting accuracy, and patient safety. Efforts to harmonize data using standardized vocabularies like SNOMED CT, LOINC, or ICD-10 are ongoing but not universally adopted. Without true semantic alignment, shared data remains vulnerable to errors and reduced clinical value. Continuous mapping, validation, and standard enforcement are necessary to close this gap.
- **Regulatory and Compliance Variations Across Countries and States:** Healthcare regulations and compliance requirements vary significantly across jurisdictions, creating challenges for organizations operating in multiple regions. What is considered compliant in one country—such as patient data sharing rules under HIPAA in the U.S.—may be restricted under GDPR in Europe or other local laws. This inconsistency complicates system design, cross-border data exchange, and multinational health IT deployments. Vendors and healthcare providers must navigate a patchwork of legal obligations, often requiring tailored solutions for each market. These differences can delay implementation timelines, increase costs, and limit the scalability of interoperable platforms. Harmonizing regulatory frameworks—or at least creating crosswalks between them—is

crucial to achieving global interoperability and supporting international collaboration in healthcare delivery and research.

8.4.6 Global and Regulatory Initiatives

- **United States:** 21st Century Cures Act: In the U.S., the 21st Century Cures Act, signed into law in 2016, is a landmark regulation that significantly advances health IT interoperability and patient empowerment. It mandates that healthcare providers and IT vendors avoid "information blocking"—practices that intentionally prevent or discourage the sharing of health data. Under this act, patients must be granted easy and secure access to their electronic health information, including through APIs compatible with modern standards like FHIR. It also promotes the development of a nationwide health information network, improving care coordination and patient engagement. The Office of the National Coordinator for Health IT (ONC) is responsible for enforcing the act and ensuring that EHR vendors meet interoperability requirements. This law is a major driver in accelerating the use of standards-based, patient-centered data exchange across the U.S. healthcare system.
- **European Union:** European Health Data Space (EHDS): The European Health Data Space (EHDS) is a major initiative by the European Union aimed at establishing a unified framework for the secure and ethical use of health data across member states. EHDS seeks to give EU citizens full control over their health data, allowing them to access and share it seamlessly across borders. It also supports the secondary use of anonymized data for research, innovation, and policy-making. The EHDS builds on the General Data Protection Regulation (GDPR) and aligns with other EU digital policies to ensure strong data protection and user rights. It encourages interoperability through common standards, formats, and infrastructures. By enabling cross-border healthcare and data access, EHDS promotes equity, continuity of care, and better outcomes across Europe.
- **Global Standards Organizations:** Several international organizations play a crucial role in developing and maintaining global health IT standards. HL7 International leads the creation of interoperability frameworks such as HL7 v2, CDA, and FHIR, widely used across the world. The International Organization for Standardization (ISO), specifically through Technical Committee 215 (ISO/TC 215 – Health Informatics), develops global health data and privacy standards to support safe and efficient health systems. Meanwhile, the World Health Organization (WHO) maintains key classification systems like ICD (International Classification of Diseases) and supports SNOMED CT in partnership with SNOMED International. These

standards organizations ensure that health information is exchanged consistently, safely, and effectively across national borders. Their collaborative efforts are essential to achieving global interoperability and enabling international public health initiatives, research, and disaster response coordination.

8.5 REIMBURSEMENT POLICIES AND DIGITAL HEALTH CODES

Reimbursement policies and digital health codes play a crucial role in the adoption, sustainability, and scaling of digital health technologies. These frameworks define how providers are paid for delivering care using digital tools such as telemedicine, remote patient monitoring (RPM), mobile health apps, AI-based diagnostics, and wearable devices. Without clear reimbursement mechanisms, even effective and innovative digital health tools may struggle to gain traction in clinical practice.

8.5.1 Overview of Digital Health Reimbursement

Reimbursement refers to financial compensation given to healthcare providers, hospitals, or organizations for delivering medical services. In digital health, this includes:

- Telehealth / Telemedicine visits
- Remote monitoring of vital signs or chronic conditions
- Asynchronous care (e.g., store-and-forward messages, e-consults)
- Mobile health (mHealth) applications
- Digital therapeutics (DTx)
- AI-powered decision support tools

Reimbursement policies vary significantly by country, payer (public vs private), and type of digital health service.

8.5.2 Digital Health Billing and Procedure Codes United States (CMS – Medicare/Medicaid + CPT Codes)

In the United States, digital health billing and procedure coding are primarily governed by the Centers for Medicare & Medicaid Services (CMS) and the American Medical Association (AMA). CMS oversees billing for federal health programs like Medicare and Medicaid, ensuring that healthcare providers are reimbursed appropriately for services, including digital and telehealth care. A key component of billing is the use of CPT (Current Procedural Terminology) codes, developed by the AMA. These standardized codes describe medical, surgical, and diagnostic services, including remote patient monitoring, virtual visits, and digital therapeutic interventions. With the growing adoption of telehealth, CMS has expanded the list of reimbursable CPT codes to cover more digital services.

Accurate coding is essential not only for reimbursement but also for data tracking, policy development, and quality reporting. CMS also supports the use of HCPCS (Healthcare Common Procedure Coding System) codes for equipment and non-physician services. Together, these coding systems help standardize digital health billing practices, promote transparency, and support value-based care initiatives (Table-8).

Table 8: Digital Health Billing and Procedure Codes

Service Type	Common CPT/HCPCS Codes	Description
Remote Patient Monitoring (RPM)	99453, 99454, 99457, 99458	For setup, data transmission, and interactive communication.
Chronic Care Management (CCM)	99490, 99487	Coordinated care for patients with multiple chronic conditions.
Remote Therapeutic Monitoring (RTM)	98975–98978	For non-physiological data like medication adherence or musculoskeletal health.
Telehealth Visits	99201–99215 (with modifiers), G2012, G2251	Office visit codes used with telehealth modifiers.
Behavioral Health Integration	99484, 99492–99494	Covers digital care coordination for mental health services.

Note: These codes are often billable to Medicare, Medicaid, and commercial payers depending on regional policy and payer contracts.

8.5.3 European and Global Reimbursement Models

Globally, countries are developing diverse reimbursement models to integrate digital health into their public healthcare systems. In Germany, the innovative DiGA Fast-Track allows approved digital health apps—like those for mental health or chronic disease management—to be prescribed by doctors and reimbursed by statutory health insurance, provided they demonstrate clinical benefit. France evaluates digital tools through its national health authority, Haute Autorité de Santé (HAS), and may include them in public insurance coverage if they meet safety and effectiveness criteria. The UK's National Health Service (NHS) uses an Evidence Standards Framework for Digital Health to assess digital tools, with local Clinical Commissioning Groups (CCGs) deciding on funding based on regional needs. In Canada, reimbursement policies vary by province, with regions like Ontario Health offering support for remote patient monitoring (RPM) and virtual care through targeted programs. Australia includes telehealth consultations and some digital monitoring tools under the Medicare Benefits Schedule (MBS), especially for rural and underserved areas. These models reflect a global trend toward formalizing and funding digital health as part of mainstream care, with growing emphasis on evidence, regulation, and patient benefit (Table-9).

Table 9: Country and Approach to Reimbursement

Country/Region	Approach to Reimbursement
Germany	DiGA Fast-Track: Allows digital health apps (with evidence of benefit) to be reimbursed by statutory health insurance.
France	Uses Haute Autorité de Santé (HAS) evaluation for digital tools and may cover under public health insurance.
UK (NHS)	Emphasizes Evidence Standards Framework for Digital Health, and regional CCGs can approve funding.
Canada	Provincial systems like Ontario Health support RPM and virtual care; reimbursement varies.
Australia	Covers telehealth and some digital monitoring under Medicare Benefits Schedule (MBS).

8.5.4 Criteria for Reimbursement Approval

To qualify for reimbursement, digital health tools often need to demonstrate:

- Clinical effectiveness
- Safety and data privacy compliance
- Cost-effectiveness
- Regulatory approval (e.g., FDA clearance, CE marking)
- Interoperability with existing health IT systems
- Evidence of improving access, outcomes, or efficiency

8.5.5 Emerging Trends in Digital Health Reimbursement

- **Value-Based Care (VBC):** Payment models that reward outcomes instead of service volume—favor digital tools that prevent complications or reduce admissions.
- **Bundled Payments:** Tools included as part of a broader care package (e.g., cardiac rehab or diabetes care bundle).
- **Pay-for-performance models:** Incentives for digital tools that track and improve key health metrics.
- **Reimbursement for AI Tools:** Still emerging; models being piloted for radiology, pathology, and triage tools.
- **Subscription models for DTx:** Some payers consider SaaS-like subscription reimbursement for validated digital therapeutics.

8.5.6 Barriers and Challenges

- **Fragmented Policies Across Payers and Regions:** One major challenge in digital health reimbursement is the lack of unified policies across different payers, regions, and healthcare systems. In countries like the

U.S., each private insurer, Medicare, and Medicaid program may have its own rules regarding what digital services are covered and how they're reimbursed. Similarly, in countries with decentralized health systems like Canada, reimbursement criteria vary widely between provinces. This fragmentation creates confusion for providers and developers trying to scale digital health solutions. It also makes it difficult to ensure consistent access to services across populations. The lack of harmonization can delay innovation, as companies must navigate multiple approval pathways and coverage policies. Patients may experience disparities in access depending on geography or insurance type. Uniform, national-level policies could help streamline adoption and ensure equity.

- **Lack of Standardized Codes for Some Emerging Technologies:** Many emerging digital health solutions, including AI diagnostics, digital therapeutics, and advanced wearables, lack dedicated CPT, HCPCS, or equivalent codes for billing. Without standardized procedure codes, it becomes difficult for providers to submit claims, and payers are often reluctant to reimburse for unclassified services. This creates a major bottleneck for the commercial adoption of innovative tools, even if they show clinical promise. Some countries are starting to adapt, but the process of establishing new codes is often slow and bureaucratic. This gap can deter developers from entering the market and limit healthcare organizations from offering cutting-edge care. Coding frameworks need to evolve in tandem with technology to support rapid yet evidence-based innovation.
- **Delays in Evidence Generation for Newer Tools (Especially AI or Wearables):** Payers typically require solid clinical evidence to reimburse any medical intervention, and digital tools are no exception. However, gathering long-term, high-quality evidence for technologies like AI algorithms, mobile apps, or wearable devices can be time-consuming and expensive. Many of these tools iterate rapidly, making traditional randomized controlled trials (RCTs) difficult to apply. As a result, promising technologies may remain unreimbursed or only partially funded due to a lack of formal evidence, even if early data and real-world usage indicate benefit. This delay slows down adoption and leaves innovators in a catch-22 situation: they need evidence for reimbursement, but they need reimbursement to generate large-scale evidence. Alternative evaluation methods, like adaptive trials and real-world data collection, are increasingly being explored to bridge this gap.

- **Administrative Burden of Billing and Documentation:** Digital health services often add layers of complexity to existing billing workflows, creating a significant administrative burden for providers. Each digital interaction—whether a telehealth visit, remote monitoring check-in, or asynchronous consultation—requires proper coding, documentation, and sometimes justification for medical necessity. The variety of payer policies and evolving reimbursement criteria adds further confusion. Providers must also ensure compliance with regulatory requirements and data reporting standards. These tasks consume valuable clinical time and resources, often requiring specialized staff or software. The additional paperwork can discourage healthcare professionals from fully adopting digital tools, especially in smaller practices. Streamlining billing processes and automating documentation through digital platforms could help reduce this friction and improve uptake.
- **Privacy and Liability Concerns Around Remote Care and Data Sharing:** Remote care delivery and digital data sharing raise complex privacy, security, and liability issues. With more patient information flowing across platforms and devices—often outside traditional clinical settings—the risk of data breaches, misuse, or unauthorized access increases. Regulations like HIPAA, GDPR, and various national laws impose strict data protection standards, but compliance is not always straightforward for digital health startups or even large providers. In addition, questions of clinical liability arise: who is responsible if an AI tool gives a wrong recommendation, or a remote monitoring alert is missed? These legal uncertainties can make providers hesitant to adopt remote care technologies at scale. Ensuring robust cybersecurity, clear accountability frameworks, and well-defined consent models is essential for building trust and ensuring the safe expansion of digital health.

8.5.7 Future Directions

- Development of international reimbursement frameworks for digital health.
- Expanded CPT and HCPCS codes for AI, virtual reality, and mental health apps.
- Faster reimbursement pathways for high-need tools (e.g., pandemic response, rural access).
- Patient-centered payment models, including app-based reimbursement via health savings accounts (HSAs).

Reimbursement policies and digital health coding systems are critical enablers of innovation in healthcare. By aligning financial incentives with technology adoption, they ensure that clinicians are supported in using tools that improve patient care. Policymakers, payers, and innovators must work together to build flexible, evidence-based, and equitable reimbursement models to support the future of digital health.

9 Chapter IMPLEMENTATION AND ADOPTION CHALLENGES

9.0 INTRODUCTION: AN OVERVIEW

The successful implementation and adoption of digital health solutions hinge on a complex interplay of technological, organizational, regulatory, financial, and human factors. Technical barriers like outdated infrastructure, lack of interoperability, and inconsistent data standards often slow down integration. Organizational resistance, limited digital literacy, and inadequate training further hinder smooth transitions. Financial constraints and fragmented reimbursement models reduce incentives for providers to adopt new tools. Regulatory uncertainty, especially around emerging technologies like AI, adds additional layers of complexity. Moreover, patient access, engagement, and equity must be addressed to prevent widening the digital divide. Overcoming these challenges requires a unified and strategic effort from governments, healthcare providers, technology vendors, payers, and patients alike. Policy alignment, investment in infrastructure and training, and clear regulatory pathways are essential. Only through such coordinated collaboration can digital health evolve from isolated innovations into fully integrated, scalable systems that enhance care quality, improve health outcomes, and ensure equitable access across all populations.

As digital health technologies continue to evolve, their successful implementation and adoption remain key challenges for healthcare systems around the world. While the potential of digital tools—such as telemedicine, AI-based diagnostics, remote patient monitoring, electronic health records (EHRs), and mobile health apps—is widely recognized, turning that potential into real-world clinical value is often complex and uneven. At the heart of the issue is the fragmentation of health IT infrastructure. Many healthcare providers still rely on outdated legacy systems that are incompatible with modern standards like FHIR and lack the flexibility needed to integrate newer technologies. Upgrading these systems requires significant financial investment, technical capacity, and institutional commitment—resources that are often in short supply, particularly in underfunded settings. Equally challenging is the lack of standardization across healthcare organizations, vendors, and regulatory bodies. Inconsistent adoption of interoperability standards (such as HL7, DICOM, SNOMED, and ICD) creates communication gaps between systems, complicating workflows and leading to duplicated tests, incomplete patient records, and administrative inefficiencies. These inconsistencies hinder smooth data exchange and make large-scale implementation difficult.

Workforce readiness also plays a crucial role in digital health adoption. Clinicians and support staff often face steep learning curves when using new systems, especially if training is inadequate or poorly supported. Resistance to change, digital literacy gaps, and concerns over increased workloads can slow or even block technology uptake. In some cases, healthcare professionals may distrust AI or automation tools, fearing a loss of clinical judgment or job security.

Patient engagement and equity present another major hurdle. While some patients are eager to use mobile apps or telehealth platforms, others—especially older adults, individuals with disabilities, or those in rural and underserved areas—may lack access to the necessary devices, internet connectivity, or digital literacy. This creates a digital divide, limiting the reach and impact of new healthcare models and raising concerns about inclusivity and health equity. Reimbursement and funding models also lag behind the pace of innovation. In many countries, digital health tools are not adequately supported by insurance providers, public health systems, or government reimbursement programs. Lack of financial incentives can deter healthcare organizations from adopting these solutions, even when they show clinical promise. For developers, unpredictable revenue models make it harder to scale their products or attract investment. Furthermore, regulatory frameworks are often slow to evolve and fragmented across jurisdictions. Navigating the complex landscape of approvals, certifications, and compliance standards can be time-consuming and costly for innovators (Fig. 1). The delay in establishing clear guidelines—particularly for emerging areas like AI, digital therapeutics, and remote monitoring—creates uncertainty and risk, further stalling adoption. Privacy, data security, and legal liability are persistent concerns.

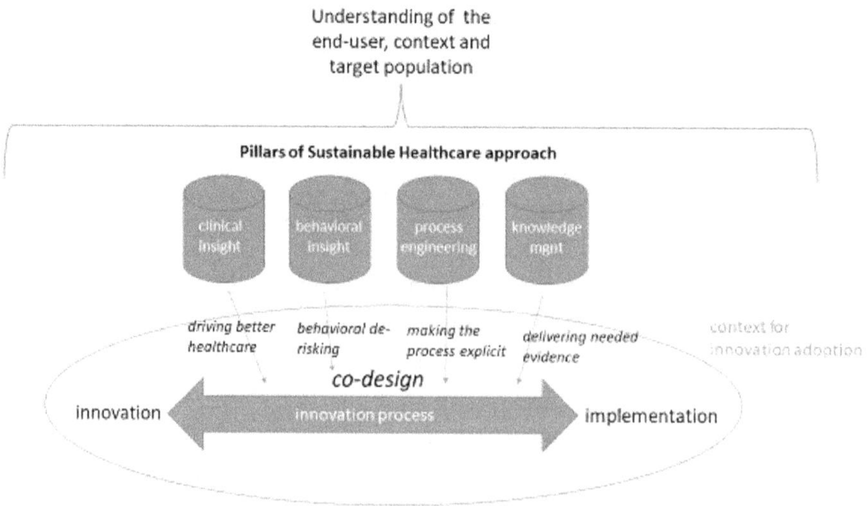

Fig. 1 Making Digital Health "Solutions" Sustainable in Healthcare Systems

As digital health relies on the collection, exchange, and analysis of sensitive personal health information, robust safeguards are essential. However, differing interpretations of laws like HIPAA or GDPR, combined with evolving threats like cyberattacks, make compliance challenging. Providers and patients alike worry about data breaches, misuse, and accountability in remote or automated care scenarios. Finally, there is the issue of evidence. Health systems and payers require proof of safety, efficacy, and cost-effectiveness before approving or reimbursing digital tools. Yet generating high-quality clinical evidence for rapidly evolving technologies is difficult. Traditional research methods may not apply to agile software, apps, or AI algorithms that are updated frequently. This delay in evidence generation slows adoption and limits integration into clinical workflows.

9.1 CLINICIAN RESISTANCE AND TRAINING GAPS:

9.1.1 Resistance to Change:

dopting new digital health technologies often disrupts established clinical routines, leading to hesitation among clinicians. Many fear that these tools may complicate workflows or require significant adjustments in how care is delivered. The lack of clarity about long-term benefits further fuels resistance. Past negative experiences with poorly designed systems also create skepticism. Change fatigue, especially in high-pressure environments, adds to the reluctance. Some clinicians also worry that digital tools could depersonalize patient care. Without strong leadership and clear communication of benefits, resistance tends to persist. To overcome this, change management strategies must be applied. Active clinician involvement and success stories from peers can help shift perceptions. Building trust is critical for meaningful adoption.

9.1.2 Lack of Digital Literacy

Not all clinicians possess the same level of comfort or familiarity with digital technologies. For those less tech-savvy, navigating complex health IT systems can be intimidating and error-prone. This lack of confidence may lead to underuse of available tools or increased reliance on support staff. In high-stakes clinical settings, hesitation in using unfamiliar systems can directly impact patient safety. Furthermore, without basic digital skills, clinicians may not fully benefit from advanced functionalities like clinical decision support or remote monitoring. Institutions often overlook the need to assess digital competency before rollout. A structured digital literacy training framework is essential. Continuous support and tailored education can close the gap. Bridging digital literacy is foundational to successful implementation.

9.1.3 Inadequate Training and Support

A common pitfall in digital health adoption is the absence of well-structured, role-specific training. Many training sessions are too generic, rushed, or delivered without real-world clinical context. As a result, clinicians are left unprepared to integrate new tools into their daily practice. Without adequate onboarding, confidence and proficiency remain low. Furthermore, limited post-training support makes it difficult for staff to troubleshoot problems independently. This leads to frustration and contributes to technology abandonment. Effective training should include hands-on practice, simulation, and access to live support. Training must also be an ongoing process—not a one-time event. Investing in high-quality, clinician-centered education significantly boosts adoption rates.

9.1.4 Fear of Increased Workload

Clinicians often view digital systems as adding administrative burden rather than reducing it. Many EHR platforms, for example, are notorious for requiring excessive clicks, documentation steps, or duplicate entries. This perceived inefficiency fuels the belief that digital tools detract from patient care time. Concerns over screen fatigue and burnout are also common. In the absence of workflow-optimized designs, clinicians may resist engaging with the tools altogether. Early involvement in system design can help ensure usability and relevance. Additionally, integrating automation features can reduce documentation time. Addressing workload fears openly and demonstrating time-saving benefits is essential to earning clinician buy-in.

9.1.5 Concerns Over Clinical Autonomy

Some clinicians worry that digital health tools—particularly AI, algorithms, or decision-support systems—could undermine their clinical judgment. There's fear that automated suggestions might replace nuanced decision-making, reducing their role to that of a data interpreter. This can lead to distrust in the technology and minimal reliance on its recommendations. Moreover, concerns over liability arise when clinicians feel pressured to follow system-generated advice. Clear boundaries need to be established: technology should support, not dictate, clinical decisions. Training should emphasize how to interpret digital insights alongside clinical experience. Ensuring transparency in how AI tools generate outputs can also boost confidence and autonomy.

9.1.6 Lack of Involvement in Implementation

When clinicians are excluded from the design, selection, or testing of digital health tools, systems often fail to meet real-world needs. This disconnect results in tools that are either impractical or inefficient for daily use. Clinician engagement during early stages of development ensures that systems align with workflow realities and patient care goals. Lack of involvement can also lead to a sense of imposition rather than collaboration. Inclusive design processes promote a sense of ownership, improving satisfaction and usage rates. Institutions should form multidisciplinary implementation teams with active clinician participation. Feedback loops should remain open post-deployment to allow for refinements. Adoption thrives when clinicians help shape the tools they use.

9.1.7 Limited Time for Learning

Time is a precious commodity in clinical environments, and packed schedules often leave little room for training or skill-building. As a result, many clinicians adopt only the bare minimum required to operate digital tools, leaving advanced features underused. Without dedicated time for exploration, systems remain foreign and difficult to navigate. This "learn-on-the-go" approach compromises both safety and efficiency. Institutions must prioritize protected training time and integrate learning into normal workflows. Micro-learning, e-modules, and just-in-time resources can offer flexibility. Peer-led sessions or on-the-floor digital champions can also bridge the knowledge gap in real time. A culture that values ongoing learning leads to deeper, more confident adoption.

9.1.8 Variable Training Quality Across Institutions

Training programs differ widely between hospitals, health systems, and even departments, leading to inconsistent skill levels among clinicians. Some receive comprehensive onboarding with simulations and live support, while others are handed a user manual with little explanation. This inconsistency causes uneven adoption, inefficiencies, and user frustration. A standard, competency based training framework can address these gaps. Certification pathways and refresher courses can ensure that all users maintain a baseline level of proficiency. National or regional guidelines for digital health training could help create consistency. Institutions must also evaluate the effectiveness of their training programs regularly and update them based on feedback and system updates.

9.1.9 Trust and Confidence Issues

Trust is foundational to adoption. Clinicians who have experienced system crashes, data loss, or poorly designed interfaces are often skeptical of digital tools. Concerns over data accuracy, patient safety, and error rates reduce confidence in using these systems during critical moments. Rebuilding trust requires demonstrating system reliability and clinical relevance over time. Transparent communication about system limitations, update cycles, and performance improvements helps manage expectations. Including clinician feedback in post-implementation reviews can also strengthen confidence. Vendors and IT teams must commit to user-centered design and responsive technical support. Trust grows when clinicians see consistent performance and meaningful results.

9.1.10 Need for Ongoing Professional Development

Digital health is a fast-moving field, and static, one-time training is not enough. Clinicians need continuous opportunities to learn about system upgrades, new features, evolving standards, and emerging technologies. Without structured ongoing education, users fall behind and risk using outdated practices. Professional development programs should be integrated into institutional learning strategies and aligned with clinical roles. Certifications, CME credits, or gamified learning can incentivize participation. Importantly, training should be practical, concise, and directly tied to improving patient care. Regularly updating digital literacy ensures that clinicians remain confident, competent, and empowered to deliver high-quality care in a digital-first environment.

9.2 PATIENT ENGAGEMENT AND USABILITY BARRIERS

9.2.1 Digital Literacy Gaps Among Patients

A significant number of patients, especially elderly individuals or those with limited formal education, struggle with basic digital skills. Many cannot comfortably use mobile apps, patient portals, or connected devices. This gap prevents full participation in digital care models and increases dependency on in-person support. Addressing this requires user-friendly design and targeted digital literacy programs.

9.2.2 Limited Access to Devices and Internet

Access to smartphones, tablets, or high-speed internet is still unequal—especially in rural, low-income, or marginalized communities. Without reliable connectivity, patients cannot benefit from telehealth, remote monitoring, or digital therapeutics. Expanding digital infrastructure and device affordability is critical to bridging this gap and achieving equitable digital health access.

9.2.3 Language and Cultural Barriers

Many digital health tools are designed primarily in English or dominant national languages, excluding non-native speakers. Additionally, cultural differences in health beliefs, communication styles, or privacy expectations can hinder engagement. Multilingual platforms, culturally sensitive content, and community-driven outreach improve inclusivity and trust.

9.2.4 Poor User Interface (UI) and Experience (UX) Design

Complex, cluttered, or unintuitive app and portal designs often discourage patient use. If interfaces are not simple, accessible, and responsive across devices, users may abandon them. Digital health tools must prioritize usability, accessibility standards (e.g., for vision or mobility impairments), and iterative design based on real patient feedback.

9.2.5 Privacy and Data Security Concerns

Patients may hesitate to engage with digital platforms due to fears about data breaches, misuse of personal information, or surveillance. High-profile cybersecurity incidents increase public skepticism. Transparent data policies, robust encryption, and clear consent mechanisms are necessary to build confidence in digital care.

9.2.6 Lack of Motivation or Perceived Benefit:

Some patients do not see a clear advantage to using digital health tools, especially if they feel their condition is manageable or the tool does not align with their personal preferences. To increase adoption, tools must demonstrate value—such as improved outcomes, convenience, or cost savings—and promote behavioral change through engagement strategies.

9.2.7 Overload of Health Apps and Portals

Patients often face a fragmented experience—multiple logins, different platforms for labs, appointments, prescriptions, and messaging. This lack of integration causes confusion and fatigue. Unified systems, single sign-on solutions, and platform consolidation enhance usability and encourage long-term engagement.

9.2.8 Inconsistent Patient Onboarding and Education

Without proper onboarding, patients may not understand how to use digital tools or what benefits to expect. Providing guided tutorials, user manuals, videos, and access to help desks or digital navigators helps patients get started and stay engaged. Education should be ongoing, especially when new features are introduced.

9.2.9 Low Engagement in Chronic and Preventive Care

Digital health tools are often underused in chronic disease management and preventive care settings, where long-term engagement is critical. Patients may start using apps but stop when immediate improvements are not seen. Gamification, personalized feedback, and care team involvement can help sustain long-term interaction.

9.2.10 Accessibility Challenges for Special Populations

Patients with disabilities, cognitive impairments, or low vision often face barriers when using standard digital platforms. Lack of assistive technology integration, voice navigation, or screen reader compatibility can exclude them. Inclusive design and compliance with accessibility guidelines (e.g., WCAG) are essential for ensuring universal access (Table-1).

Table-1 : Concise summary of the Patient Engagement and Usability Barriers

S.No	Barrier	Summary Description
1	Digital Literacy Gaps	Many patients, especially older adults or less educated individuals, lack basic skills to use digital tools.
2	Limited Access to Devices and Internet	Rural and low-income populations often lack smartphones or internet, limiting digital health access.
3	Language and Cultural Barriers	Language differences and cultural beliefs can hinder tool usage and patient trust.
4	Poor UI/UX Design	Complex or inaccessible interfaces discourage patient use and reduce engagement.
5	Privacy and Data Security Concerns	Fear of data misuse or cyber threats discourages patient trust in digital health platforms.
6	Lack of Motivation or Perceived Benefit	Some patients don't see value in digital tools, especially for non-urgent or manageable conditions.
7	Overload of Health Apps and Portals	Multiple, unintegrated systems overwhelm patients, leading to confusion and app fatigue.
8	Inconsistent Onboarding and Education	Lack of proper guidance or tutorials limits understanding and consistent tool usage.
9	Low Engagement in Chronic/Preventive Care	Patients often drop off over time due to lack of results or motivation; ongoing support is needed.
10	Accessibility Challenges for Special Populations	Patients with disabilities face usability issues due to lack of inclusive design or assistive tech support.

9.3 INFRASTRUCTURE GAPS IN LOW-RESOURCE SETTINGS

9.3.1 Limited Internet Connectivity

Many low-resource regions struggle with poor or unreliable internet access, which significantly restricts their ability to leverage modern digital health technologies. This lack of connectivity impacts essential services like telemedicine, electronic health record (EHR) access, and real-time data sharing among healthcare providers. Without stable internet, cloud-based platforms become unusable, leaving providers and patients disconnected from vital health information and support systems. This digital divide often results in increased health disparities between urban and rural populations. Bridging this gap requires investments in infrastructure development, including expanding broadband coverage to underserved areas and exploring alternative connectivity solutions such as satellite internet or community Wi-Fi networks.

9.3.2 Inadequate Hardware Availability

Healthcare facilities in underserved settings frequently lack adequate hardware like computers, tablets, and smartphones necessary for digital health applications. Even when devices are available, many are outdated or malfunctioning, reducing their utility in clinical environments. This shortage hinders the implementation of technologies such as electronic health records, telehealth consultations, and mobile health monitoring. The absence of proper equipment also limits training opportunities for healthcare workers and slows the digitization of patient care. Addressing this issue requires targeted funding for procurement, sustainable maintenance programs, and partnerships to supply affordable, quality hardware suited for resource-constrained environments.

9.3.3 Power Supply Instability

Unstable or intermittent electricity supply is a major barrier to digital health adoption in many low-resource areas. Frequent power outages disrupt critical health IT systems, cause data loss, and prevent continuous operation of devices like patient monitors and servers. Healthcare facilities without reliable power may have to rely on backup generators or batteries, which are costly and sometimes unavailable. This unreliability limits the feasibility of deploying real-time monitoring, automated alerts, and cloud-based services. To mitigate this, investments in renewable energy sources such as solar power, along with battery storage solutions, can provide more consistent electricity and support the digital health infrastructure sustainably.

9.3.4 Lack of Skilled IT Personnel

Low-resource settings often face a shortage of qualified IT professionals who can install, maintain, and troubleshoot health information systems. This skills gap results in frequent system failures, prolonged downtimes, and a lack of timely technical support for digital tools. Without local expertise, healthcare providers may become frustrated or unable to fully utilize digital platforms. The situation is worsened by brain drain, where trained personnel migrate to better-resourced areas. Addressing this challenge requires investment in specialized training programs, capacity-building initiatives, and retention strategies to build a sustainable workforce capable of supporting digital health technologies in underserved regions.

9.3.5 Insufficient Data Storage and Backup Facilities

Many healthcare facilities in low-resource areas lack robust infrastructure for secure and reliable data storage and backup. This leads to reliance on paper-based records or unstable digital systems prone to data loss, which undermines patient care continuity and health system efficiency. Inadequate storage also compromises data security and privacy, increasing the risk of unauthorized access or accidental breaches. The absence of proper backup mechanisms leaves critical health information vulnerable in the event of system failures or disasters. To improve this, investment is needed in secure, scalable storage solutions—potentially cloud-based—and protocols for regular data backup and disaster recovery.

9.3.6 Financial Constraints and Funding Limitations

Financial limitations are a major hurdle in establishing and sustaining digital health infrastructure in low-resource settings. Restricted budgets often prevent healthcare facilities from acquiring necessary hardware, software licenses, and maintenance services. Many digital health projects rely heavily on short-term grants or donor funding, which can lead to instability and difficulties in scaling or sustaining initiatives long term. Ongoing operational costs such as internet service fees and staff training also strain limited resources. Sustainable financing models, including government budget allocations, public-private partnerships, and innovative funding mechanisms, are essential to support enduring digital health infrastructure.

9.3.7 Poor Integration of Systems

Health information systems in low-resource settings are often fragmented, with various digital platforms developed independently without interoperability. This siloed approach leads to duplicated efforts, redundant data entry, and challenges in sharing information across different care settings. Lack of system integration reduces overall efficiency, increases administrative burden, and complicates comprehensive patient management. Furthermore, it hinders data aggregation necessary for public health surveillance and decision-making. Achieving interoperability through adoption of standards, unified platforms, and collaborative governance is critical to overcoming these integration challenges and optimizing health outcomes.

9.3.8 Security and Privacy Infrastructure Deficits

Many low-resource healthcare environments lack adequate cybersecurity infrastructure, such as firewalls, encryption technologies, and secure networks, leaving digital health systems vulnerable to breaches and data theft. This insecurity undermines patient confidentiality and erodes trust in digital platforms, deterring adoption by both providers and patients. The absence of robust privacy policies and staff training on data protection further exacerbates these risks. To build a secure digital health ecosystem, investments are needed in cybersecurity technologies, policy frameworks, and ongoing education for healthcare workers on best practices for data privacy and security.

9.3.9 Limited Access to Training and Capacity Building

Healthcare workers in low-resource settings often have limited opportunities to receive training on new digital health tools due to shortages of trainers, infrastructure, and educational resources. This training gap restricts their ability to effectively use digital platforms, leading to underutilization or misuse of technology. Without ongoing capacity building, staff may struggle with troubleshooting and adapting to updates, negatively impacting patient care. Developing localized, context-specific training programs, utilizing remote learning technologies, and fostering peer support networks can enhance workforce competence and confidence in digital health adoption.

9.3.10 Geographic and Environmental Challenges

Remote and rural areas face unique geographic and environmental barriers that complicate digital health implementation. Difficult terrain, poor road infrastructure, and extreme weather conditions hinder delivery, installation, and maintenance of digital health equipment. These challenges also limit access to centralized technical support and supply chains for replacement parts or upgrades. Geographic isolation increases operational costs and can delay timely responses to system failures. Tailored strategies such as mobile health units, community-based support, and ruggedized equipment designed for harsh environments are necessary to overcome these obstacles and expand digital health reach.

9.4 TECHNICAL LIMITATIONS AND DEVICE RELIABILITY

9.4.1 Limited Processing Power and Storage Capacity

Many digital health devices, especially those designed for portability and wearability, face significant constraints in processing power and data storage. These devices often rely on small, energy-efficient processors to conserve battery life, which limits their ability to perform complex computations or advanced analytics locally. Similarly, limited onboard storage means that large volumes of health data — such as continuous biometric monitoring or high-resolution images — cannot be saved on the device for long periods. This limitation necessitates frequent data offloading to external servers or cloud platforms for processing and storage. However, in many healthcare settings, especially rural or low-resource environments, stable internet connectivity is not guaranteed, which complicates real-time data transfer and synchronization. Consequently, these constraints restrict device functionality and responsiveness, potentially impacting timely clinical decision-making. Device manufacturers must balance power consumption, processing capability, and storage to optimize usability without sacrificing critical performance.

9.4.2 Battery Life Constraints

Battery life remains one of the most pressing technical challenges for mobile and wearable digital health devices. Continuous operation of sensors, wireless communication modules, and data processing tasks demands substantial energy. However, current battery technologies often provide limited capacity, leading to devices that require frequent recharging or battery replacements. This dependency disrupts continuous patient monitoring and can lead to gaps in data collection, especially in chronic disease management or remote patient surveillance where uninterrupted data is vital. The inconvenience of charging can also decrease user adherence and satisfaction, as patients or healthcare workers may neglect or delay recharging. In remote or resource-poor areas, inconsistent access to electricity exacerbates this issue, making it difficult to maintain device operability. Advances in low-power electronics, energy harvesting techniques, and more efficient battery designs are critical to improving the autonomy and reliability of digital health devices.

9.4.3 Device Durability and Environmental Resistance

Digital health devices must operate reliably in a wide range of real-world environments, which can be unpredictable and harsh. Exposure to dust, moisture, extreme temperatures, and physical shocks is common in clinical, home care, and community settings. Devices lacking sufficient ruggedness or environmental sealing are prone to damage, malfunction, or reduced lifespan under these conditions. For example, water ingress can corrode internal components, and temperature fluctuations may impair sensor accuracy or battery performance. Frequent device failures increase maintenance costs and downtime, reducing overall system effectiveness and increasing the burden on healthcare providers and patients. Robust design standards, including protective casings, waterproofing, shock absorption, and thermal management, are essential to ensure longevity and consistent performance. Without these considerations, device reliability suffers, undermining user confidence and adoption rates.

9.4.4 Software Bugs and System Crashes

Software reliability is crucial for digital health devices that often perform critical monitoring or decision support functions. However, software bugs, glitches, or compatibility conflicts can lead to system crashes or erratic behavior, interrupting clinical workflows and potentially jeopardizing patient safety. Inconsistent performance or unexpected downtime frustrates users and erodes trust in the technology. The complexity of healthcare environments, with diverse hardware and software platforms, complicates software development and testing. Ensuring reliable performance requires thorough and ongoing quality assurance processes, including extensive pre-deployment testing, user acceptance testing, and post-launch monitoring for issues. Timely software updates, patches, and well-managed version control help address emerging bugs and security vulnerabilities. Additionally, effective communication channels for reporting and resolving software problems are necessary to maintain system integrity and user confidence.

9.4.5 Interoperability Issues

Interoperability remains a fundamental challenge for digital health devices integrating into complex healthcare ecosystems. Devices may use proprietary data formats, communication protocols, or interfaces that are incompatible with electronic health records (EHRs) or other clinical systems. This fragmentation leads to isolated data silos, manual data entry, and duplication of effort, undermining care coordination and data-driven decision-making. Lack of adherence to established interoperability standards such as HL7 FHIR, DICOM, or IEEE protocols further complicates seamless data exchange. Without interoperability, the potential benefits of comprehensive, longitudinal health data aggregation are lost, limiting insights into patient outcomes and public health trends. Addressing interoperability requires collaborative efforts among manufacturers, standards bodies, and healthcare organizations to adopt common frameworks and ensure that devices support standardized data exchange and integration capabilities.

9.4.6 Calibration and Accuracy Challenges

Medical devices used in diagnostics and monitoring must provide accurate and reliable measurements to support clinical decisions. Many such devices require regular calibration to maintain measurement precision over time. Inadequate calibration protocols or lack of access to skilled personnel can lead to drift or inaccuracies, resulting in incorrect data that may compromise patient safety or treatment efficacy. In low-resource settings, calibration equipment may be unavailable or too costly, exacerbating this problem. Additionally, environmental factors such as temperature, humidity, or mechanical wear can affect sensor accuracy. Ensuring proper calibration involves establishing standardized procedures, training healthcare workers, and incorporating self-calibration or automated calibration features into devices where possible. Without consistent accuracy assurance, device reliability is diminished, reducing clinical utility and acceptance.

9.4.7 Limited Scalability

Some digital health devices and platforms are initially designed for pilot projects or small-scale deployments. These solutions often lack the architectural flexibility, robustness, or support infrastructure needed to scale effectively across larger patient populations or broader geographic areas. Scaling issues include hardware supply chain constraints, increased demand on data storage and processing, user support challenges, and higher maintenance requirements. Without scalability, promising innovations cannot achieve widespread impact or sustain long-term health system improvements. Planning for scalability requires early consideration of infrastructure needs, modular designs, cloud-based services, and interoperability standards. Failure to do so risks fragmentation, inefficiency, and duplication as multiple isolated systems proliferate rather than converging into cohesive solutions.

9.4.8 Security Vulnerabilities

Security is a critical aspect of digital health device reliability, as these devices handle sensitive personal health information. Many devices suffer from technical limitations such as weak encryption, unsecured wireless transmissions, or poor authentication mechanisms. These vulnerabilities expose systems to risks including data breaches, unauthorized access, and tampering, which can lead to privacy violations or compromised clinical data integrity. Cybersecurity threats also undermine user trust and may result in regulatory penalties. Addressing these limitations requires implementing strong security protocols at the hardware and software levels, including end-to-end encryption, multi-factor authentication, and regular security audits. Furthermore, manufacturers must stay vigilant against emerging threats and promptly update devices to mitigate vulnerabilities.

9.4.9 Lack of Standardized Testing and Certification

The digital health device market suffers from inconsistent regulatory oversight and a lack of standardized testing or certification frameworks. This inconsistency results in a wide range of product quality, reliability, and safety levels. Without rigorous validation, healthcare providers may face challenges in selecting trustworthy devices, leading to skepticism and reluctance to adopt new technologies. Standardized testing protocols evaluate device accuracy, interoperability, security, usability, and durability. Certification from recognized bodies assures users and regulators of compliance with essential quality and safety benchmarks. Establishing and enforcing these standards globally would facilitate market transparency, encourage innovation, and protect patients. Without this, fragmentation persists, limiting trust and scalability.

9.4.10 Maintenance and Technical Support Limitations

Effective maintenance and timely technical support are vital to sustaining device reliability and user confidence. Many healthcare settings, especially in remote or low-resource areas, lack sufficient technical infrastructure and skilled personnel to manage device upkeep. Delays in repairs or software updates result in prolonged downtime, lost data, and workflow interruptions. The absence of local support networks further complicates troubleshooting and increases dependency on centralized or remote assistance, which may not be promptly available. To ensure continuous operation, manufacturers and healthcare organizations must develop robust support frameworks, including training programs for local technicians, remote monitoring capabilities, and clear escalation procedures. A proactive approach to maintenance reduces device failures and prolongs lifespan, improving overall system resilience and user satisfaction.

9.5 Change Management in Healthcare Systems

9.5.1 Importance of Change Management

In healthcare, change management is not just about adopting new technologies but ensuring they improve patient care without overwhelming staff. With multiple roles, departments, and regulatory constraints, unstructured change can create confusion, inefficiency, or even clinical risk. A well-planned change management strategy helps identify potential disruptions, align stakeholders with shared goals, and guide transitions smoothly. It involves setting realistic timelines, managing expectations, and fostering collaboration across departments. Change must be treated as a human process, not just a technical one. Organizations that ignore structured change management often experience tool rejection, wasted investments, and stagnation. Effective change practices also encourage a proactive mindset toward continuous improvement. Ultimately, it acts as the bridge between innovation and sustainable impact in healthcare delivery.

9.5.2 Leadership Commitment and Sponsorship

Leadership buy-in is foundational to any successful transformation. Executives and clinical leaders must not only approve change but visibly support and participate in the process. Their involvement provides strategic direction and legitimizes the effort among staff. When leaders consistently communicate the vision and demonstrate commitment through actions—such as attending training or addressing concerns—it builds trust. They also have the authority to allocate necessary resources like time, funding, and personnel. Without strong sponsorship, change efforts risk losing momentum or being deprioritized amid operational pressures. Leaders must champion the change through every phase, reinforcing it as an organizational priority. Empowering mid-level managers as change agents also amplifies leadership's reach and influence.

9.5.3 Stakeholder Engagement

Engaging the right stakeholders early ensures the change reflects real-world needs and challenges. Frontline clinicians, nurses, administrators, IT personnel, and even patients bring diverse perspectives that can shape more practical, acceptable solutions. Involving them from the planning stage fosters a sense of ownership and reduces resistance. Engagement also surfaces hidden barriers, such as unspoken workflow dependencies or cultural norms, that could derail implementation. Co-design workshops, pilot testing, and regular check-ins keep stakeholders involved and valued. This participatory approach builds transparency and accountability, increasing the likelihood of successful adoption. It also promotes alignment across silos, which is crucial in complex healthcare environments.

9.5.4 Clear Communication

Poor communication is a leading cause of failure in change initiatives. Effective change management demands timely, transparent, and tailored communication to all affected groups. Staff must understand why the change is happening, how it affects them, what support is available, and when key milestones will occur. Consistent messaging from leadership and change teams helps eliminate misinformation and uncertainty. Communication channels should be varied—emails, meetings, intranet updates, posters, or one-on-one sessions—to reach different audiences effectively. It's also important to create opportunities for two-way dialogue, where staff can ask questions and voice concerns. Clarity and openness build trust and readiness for change.

9.5.5 Training and Education

Comprehensive training is vital to building user competence and confidence in new systems or processes. Training should be role-specific, interactive, and ideally integrated into actual clinical scenarios. Simulation-based learning, live demonstrations, and hands-on workshops are more effective than passive presentations. Training must go beyond basic use; it should help users understand how the change fits into their workflow and improves outcomes. Post-implementation support, such as on-site coaching or digital help tools, reinforces learning. Offering refresher sessions ensures retention and accommodates late adopters or new staff. Ultimately, strong education programs empower users and reduce early-phase friction or misuse.

9.5.6 Addressing Resistance and Barriers

Resistance to change is natural, especially in high-pressure environments like healthcare where stability is valued. Identifying the root causes—fear of incompetence, workload increase, loss of autonomy, or previous bad experiences—is essential. A proactive strategy includes listening sessions, anonymous surveys, and one-on-one conversations to understand concerns. Designating peer "change champions" who support and mentor others is highly effective. Offering small wins early in the process helps shift attitudes positively. Respecting individual emotions and providing reassurance and empathy is just as important as technical readiness. The goal is not to eliminate resistance, but to acknowledge, address, and transform it into constructive feedback.

9.5.7 Workflow Integration

For any digital or procedural change to succeed, it must be thoughtfully integrated into existing workflows—or accompanied by realistic workflow redesign. If new systems are seen as adding steps, creating duplication, or disrupting routines, users will reject them. Change teams must map out current processes, identify pain points, and test how the new approach fits into actual work patterns. Involving end users in this mapping ensures that proposed changes are practical and sustainable. Workflow alignment minimizes disruption, enhances efficiency, and improves user satisfaction. Seamless integration is a hallmark of well-managed change and a predictor of long-term success.

9.5.8. Monitoring and Feedback Mechanisms

Monitoring progress during and after implementation allows organizations to detect adoption challenges early and course-correct. Key metrics may include user login frequency, error rates, time-on-task, or patient outcomes. Just as important is capturing qualitative feedback—staff satisfaction, perceived ease-of-use, and confidence levels. Regular feedback loops through surveys, debrief meetings, or digital dashboards ensure that frontline experiences inform ongoing refinements. This continuous improvement model makes change feel dynamic and responsive rather than top-down. Establishing a safe space for feedback encourages honest input, which is crucial for evolving the change strategy and supporting long-term user engagement.

9.5.9 Sustaining Change

Sustaining change means embedding new processes and technologies into the daily fabric of healthcare delivery. After initial rollout, systems can drift back to old habits if ongoing reinforcement is absent. This requires institutionalizing new practices through updated policies, standard operating procedures, and job descriptions. Recognition and rewards for successful adoption can further motivate staff. Creating structures for ongoing support, such as a digital help desk or learning community, ensures users stay competent as systems evolve. Leadership must continue to monitor outcomes and emphasize accountability. Sustaining change is not a one-time effort—it requires vigilance and reinforcement over time.

9.5.10 Cultural Transformation

At its core, change management is about transforming culture. A culture that embraces innovation, collaboration, and continuous learning is more adaptable to future change. This shift takes time and effort, involving both mindset and behaviour change. Leaders must champion a "fail fast, learn faster" ethos and encourage experimentation without fear of blame. Promoting cross-disciplinary collaboration and recognizing innovative efforts nurtures this adaptive culture. Storytelling—sharing examples of success and lessons learned—also helps spread enthusiasm and normalize change. Culture change isn't just the end goal—it's the ongoing context in which all future changes occur (Table-2).

Table-2: Summary of Change Management in Healthcare Systems

Heading	Summary
Importance of Change Management	A structured approach is essential to guide transitions, reduce confusion, align stakeholders, and embed new technologies without disrupting patient care. Change must be human-centered and continuous.
Leadership Commitment and Sponsorship	Strong, visible leadership ensures prioritization, resource allocation, and trust-building, which are crucial for successful and sustained change.
Stakeholder Engagement	Involving clinicians, staff, IT, and patients early in the process fosters ownership, uncovers hidden challenges, and improves adoption success.
Clear Communication	Timely, transparent, and audience-specific communication helps manage expectations, reduces misinformation, and prepares staff for change.
Training and Education	Role-specific, hands-on training increases user confidence and effectiveness, while ongoing support and refreshers ensure long-term competency.
Addressing Resistance and Barriers	Understanding root causes of resistance and offering empathy, peer support, and small wins helps convert opposition into constructive feedback.
Workflow Integration	Successful implementation requires aligning or redesigning workflows so that new tools complement rather than disrupt existing practices.
Monitoring and Feedback Mechanisms	Tracking adoption metrics and collecting staff feedback ensures early issue detection, continuous improvement, and responsive adaptation.
Sustaining Change	Embedding change through updated policies, support systems, and rewards maintains long-term use and avoids regression to old habits.
Cultural Transformation	Encouraging innovation, learning, and collaboration creates a flexible culture that can adapt to future change and supports ongoing transformation.

10 Chapter

FUTURE OF DIGITAL HEALTH MONITORING

10.0 INTRODUCTION: AN OVERVIEW

The healthcare landscape is undergoing a profound transformation, fueled by the integration of cutting-edge technologies into patient care, diagnostics, and disease prevention. At the forefront of this transformation is digital health monitoring—a rapidly evolving domain that leverages wearable sensors, mobile apps, artificial intelligence (AI), cloud computing, and big data analytics to track and enhance individual health in real time. As global populations age, chronic diseases rise, and the demand for personalized care grows, digital health solutions are becoming not just complementary, but essential tools in modern medicine. Digital health monitoring represents a shift from reactive, clinic-based treatment models to proactive, patient-centered care. Today, individuals can measure vital signs, detect early signs of illness, and manage chronic conditions through smartwatches, biosensors, and smartphone-integrated platforms. These tools are bridging the gap between patients and providers, enabling continuous care beyond the walls of hospitals and clinics. From glucose monitors for diabetics to wearable ECG devices for cardiac patients, digital monitoring tools are empowering people to take control of their own health in ways never before possible. The widespread adoption of remote patient monitoring (RPM) during the COVID-19 pandemic acted as a major catalyst, proving that decentralized care is both feasible and beneficial. Health professionals began to harness telehealth platforms and IoT-connected devices to monitor symptoms, adjust treatments, and maintain continuity of care—even under lockdown. This experience showcased not only the value of digital tools, but also the urgent need to embed them more deeply into mainstream healthcare systems (Fig. 1).

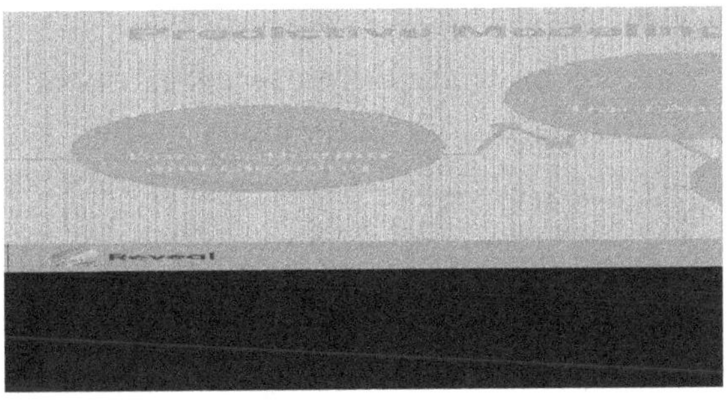

Fig. 1 The Hey Features of Digital Health

Simultaneously, advancements in AI and machine learning are redefining how health data is interpreted. Algorithms can now detect anomalies in heart rhythms, predict flare-ups in chronic conditions, or suggest medication adjustments—often before human clinicians might recognize the signs. As digital devices generate vast volumes of continuous health data, these AI-driven insights will become crucial in identifying patterns, forecasting risk, and supporting evidence-based interventions.

Another emerging frontier is personalized medicine, which relies heavily on continuous data from digital health monitoring systems. Real-time data feeds can help tailor treatments based on individual physiology, lifestyle habits, and genetic profiles. Combined with AI, this offers a future where treatments are dynamically adapted to each patient's needs—a leap forward from the one-size-fits-all approach of the past. Moreover, digital health monitoring is beginning to intersect with mental health, leveraging mobile sensors and behavioral tracking to detect stress, anxiety, or depressive episodes. Passive data—like changes in voice tone, sleep patterns, or screen usage—can provide early indicators of mental health concerns, enabling interventions before crises emerge. Despite these advances, the road ahead involves critical challenges. Issues around data privacy, cybersecurity, regulatory frameworks, equitable access, and interoperability remain significant hurdles. As devices become more complex and interconnected, safeguarding sensitive health information and ensuring ethical use of AI-driven diagnostics becomes imperative. Equally important is ensuring that digital health tools do not exacerbate existing health inequities due to cost, digital literacy, or geographic barriers.

Nevertheless, the momentum is undeniable. Governments, startups, and tech giants alike are investing in digital health infrastructure, building ecosystems where wearable tech, cloud-based platforms, and clinical-grade sensors can work together to support healthier lives. The convergence of disciplines—healthcare, engineering, data science, and behavioral psychology—is creating a fertile ground for innovation in health monitoring. In this chapter, we delve into the evolving landscape of digital health monitoring, exploring its key technologies, trends, benefits, and challenges. From predictive analytics and sensor miniaturization to regulatory evolution and patient empowerment, we examine how digital health monitoring is shaping the future of care—making it more intelligent, accessible, personalized, and continuous. As we step into an era where healthcare is increasingly digitized, data-driven, and decentralized, understanding this transformation is crucial for policymakers, clinicians, technologists, and patients alike.

10.1 PREDICTIVE AND PREVENTIVE HEALTH MODELS

The traditional healthcare model has long operated on a reactive basis—intervening only after symptoms appear or diseases progress to critical stages. However, advances in digital technology and data science are driving a fundamental shift toward a more proactive, preventive approach. Rather than waiting for illness to occur, modern healthcare systems are increasingly focused on anticipating health issues and intervening early to prevent their onset or mitigate their severity. This shift is being powered by a range of digital tools, including wearable devices, mobile health applications, remote monitoring systems, and AI-driven analytics platforms. These technologies continuously collect and analyze data such as heart rate, glucose levels, physical activity, sleep patterns, and even emotional states. With this real-time data, healthcare providers can now detect subtle physiological changes that may signal the early stages of disease, long before symptoms are visible to the patient or clinician.

Data-driven models, particularly those built on machine learning algorithms, are central to predictive health. By processing vast amounts of historical and real-time data, these models can identify patterns and correlations that may indicate future health risks. For example, predictive analytics can flag individuals at high risk of developing conditions like diabetes, cardiovascular disease, or depression based on lifestyle factors, genetic markers, and biometrics. This enables tailored preventive interventions, such as personalized diet plans, medication adjustments, or behavioral coaching, aimed at avoiding the disease altogether or slowing its progression.

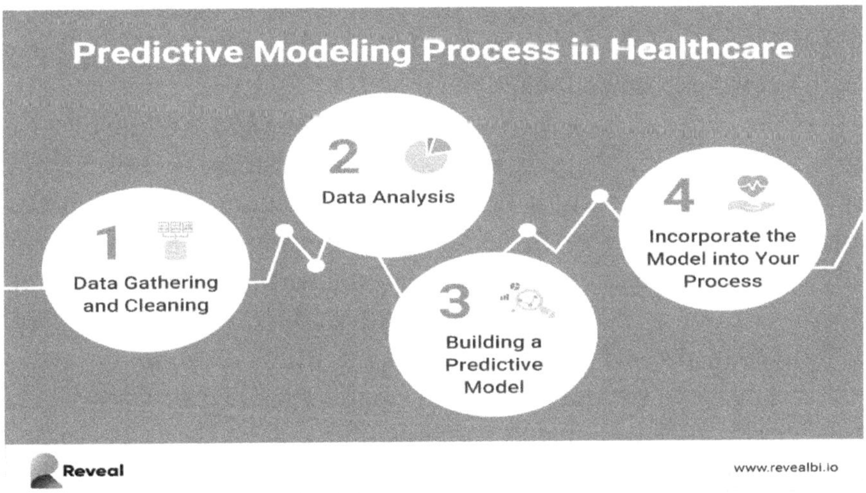

Fig. 2 Predictive Modeling Process in Healthcare

Ultimately, predictive and preventive health represents a paradigm shift in how we think about wellness—one that is centered on maintaining health rather than treating illness. It empowers individuals to take a more active role in their well-being while allowing healthcare systems to deliver smarter, more efficient, and more targeted care.

10.1.2 Role of Artificial Intelligence and Machine Learning

Artificial Intelligence (AI) and Machine Learning (ML) are revolutionizing digital health monitoring by enabling the intelligent analysis of massive and complex health datasets. These technologies allow systems to uncover patterns, correlations, and predictive insights that would be impossible for humans to detect manually. With continuous data being collected from wearable devices, electronic health records (EHRs), imaging systems, and genetic profiles, AI and ML can transform raw data into meaningful clinical predictions, making healthcare more proactive, personalized, and precise. AI algorithms process various types of structured and unstructured data—such as ECG signals, blood pressure trends, lab results, imaging scans, and even voice or gait patterns—to detect early signs of disease or health deterioration. For example, AI models trained on ECG data can identify subtle irregularities that signal an increased risk of heart disease, often before symptoms manifest. Similarly, ML algorithms can analyze a person's lifestyle factors—including physical activity, diet, sleep patterns, and stress levels—to predict the likelihood of developing conditions like type 2 diabetes or obesity. This capability enables healthcare providers to intervene earlier and personalize treatment plans based on an individual's specific risk profile. Two fundamental approaches in ML—supervised and unsupervised learning—are widely used in health prediction. Supervised learning involves training algorithms on labeled datasets, where the outcome (such as the presence of disease) is already known. The model learns to associate input features (like cholesterol levels, age, or glucose levels) with known outcomes, making it suitable for risk prediction and diagnostic applications. In contrast, unsupervised learning is used on unlabeled data to discover hidden patterns or groupings, which is useful for identifying unknown disease subtypes, patient stratification, or detecting anomalies in health behavior without predefined categories. In real-world applications, AI-driven systems are now being used to predict hospital readmissions, identify patients at risk of sepsis, monitor progression of neurodegenerative diseases, and optimize medication dosages. Moreover, natural language processing (NLP), a subfield of AI, is being used to extract insights from physician notes, patient feedback, and clinical reports, further enriching predictive models with qualitative data. The power of AI and ML lies not only in their analytical speed but also in their ability to continuously learn and improve as new data becomes available. As these technologies become more integrated into healthcare delivery systems, they hold the promise of reducing diagnostic errors, lowering costs, and improving patient outcomes by transforming raw health data into actionable foresight.

10.1.3 Use of Wearables and IoT Devices

Wearable technology and Internet of Things (IoT) devices have become essential tools in modern digital health monitoring, enabling real-time tracking of vital health indicators outside of clinical settings. Devices such as smartwatches, fitness bands, biosensors, and smart rings are now widely used to collect continuous physiological data, helping both individuals and healthcare providers monitor and manage health more proactively. These devices are equipped with sensors capable of tracking a wide range of biometric parameters, including heart rate, respiratory rate, blood oxygen saturation (SpO_2), body temperature, glucose levels, and sleep quality. For instance, smartwatches can continuously monitor heart rate variability and detect irregular rhythms that may indicate arrhythmias, while wearable glucose monitors provide real-time feedback to diabetic patients on their blood sugar levels. Sleep trackers assess sleep cycles, REM stages, and disturbances, helping users optimize rest and recovery, which is vital for overall health. The key advantage of wearable and IoT devices is their ability to generate continuous, real-time health data. Unlike traditional episodic medical checkups, these tools offer round-the-clock insights into a person's physiological state. This constant data stream enables early detection of abnormalities and timely alerts for potential health issues. For example, a sudden drop in oxygen saturation or a spike in heart rate can trigger immediate notifications to both the user and healthcare providers, prompting rapid intervention and potentially preventing medical emergencies. Moreover, by aggregating and analyzing data over time, these devices can help identify long-term trends and patterns in a person's health, making them valuable for chronic disease management. Conditions such as hypertension, diabetes, and sleep apnea can be monitored more effectively through personalized digital feedback loops. Integration with smartphone apps and cloud-based platforms allows this data to be easily shared with medical professionals, supporting more informed decision-making during consultations or remote care sessions. In addition to clinical benefits, wearables also play a motivational role by promoting healthier lifestyles. Many devices offer activity tracking, goal-setting, and behavioral nudges that encourage users to stay active, hydrated, or mindful. As technology continues to advance, wearable sensors are becoming smaller, more accurate, and capable of monitoring an expanding range of health metrics, further strengthening their role in preventive healthcare.

10.1.4 Risk Stratification and Population Health Management

Risk stratification is a critical component of modern healthcare that uses digital tools to categorize patients based on their likelihood of developing certain health conditions or experiencing adverse outcomes. Through the analysis of electronic health records (EHRs), wearable device data, genetic information, and lifestyle factors, advanced algorithms can identify patients who fall into low, moderate, or high-risk categories. This process allows healthcare providers to prioritize care for those who need it most, improving both efficiency and clinical outcomes. Digital health technologies play a central role in enabling this stratification. Machine learning models can process vast volumes of patient data and uncover hidden risk factors that may not be immediately obvious through traditional clinical assessments. For example, a predictive algorithm might flag a middle-aged patient with slightly elevated blood pressure, poor sleep patterns, and a sedentary lifestyle as high risk for cardiovascular disease—even if current symptoms are minimal. Grouping patients in this way allows clinicians to design care pathways that are customized to each risk tier, ensuring that preventive measures and treatments are directed where they will be most effective.

This targeted approach enhances resource optimization, a key goal in healthcare systems worldwide. Rather than allocating equal resources across an entire population, health services can focus intensive monitoring, specialist referrals, or intervention programs on high-risk patients, while offering general wellness programs to lower-risk groups. This reduces unnecessary hospitalizations, minimizes healthcare costs, and prevents clinical burnout by aligning services with actual patient needs. Risk stratification also strengthens chronic disease management, particularly in large or aging populations. Patients with chronic conditions like diabetes, heart failure, or COPD can be continuously monitored through digital platforms, allowing for early detection of complications or declining health status. Personalized care plans, medication adjustments, and behavioral interventions can be deployed proactively, helping patients maintain stability and avoid emergency care. At a population level, these insights are invaluable for public health planning. Health systems can use aggregated, anonymized data to identify trends across regions or demographics, guiding policies and preventive campaigns. As digital tools and AI become more refined, risk stratification will become even more precise—enabling truly personalized, population-scale health management.

10.1.5 Genomics and Personalized Risk Prediction

The integration of genomic data with digital health monitoring is ushering in a new era of personalized risk prediction in medicine. By analyzing an individual's DNA alongside physiological and lifestyle data, healthcare providers can now assess inherited health risks with unprecedented accuracy. This fusion of genetics and digital health enables a more tailored approach to prevention, diagnosis, and long-term care planning. Through AI-powered gene analysis, patterns and mutations within the human genome can be identified and matched to known disease associations. For example, individuals with specific mutations in the BRCA1 or BRCA2 genes are at significantly increased risk for breast and ovarian cancers. AI algorithms can quickly detect these mutations and contextualize them with real-time health data—such as hormonal levels, menstrual history, or family history—collected via digital health platforms. This combined analysis leads to earlier risk detection, long before symptoms appear, allowing for proactive medical and lifestyle interventions.

The potential of genomics extends to a wide range of hereditary conditions, including cardiovascular diseases, certain types of diabetes, neurodegenerative disorders like Huntington's or Alzheimer's, and rare genetic syndromes. Predictive models built on large genomic datasets can identify correlations between specific genetic variants and disease predispositions. When this genomic information is integrated with wearable sensor data, electronic health records, and personal health apps, a more dynamic and accurate picture of future health risks emerges. Crucially, this integration supports the development of individualized prevention plans. A BRCA-positive individual, for instance, may be advised to undergo more frequent screenings, make specific dietary or hormonal adjustments, or consider preventive surgeries. Someone with a genetic predisposition to type 2 diabetes could receive customized nutritional guidance and exercise routines based on both their genotype and real-time metabolic readings from wearable devices. As sequencing costs decline and consumer genomics services expand, more individuals are gaining access to their genetic data. When paired with continuous digital monitoring and AI analysis, this information empowers people to take preemptive control of their health. In the long term, this approach has the potential to shift healthcare from a reactive model to a truly predictive, preventive, and personalized system, where care is uniquely shaped around each individual's genetic blueprint.

10.1.6 Behavioral and Lifestyle Monitoring

Behavioral and lifestyle monitoring is becoming an integral part of digital health, leveraging mobile apps and smart devices to help individuals manage their day-to-day habits that directly influence long-term well-being. These tools allow users to track critical aspects of health such as diet, physical activity, sleep patterns, medication adherence, hydration, and even mood. By consistently collecting behavioral data, digital platforms can identify trends that contribute to both physical and mental health outcomes. Mobile health apps now offer seamless integration with wearables, enabling automatic tracking of steps, calories burned, heart rate variability, and sleep cycles. Users can manually log meals, mood shifts, medication intake, and symptoms, while some platforms use voice, motion, or facial recognition to monitor behaviors passively. For mental health, apps often prompt self-reflection through guided journals or stress-level check-ins, helping users stay emotionally aware and engaged with their wellness goals. One of the most impactful advancements in this field is the use of AI-driven nudges and feedback loops to promote healthier behaviors. Based on collected data, these systems send personalized recommendations, reminders, or motivational messages at strategic times. For instance, if an app detects a sedentary period or poor sleep quality, it might suggest a walk, breathing exercise, or a change in evening routines. These subtle prompts create continuous engagement and habit reinforcement without overwhelming the user. Behavioral monitoring also plays a critical role in early detection of mental and behavioral health issues. AI algorithms can analyze speech tone, social withdrawal patterns, erratic sleep, or reduced physical activity as indicators of depression or anxiety. In substance use recovery, digital platforms may detect warning signs of relapse—such as missed medication, social isolation, or irregular check-ins—and alert support networks or care teams in real time. This proactive approach not only improves individual health outcomes but also enables clinicians and caregivers to intervene before conditions escalate. By recognizing deviations from healthy patterns early, digital health tools offer a powerful method for preventive mental health care and long-term lifestyle management. As these technologies become more personalized and context-aware, behavioral monitoring will continue to enhance the way we understand, manage, and sustain health in everyday life.

10.1.7 Predictive Modeling in Chronic Disease Management

Predictive modeling is transforming the management of chronic diseases such as asthma, chronic obstructive pulmonary disease (COPD), diabetes, and hypertension by enabling early identification of disease exacerbations and timely intervention. These long-term conditions often have fluctuating symptoms and unpredictable flare-ups that can lead to emergency room visits or hospital admissions if not managed proactively. By analyzing continuous health data collected through wearables, IoT devices, and electronic health records, predictive models use algorithms to forecast when a patient's condition might worsen, allowing healthcare providers to act before serious complications arise. For example, in asthma and COPD, predictive analytics can monitor changes in lung function, oxygen saturation, and environmental factors such as air quality or allergen exposure. These insights can trigger alerts that help patients adjust their medication or seek medical advice promptly. Similarly, in diabetes management, models analyze blood glucose trends, physical activity, and dietary habits to predict dangerous hypo- or hyperglycemic events. For hypertension, continuous monitoring of blood pressure combined with lifestyle data allows for early detection of elevated risks, prompting preemptive care. These real-time predictions enable timely interventions, including medication adjustments, lifestyle recommendations, or teleconsultations with healthcare providers. Patients can receive personalized alerts or coaching to modify behaviors or adhere to treatment plans, reducing the likelihood of severe exacerbations. Telemedicine platforms further support remote consultations, allowing clinicians to review patient data instantly and provide guidance without the need for an in-person visit, which is especially beneficial for individuals in rural or underserved areas. The impact of predictive modeling in chronic disease management is profound. By anticipating health deterioration, these technologies significantly reduce emergency room visits and hospital admissions, easing the burden on healthcare systems while improving patient quality of life. Early intervention not only lowers healthcare costs but also decreases the risk of complications and mortality. As data collection and AI capabilities continue to advance, predictive modeling will become even more accurate and integrated into routine chronic care, fostering a shift toward proactive, patient-centered disease management.

10.1.8 Preventive Care in Remote and Rural Areas

Preventive care in remote and rural areas faces significant challenges due to limited access to healthcare facilities, shortage of medical professionals, and infrastructural barriers. Digital health monitoring offers a promising solution to bridge these healthcare access gaps, enabling continuous health tracking and early disease detection even in underserved regions. Through mobile health technologies and IoT devices, patients can be monitored remotely, reducing the need for frequent travel to distant clinics and hospitals. One of the most effective approaches in these settings is empowering community health workers (CHWs) with mobile diagnostic tools. These workers, often the first point of contact in rural healthcare, are equipped with smartphones, portable sensors, and point-of-care testing devices that allow them to gather vital signs, screen for chronic conditions, and collect relevant health data onsite. This information is then transmitted in real-time to centralized healthcare providers or AI systems for analysis, ensuring that critical insights reach medical experts without delay. AI-driven platforms play a crucial role by providing triaging and escalation support in low-resource settings. Algorithms analyze incoming patient data to identify high-risk cases and prioritize urgent care needs. This intelligent triage system helps in managing limited medical resources efficiently by directing patients to appropriate levels of care, whether it's immediate hospital referral or community-based intervention. For instance, an AI system can flag symptoms suggestive of an impending stroke or heart attack, prompting rapid action from healthcare teams. Additionally, digital platforms facilitate teleconsultations, allowing rural patients to connect with specialists and receive guidance without leaving their communities. Preventive health education and behavior change communication can also be delivered through mobile apps, SMS, or voice calls, addressing cultural and literacy barriers. By integrating digital monitoring, mobile diagnostics, and AI-based triage, preventive care in remote and rural areas becomes more accessible, timely, and effective. This integrated approach not only improves individual health outcomes but also strengthens public health infrastructure, reduces disease burden, and advances health equity across geographic and socioeconomic divides.

10.1.9 Ethical and Privacy Concerns

As digital health monitoring and predictive analytics become increasingly integrated into healthcare, significant ethical and privacy concerns arise, demanding careful attention from developers, clinicians, policymakers, and patients alike. One of the foremost issues is data ownership: health data collected from wearables, apps, and medical records often involve sensitive personal information. Questions emerge about who owns this data—the individual, the healthcare provider, or the technology company—and how it can be used, shared, or monetized. Without clear ownership rights and transparent consent mechanisms, patients risk losing control over their own health information. Informed consent is another critical challenge, especially when complex AI algorithms are involved. Patients must fully understand what data is being collected, how it will be used, and the potential risks and benefits of predictive health models. However, the technical complexity of AI systems can make this difficult, leading to concerns about whether consent is truly informed or merely procedural. Algorithmic bias is a pressing ethical issue as well. AI and machine learning models can inadvertently perpetuate or amplify existing disparities if they are trained on biased or unrepresentative datasets. For example, predictive models that do not include diverse populations may produce inaccurate risk assessments for minority groups, leading to unequal treatment and exacerbating health inequities. Addressing this requires rigorous testing, diverse data inclusion, and ongoing monitoring for fairness. The importance of explainable AI in healthcare cannot be overstated. Clinicians and patients need to understand the rationale behind AI-driven decisions and predictions to trust and effectively use these tools. Explainability enhances transparency, accountability, and facilitates shared decision-making, which is crucial in clinical contexts where lives and well-being are at stake. Furthermore, regulatory considerations play a pivotal role in shaping the ethical use of predictive diagnostics. Governments and health authorities worldwide are working to develop guidelines and frameworks that balance innovation with patient safety, privacy protection, and data security. Regulations such as GDPR in Europe and HIPAA in the United States set standards for data handling, but rapid technological advances require continuous updates to policies. Ultimately, addressing these ethical and privacy concerns is essential to ensure that digital health technologies are developed and deployed in ways that respect patient rights, promote equity, and foster trust. Only then can the full potential of predictive and preventive health models be realized in a responsible and sustainable manner.

10.1.10 Challenges and Limitations

Despite the promising advances in digital health monitoring and predictive modeling, several challenges and limitations hinder their widespread and effective adoption. One of the primary obstacles is data quality. Health data collected from various sources such as wearables, mobile apps, and electronic health records can be inconsistent, incomplete, or noisy. Poor data quality undermines the accuracy of predictive models and can lead to unreliable or misleading health assessments. Alongside this, the lack of interoperability between different health systems, devices, and platforms creates significant barriers to seamless data integration. Fragmented data silos prevent comprehensive analysis, limiting the potential of holistic and coordinated care. Infrastructure gaps, especially in rural and low-resource settings, further complicate the deployment of digital health technologies. Reliable internet access, electricity, and technical support are essential for continuous monitoring and timely data transmission but are not universally available. These infrastructural challenges restrict the benefits of digital health to more developed regions, exacerbating existing health inequities. The digital divide remains a profound issue, as marginalized populations may lack access to smartphones, wearable devices, or the digital literacy required to engage with health technologies effectively. This divide risks widening health disparities if preventive and predictive tools primarily serve tech-savvy or wealthier individuals, leaving vulnerable groups behind. Another significant concern is the potential over-reliance on AI-driven predictions without sufficient clinical judgment. While predictive models can provide valuable insights, they should complement—not replace—the expertise of healthcare professionals. Blind trust in algorithmic outputs can lead to diagnostic errors or inappropriate treatments, particularly when models fail to account for complex patient nuances or rare conditions. Ensuring that AI serves as a decision-support tool rather than an autonomous decision-maker is critical for patient safety.

Moreover, ethical, legal, and privacy issues related to data handling and algorithm transparency add layers of complexity. Addressing these challenges requires ongoing collaboration between technologists, clinicians, policymakers, and patients to develop standards, enhance infrastructure, promote equitable access, and maintain the essential human element in healthcare delivery.

10.1.11 Future Outlook

The future of digital health monitoring is poised for remarkable growth, driven by emerging technologies and evolving healthcare paradigms. One significant trend is the integration of health monitoring systems with smart home technology. Sensors embedded in everyday home environments—such as smart mirrors, beds, and refrigerators—will seamlessly collect health data, offering continuous, non-intrusive monitoring of vital signs, activity levels, and even medication adherence. Coupled with voice assistants and IoT devices, this integration will create a connected ecosystem that supports personalized health management and early intervention without requiring active user engagement. Another exciting development is the use of augmented reality (AR) and virtual reality (VR) in remote monitoring and telemedicine. AR can provide healthcare professionals with enhanced visualization tools during remote consultations, enabling detailed examinations and guided interventions even at a distance. For patients, VR-based therapeutic programs will support rehabilitation, mental health care, and chronic disease management, making healthcare more interactive and accessible. On a broader scale, the future of digital health points toward precision public health, which combines individual-level data from wearables and genomics with population-level epidemiological and environmental information. This fusion enables more targeted and effective public health strategies by identifying at-risk communities, forecasting disease outbreaks, and optimizing resource allocation. By harnessing big data analytics, AI, and geospatial information, health systems will shift from reactive responses to proactive prevention on a population scale. The overarching vision for the future is a world where health crises—whether chronic disease exacerbations, infectious outbreaks, or mental health emergencies—are predicted and prevented before they manifest. Continuous data streams, AI-driven predictive models, and integrated care networks will empower individuals and healthcare providers alike to maintain optimal health and rapidly address emerging risks. This transformative approach promises to reduce healthcare costs, improve quality of life, and move society closer to achieving universal, equitable health outcomes.

10.2 INTEGRATION WITH GENOMICS AND DIGITAL TWINS:

10.2.1 Genomics and Digital Twins

Genomics is the study of an individual's complete set of DNA, including all of its genes, which provides critical insights into hereditary risks and disease predispositions. Digital twin technology refers to the creation of a dynamic, virtual replica of a physical entity—in healthcare, this means modeling a patient's biological and physiological characteristics in a digital environment. The synergy between genomics and digital twins lies in combining detailed genetic information with real-time physiological data to build highly personalized virtual patient models. These models simulate how diseases may develop or respond to treatments unique to each individual's genetic makeup. By integrating genomics into digital twins, healthcare providers can move beyond generalized care to deliver precision medicine tailored specifically to the patient's biology. This fusion enhances predictive accuracy, enables customized interventions, and supports continuous health monitoring. Overall, genomics and digital twin integration represent a significant step toward truly personalized healthcare.

10.2.2 Role of Genomic Data in Personalized Medicine

Genomic sequencing decodes the genetic blueprint of an individual, revealing variants linked to diseases and drug responses. This data plays a vital role in personalized medicine by informing risk prediction models that identify individuals prone to conditions like cancer, cardiovascular diseases, or rare genetic disorders. Treatment customization based on genomic information can optimize drug selection and dosing, improving efficacy and minimizing adverse effects. For example, pharmacogenomics uses gene data to determine how a patient metabolizes medications, guiding tailored prescriptions. Additionally, gene-based diagnostics enable early detection of hereditary cancers or genetic syndromes, allowing preventive measures. Therapies like gene editing and targeted biologics are developed based on specific genetic mutations, further advancing personalized care. Genomic data empowers clinicians to design precise, patient-centric treatment plans that maximize outcomes and minimize risks.

10.2.3 Digital Twins

Concept and Applications: Digital twins are sophisticated virtual models that replicate the biological and physiological states of individuals, continuously updated with real-world health data. These replicas allow healthcare professionals to simulate and analyze disease progression, predict treatment responses, and evaluate intervention strategies without risking patient safety. For example, a digital twin of a heart could simulate how different medications affect cardiac function or how lifestyle changes impact disease outcomes. Applications extend to chronic disease management, surgical planning, and rehabilitation monitoring, enabling more informed clinical decisions. By using digital twins, clinicians can anticipate complications, test therapies virtually, and personalize care protocols. This technology facilitates proactive, data-driven healthcare and supports more precise and adaptive treatment approaches.

10.2.4 Integration of Genomic Data into Digital Twins

Integrating genomic data into digital twins significantly enhances their accuracy and predictive power. Genetic information provides the foundational layer for modeling an individual's unique biological makeup, influencing how diseases develop and respond to treatment. By embedding genomic variants, mutations, and gene expression profiles into the virtual model, digital twins can simulate hereditary disease risks and anticipate patient-specific health trajectories. This integration enables more precise identification of vulnerabilities and opportunities for preventive care. For instance, a digital twin incorporating BRCA gene mutations could simulate breast cancer risk and guide personalized screening schedules. The combined model supports tailored interventions, ranging from lifestyle modifications to targeted therapies, ensuring more effective and timely healthcare delivery.

10.2.5 Predictive Modeling Using Genomic-Enhanced Digital Twins

AI-driven predictive modeling leverages genomic-enhanced digital twins to forecast individual health trajectories with high precision. These models simulate complex interactions between genetics, environment, and lifestyle, predicting the onset or progression of diseases such as cancer, diabetes, and cardiovascular conditions. For example, digital twins of cancer patients integrated with genomic data can help predict tumor growth and response to chemotherapy, enabling personalized treatment adjustments. Similarly, in chronic disease management, these simulations can identify early warning signs of exacerbations, guiding proactive interventions. By combining rich genetic data with continuous physiological monitoring, predictive models offer dynamic, real-time insights that improve patient outcomes and reduce healthcare costs. Case studies demonstrate that this approach enhances precision, early detection, and treatment personalization.

10.2.6 Challenges in Integration

Despite its potential, integrating genomics with digital twins faces significant challenges. The complexity of combining vast genomic datasets with real-time physiological data requires advanced computational power and sophisticated algorithms. Data standardization and interoperability issues complicate seamless integration across diverse platforms and devices. Privacy and security concerns are paramount, as combining sensitive genetic and health data increases risks of unauthorized access and misuse. Ethical considerations also arise, including informed consent, data ownership, and potential discrimination based on genetic information. Additionally, ensuring model transparency and explainability is critical to gain clinician and patient trust. Overcoming these challenges demands interdisciplinary collaboration, robust data governance, and continuous technological innovation.

10.2.7 Future Directions and Innovations

Future advancements in genomics and digital twins will focus on integrating multi-omics data—such as transcriptomics, proteomics, and metabolomics—with real-time digital twin models, offering a more comprehensive view of health. The development of real-time digital twins linked with continuous monitoring devices will enable adaptive, personalized healthcare that evolves with the patient's condition. Advances in AI and machine learning will improve predictive accuracy, decision support, and automated intervention recommendations. Emerging technologies like quantum computing may address computational challenges. The vision is to create fully personalized, adaptive healthcare ecosystems where genomic and physiological data seamlessly inform prevention, diagnosis, and treatment. This integration will transform medicine, shifting it towards highly predictive, preventive, and precise care.

10.3 AI-DRIVEN PERSONAL HEALTH ASSISTANTS

10.3.1 Introduction to AI Health Assistants

AI-driven personal health assistants are intelligent digital tools designed to help individuals manage various aspects of their health. These assistants may be voice-based (like Alexa or Google Assistant), app-based (such as health chatbots), or embedded in wearable devices. By using machine learning, natural language processing (NLP), and predictive analytics, they can offer personalized and timely support. These systems understand user queries, track behaviors, and adapt to changing health needs. Their role in modern healthcare is expanding as they become more interactive, intuitive, and context-aware. Ultimately, they bridge the gap between the individual and real-time health management.

10.3.2 Functions and Capabilities

AI health assistants perform a wide range of functions to support daily wellness. They monitor metrics like heart rate, sleep, activity levels, mood, and medication adherence. Based on this data, they provide tailored advice on diet, exercise, hydration, and rest. These assistants also set reminders, answer medical queries, and deliver evidence-based health education. Advanced models can analyze lab results, sensor inputs, or self-reported symptoms to offer diagnostic guidance. They serve as round-the-clock companions that promote proactive self-care and continuous engagement in health routines.

10.3.3 Integration with Wearables and Health Apps

Modern AI health assistants seamlessly integrate with wearable devices such as smartwatches and fitness bands. They collect continuous health data—like step count, sleep quality, and heart rate variability—for real-time analysis. When paired with mobile apps, they can also track nutrition, menstrual cycles, stress levels, or symptoms of chronic illnesses. This creates a comprehensive, unified health profile for each user. Such integration enhances personalization and supports more accurate feedback. It also ensures that no health-related information is siloed, allowing for more informed decision-making by users and providers alike.

10.3.4 Predictive and Preventive Features

AI assistants go beyond reactive support by using real-time data to predict health risks before symptoms arise. They can generate alerts for early signs of problems, such as abnormal heart rates, potential dehydration, or elevated blood pressure. These systems offer adaptive feedback loops that recommend behavioral adjustments—like increased hydration, rest, or stress reduction—before conditions worsen. Such features empower users to act early, reducing the likelihood of medical emergencies. Over time, these assistants learn user patterns, making their suggestions more accurate and timely.

10.3.5 Support for Chronic Disease Management

For individuals managing chronic conditions like diabetes, asthma, or hypertension, AI health assistants offer critical support. They remind users to take medications, attend check-ups, or measure vital signs like glucose or blood pressure. These tools also track long-term symptom trends, medication effects, and potential side effects. When anomalies arise, they can notify the patient, caregivers, or healthcare providers. This enables early intervention, potentially preventing exacerbations or hospitalizations. Overall, they support more consistent and personalized chronic disease care.

10.3.6 Personalized Mental Health Support

AI-driven assistants are increasingly being used for mental health support. Using conversational AI, they can detect emotional cues, stress indicators, and behavioral changes through interactions. They offer mindfulness exercises, mood tracking, guided breathing sessions, and journaling prompts to promote emotional well-being. When signs of anxiety or depression are detected, the assistant can gently encourage the user to seek professional help. Some platforms integrate with mental health services for quick access to therapists or hotlines. This offers discreet, immediate, and personalized support for mental well-being.

10.3.7 Ethical, Privacy, and Trust Issues

The rise of AI health assistants brings with it significant concerns around data privacy and ethics. These tools collect highly personal information, including biometric and behavioral data, raising questions about storage, consent, and third-party sharing. Many users don't fully understand how their data is processed or how decisions are made by the AI. This can lead to mistrust, especially if transparency and explainability are lacking. Ensuring compliance with privacy laws such as HIPAA or GDPR is essential. Building user trust requires robust safeguards, clear communication, and responsible AI governance.

10.3.8 Future of AI Health Assistants

The future of AI-driven health assistants lies in becoming smarter, more proactive, and emotionally intelligent. They will evolve from passive responders to active, conversational companions capable of anticipating user needs. Integration with genomics, real-time diagnostics, and full medical histories will make them powerful tools for truly personalized healthcare. These assistants may act as 24/7 health coaches, triage advisors, and early warning systems—especially useful in aging populations. Ultimately, they aim to deliver a seamless blend of prevention, prediction, and support tailored to each user's unique health journey.

10.4 NON-INVASIVE SENSORS AND AMBIENT MONITORING

10.4.1 Introduction to Non-Invasive Health Monitoring

Non-invasive health monitoring refers to the collection of physiological data without the need for needles, implants, or intrusive devices. This approach emphasizes comfort, safety, and user compliance, making it ideal for long-term and continuous use. Wearable sensors, smart textiles, and ambient technologies passively monitor health conditions like heart rate, temperature, and respiratory function. These tools reduce the burden on both patients and providers by enabling at-home care. The growing demand for less invasive monitoring reflects a shift toward preventive, user-friendly healthcare. As technology advances, non-invasive methods are becoming more accurate and widely accepted in clinical and personal use.

10.4.2 Types of Non-Invasive Sensors

Various non-invasive sensors are now available to track diverse health parameters. Optical sensors like photoplethysmography (PPG) measure heart rate and oxygen saturation through light-based detection. Electrodermal activity sensors track skin conductance to assess stress and emotional responses. Skin-contact biosensors monitor hydration levels, glucose, and respiratory rates without penetrating the skin. Innovative tools like sweat analysis patches and smart tattoos offer biochemical insight through surface readings. These technologies provide real-time data while remaining unobtrusive, encouraging regular use. The wide variety of sensor types allows for comprehensive and personalized health monitoring.

10.4.3 Ambient and Contactless Monitoring Technologies

Ambient monitoring technologies gather health information through the environment without direct contact with the body. Radar-based sensors and infrared cameras can detect breathing patterns, movement, and even heartbeats from a distance. Smart beds, mirrors, and bathroom fixtures can passively assess posture, activity, and sleep quality. Pressure-sensitive floors and smart furniture monitor mobility, helping detect falls or changes in routine, especially in elderly care. These systems offer silent, constant observation that supports safety and early detection. They're especially useful in post-operative recovery, dementia care, and sleep disorder management.

10.4.4 Data Collection and Real-Time Analytics

Non-invasive and ambient devices continuously stream data to cloud-based platforms, where it is processed using AI and analytics. These systems detect anomalies, compare trends, and deliver personalized insights or alerts. Real-time feedback helps users and clinicians make timely decisions, such as adjusting medication or seeking medical attention. Integration with smartphones and dashboards makes the information accessible and actionable. Predictive models can anticipate issues before symptoms arise, promoting preventive care. This real-time ecosystem supports better outcomes through early intervention and continuous oversight.

10.4.5 Applications in Home and Clinical Settings

Non-invasive monitoring is transforming both home care and clinical workflows. At home, it supports chronic disease management for conditions like heart failure, sleep apnea, and COPD. Patients recently discharged from hospitals benefit from passive monitoring, reducing readmission rates. In elderly and dementia care, ambient sensors enhance safety while allowing individuals to age in place independently. Hospitals use contactless sensors for infection control and remote triaging, reducing exposure risks. These technologies extend care beyond traditional settings, enabling a more decentralized, patient-centric model.

10.4.6 Advantages of Non-Invasive and Ambient Monitoring

Non-invasive and ambient systems offer significant advantages in comfort, convenience, and compliance. They allow continuous health tracking without disrupting daily life or causing discomfort, making them suitable for long-term use. These tools reduce the frequency of hospital visits and avoid invasive tests or procedures. Their passive nature increases user adherence, especially among the elderly and children. Additionally, they enable early detection of health issues, facilitating timely and proactive care. Their integration with digital health systems also supports better data-driven decision-making.

10.4.7 Limitations and Challenges

Despite their benefits, non-invasive and ambient technologies face several challenges. Accuracy can be inconsistent in uncontrolled environments with movement, lighting, or noise interference. Data privacy is a major concern, especially in ambient setups that monitor individuals in private spaces. Devices require regular calibration and maintenance to function optimally. Technical complexity may hinder adoption, particularly among older or less tech-savvy users. Integration with clinical systems and EHRs is still evolving, limiting full interoperability. Addressing these issues is essential for wider acceptance and effectiveness.

10.4.8 Future Trends and Innovations

The future of non-invasive monitoring lies in smarter, more integrated solutions. Smart fabrics and clothing embedded with biosensors will make health tracking part of everyday wear. AI-powered ambient systems will learn user behavior and adjust monitoring accordingly, offering personalized insights. Environmental data—such as air quality, light exposure, and noise—will be combined with physiological signals for holistic health analysis. These innovations aim to create seamless, invisible health monitoring systems. The long-term vision is predictive, preventive care embedded effortlessly into daily life.

10.5 DIGITAL BIOMARKERS AND REAL-TIME DIAGNOSTICS

10.5.1 Introduction to Digital Biomarkers

Digital biomarkers are objective, quantifiable physiological and behavioral data collected through digital devices, such as smartphones, wearables, and sensors. Unlike traditional biomarkers that require lab testing, digital biomarkers are continuously collected in real-world settings. They include metrics like gait speed, typing patterns, voice tone, heart rate variability, and sleep patterns. These indicators reflect underlying health conditions and changes over time. Digital biomarkers are gaining importance in both research and clinical practice. Their non-invasive nature and scalability make them suitable for large-scale population health monitoring. They are central to the future of personalized, real-time diagnostics (Fig. 3).

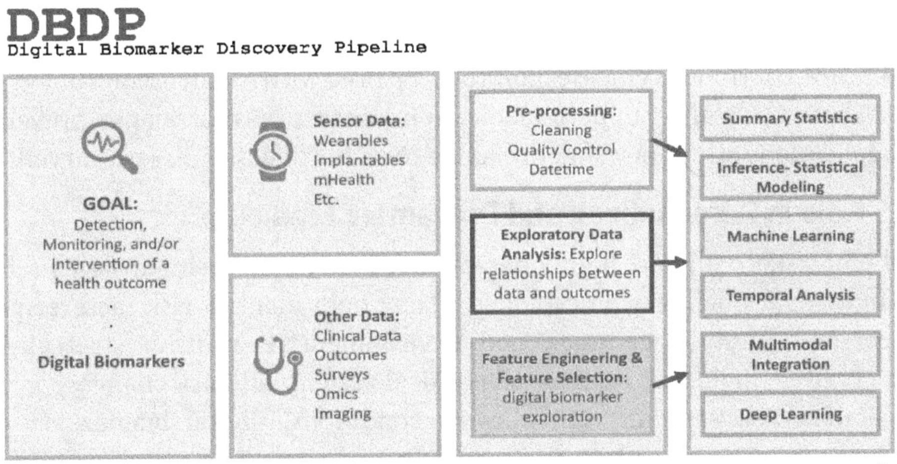

Fig.3 Digital Biomarker Discovery Pipeline

10.5.2 Types and Sources of Digital Biomarkers

Digital biomarkers are derived from various data sources, including wearable sensors, smartphone usage, smart home systems, and mobile health apps. Physiological biomarkers track heart rate, respiration, skin temperature, and movement. Behavioral biomarkers assess mood, cognition, motor function, and even social interaction patterns. Voice and speech analysis can detect neurological decline, while typing and touch patterns may signal cognitive or emotional changes. These digital signals are collected passively and continuously, allowing early detection of health deterioration. The diverse types of biomarkers enable a multidimensional view of health.

10.5.3 Real-Time Diagnostics through AI and IoT

AI and IoT technologies enable real-time analysis of digital biomarkers for early diagnosis and intervention. Continuous data collected by connected devices is processed using machine learning algorithms to detect deviations from normal patterns. This allows for immediate alerts to patients and healthcare providers when health risks emerge. For example, early signs of arrhythmia, Parkinson's, or mental health issues can be flagged based on subtle changes in biometrics. Real-time diagnostics reduce delays in care and support faster, evidence-based decisions. This shift is especially valuable for managing chronic and progressive diseases.

10.5.4 Applications in Disease Detection and Monitoring

Digital biomarkers are being used to detect and monitor conditions like Alzheimer's, depression, cardiovascular disease, and diabetes. For example, voice modulation and typing patterns may detect cognitive decline years before clinical diagnosis. Sleep disruptions and heart rate variability can signal early cardiovascular risk. In diabetes care, continuous glucose monitoring paired with AI can predict blood sugar spikes. These tools also support medication adherence and relapse prevention. Such applications offer powerful, proactive tools for ongoing disease surveillance.

10.5.5 Role in Personalized and Preventive Medicine

Digital biomarkers support highly personalized care by offering insights tailored to an individual's behavior and biology. They help identify risk factors specific to a person's lifestyle, genetics, and environment. Preventive strategies can then be crafted, including nudges for physical activity, dietary changes, or stress management. For patients with chronic conditions, digital biomarkers guide individualized treatment plans that adapt in real time. This precision approach reduces the trial-and-error nature of traditional care. Ultimately, they shift healthcare toward prevention and early intervention.

10.5.6 Regulatory and Validation Challenges

Despite their promise, digital biomarkers face challenges in validation, regulation, and clinical acceptance. Ensuring reliability and accuracy across different devices and environments is difficult. There are also concerns about standardization and reproducibility in real-world settings. Regulatory bodies like the FDA and EMA are still developing frameworks to evaluate digital biomarker tools. Ethical and privacy issues must also be addressed when handling personal and sensitive data. Without clear guidelines, clinical adoption remains slow. Robust validation and transparent governance are essential for trust and scalability.

10.5.7 Future Prospects and Innovations

The future of digital biomarkers includes greater integration with genomics, real-time diagnostics, and adaptive AI. Multi-modal biomarker systems will combine physiological, behavioral, and environmental data for holistic health insights. Innovations like smart fabrics, neuro-sensors, and digital phenotyping will deepen our understanding of disease. Digital biomarkers will also play a role in remote clinical trials and decentralized healthcare delivery. The ultimate goal is to create predictive, personalized systems that catch illness before symptoms appear. These tools will redefine health monitoring in the age of precision medicine.

10.6 ROLE OF 5G, EDGE COMPUTING, AND BLOCKCHAIN

10.6.1 Introduction to Enabling Technologies

Emerging technologies like 5G, edge computing, and blockchain are reshaping digital health ecosystems. They enable faster, safer, and smarter ways to collect, transmit, and store medical data. These technologies serve as the digital backbone for innovations such as real-time diagnostics, remote monitoring, AI-driven decision-making, and data security. As healthcare shifts toward connected, data-intensive models, traditional networks and infrastructure face challenges in scalability and speed. This trio—5G, edge computing, and blockchain—offers solutions tailored to meet these demands. Together, they support low-latency communication, localized data processing, and secure health records. Their convergence is pivotal in building a resilient and intelligent digital health infrastructure.

10.6.2 5G in Healthcare Monitoring and Diagnostics

5G networks provide ultra-high-speed and low-latency communication essential for real-time health applications. With faster data transfer rates, 5G enables remote diagnostics, live video consultations, and continuous wearable device data streaming. This is especially critical in emergency care, robotic surgery, and intensive remote monitoring. For patients in rural or underserved areas, 5G facilitates equitable access to advanced medical services. It also supports dense networks of IoT health sensors without congestion. The ability to stream high-resolution medical imaging in real time enhances decision-making speed and accuracy. In essence, 5G removes geographical and bandwidth limitations in modern healthcare.

10.6.3 Edge Computing for Real-Time Health Data Processing

Edge computing processes data close to its source—on devices or nearby servers—rather than sending everything to the cloud. This reduces latency, increases responsiveness, and improves privacy in healthcare applications. For example, wearable devices can analyze vital signs on-device to trigger alerts in seconds, even without internet connectivity. In hospitals, edge servers allow imaging systems and monitors to analyze data instantly, enhancing patient safety. It also reduces bandwidth costs and avoids cloud bottlenecks, especially when dealing with large data volumes like video or MRI scans. Edge computing supports real-time decision-making, crucial for critical care and emergency settings.

10.6.4 Blockchain for Data Security and Interoperability

Blockchain offers a decentralized and immutable ledger system to secure and manage healthcare data transparently. It ensures that patient records cannot be tampered with and allows patients to control who accesses their data. This is vital in a healthcare ecosystem where data is shared among hospitals, labs, insurers, and patients. Blockchain can also facilitate interoperability by creating standardized, trusted pathways for exchanging medical information. Smart contracts within blockchain systems can automate consent management and data-sharing rules. By reducing fraud, increasing transparency, and empowering patient ownership, blockchain enhances trust in digital health platforms.

10.6.5 Synergy of 5G, Edge, and Blockchain in Smart Health Systems

The real potential lies in integrating 5G, edge computing, and blockchain into unified health systems. A wearable device could use 5G to send vital data instantly, process it locally using edge computing, and log it securely using blockchain. In smart hospitals, this trio supports autonomous systems like AI-based diagnostics, robotic assistants, and predictive alerts. Together, they create a secure, scalable, and responsive ecosystem ideal for telemedicine, remote surgery, and chronic disease management. This synergy ensures seamless data flow, real-time analysis, and tamper-proof storage—all with minimal latency. It's a foundation for a new era of connected, intelligent healthcare (Table-1).

Table- 1: Role of 5G, Edge Computing, and Blockchain in Digital Health

Technology	Key Role in Digital Health	Applications	Benefits
5G	High-speed, low-latency communication for real-time data transmission	Remote monitoring, telemedicine, robotic surgery, real-time imaging	Faster diagnostics, improved access in remote areas, seamless data streaming
Edge Computing	Local data processing near the source (on-device or local server)	On-device AI alerts, ICU monitors, wearable health analytics	Reduced latency, improved data privacy, decreased cloud dependency
Blockchain	Secure, transparent, decentralized health data storage and sharing	Medical record management, consent tracking, clinical trials, interoperability platforms	Enhanced data security, patient ownership, tamper-proof records, automated trust mechanisms

REFERENCES

Abubakar, I. et al. The Lancet Nigeria Commission: investing in health and the future of the nation. Lancet 399, 1155–1200 (2022).

Adedinsewo, D. A. et al. Artificial intelligence guided screening for cardiomyopathies in an obstetric population: a pragmatic randomized clinical trial. Nat. Med. 30, 2897–2906 (2024).

Akar, J. G. et al. Use of remote monitoring of newly implanted cardioverter-defibrillators: insights from the patient related determinants of ICD remote monitoring (PREDICT RM) study. Circulation 128, 2372–2383 (2013).

Albarqouni L, Hoffmann T, Straus S, et al. Core competencies in evidence-based practice for health professionals: consensus statement based on a systematic review and Delphi survey. JAMA Netw Open. 2018;1(2):e180281-e180281. Lazarus JV, Romero D, Kopka CJ, et al; COVID-19 Consensus Statement Panel. A multinational Delphi consensus to end the COVID-19 public health threat. Nature. 2022;611(7935):332-345.

Appraising scientific evidence: qualitative versus quantitative research. The Association of Faculties of Medicine of Canada; undated (http://phprimer.afmc.ca/Part2-MethodsStudyingHealth/Chapter5AssessingEvidenceAndInformation/Appraisingscientificevidencequalitativeversusquantitativeresearch, accessed 6 May 2016).

Arhin, K., Oteng-Abayie, E. F. & Novignon, J. Assessing the efficiency of health systems in achieving the universal health coverage goal: evidence from Sub-Saharan Africa. Health Econ. Rev. 13, 25 (2023).

Arias López MDP, Ong BA, Borrat Frigola X, et al. Digital literacy as a new determinant of health: a scoping review. PLOS Digit Health. 2023;2(10):e0000279.

Arias López, M. D. P. et al. Digital literacy as a new determinant of health: a scoping review. PLOS Digit. Health 2, e0000279 (2023).

Armoundas, A. A. et al. Controversy in hypertension: pro-side of the argument using AI for hypertension diagnosis and management. Hypertension 82, 929–944 (2025).

Armoundas, A. A. et al. Data interoperability for ambulatory monitoring of cardiovascular disease: a scientific statement from the American Heart Association. Circ. Genom. Precis. Med. 17, e000095 (2024).

Armoundas, A. A. et al. Use of artificial intelligence in improving outcomes in heart disease: a scientific statement from the American Heart Association. Circulation 149, e1028–e1050 (2024).

Australian Medical Council Limited. Review of accreditation standards for primary medical programs (medical school standards review). July 2023. Accessed November 20, 2024.

Ayres EJ, Greer-Carney JL, Fatzinger McShane PE, Miller A, Turner P. Nutrition informatics competencies across all levels of practice: a national Delphi study. J Acad Nutr Diet. 2012;112(12):2042-2053.

Baumgartner M, Sauer C, Blagec K, Dorffner G. Digital health understanding and preparedness of medical students: a cross-sectional study. Med Educ Online. 2022;27(1):2114851.

Bazoukis, G. et al. Impact of social determinants of health on cardiovascular disease. J. Am. Heart Assoc. 14, e039031 (2025).

Bazoukis, G. et al. The inclusion of augmented intelligence in medicine: a framework for successful implementation. Cell Rep. Med. 3, 100485 (2022).

Begazo, T., Dutz, M. A. & Blimpo, M. Digital Africa: Technological Transformation for Jobs (World Bank, 2023).

Bertalan Mesko. The promise of the metaverse in cardio- vascular health. European Heart Journal, 2022; ehac231.

Bertalan Mesko. The promise of the metaverse in cardiovascular health, European Heart Journal, 2022; ehac231. https://doi.org/10.1093/eurheartj/ehac231

Bichel-Findlay J, Koch S, Mantas J, et al. Recommendations of the International Medical Informatics Association (IMIA) on education in biomedical and health informatics: second revision. Int J Med Inform. 2023;170:104908.

Blood, A. J. et al. Results of a remotely delivered hypertension and lipid program in more than 10000 patients across a diverse health care network. JAMA Cardiol. 8, 12–21 (2023).

Borges do Nascimento IJ, Abdulazeem H, Vasanthan LT, et al. Barriers and facilitators to utilizing digital health technologies by healthcare professionals. NPJ Digit Med. 2023;6(1):161.

Boriani, G. et al. Current status of reimbursement practices for remote monitoring of cardiac implantable electrical devices across Europe. Europace 24, 1875–1880 (2022).

Boriani, G. et al. Reimbursement practices for use of digital devices in atrial fibrillation and other arrhythmias: a European Heart Rhythm Association survey. Europace 24, 1834–1843 (2022).

Bradford, A. The false choice between digital regulation and innovation. Northwest. Univ. Law Rev. 119, 377–453 (2024).

Brant, L. C. C. et al. Epidemiology of cardiometabolic health in Latin America and strategies to address disparities. Nat. Rev. Cardiol. 21, 849–864 (2024).

Brockes C, Grischott T, Dutkiewicz M, Schmidt-Weitmann S. Evaluation of the education "Clinical Telemedicine/e-Health" in the curriculum of medical students at the University of Zurich. Telemed J E Health. 2017;23(11):899-904.

Bryson JM, Patton MQ, Bowman RA. Working with evaluation stakeholders: a rationale, step-wise approach and toolkit. Eval Program Plann. 2011;34(1):1–12. doi:10.1016/j.evalprogplan.2010.07.001.

Building our understanding: key concepts of evaluation – what is it and how do you do it? Atlanta (GA): United States Centers for Disease Control and Prevention, Health Communities Program; undated.

Çalışkan SA, Demir K, Karaca O. Artificial intelligence in medical education curriculum: an e-Delphi study for competencies. PLoS One. 2022;17(7):e0271872.

Carroll C, Patterson M, Wood S, Booth A, Rick J, Balain S. A conceptual framework for implementation fidelity. Implementation Science. 2007;2:40.

Chen Yan, Lin Wei, Chen Gang. On Application of Metaverse in Medical Education via Platform of Medical Electronic Journals: A Case Study of Journal of Trauma and Emergency Electronic Version, 2022. SSRN: https:// ssrn.com/ abstract=4052566 or http://dx.doi.org/10.2139/ ssrn.4052566

Chidambaram, S. et al. An introduction to digital determinants of health. PLOS Digit. Health 3, e0000346 (2024).

Chowdhury, S. R., Sunna, T. C. & Ahmed, S. Telemedicine is an important aspect of healthcare services amid COVID-19 outbreak: its barriers in Bangladesh and strategies to overcome. Int. J. Health Plann. Manag. 36, 4–12 (2021).

Churchwell, K. et al. Call to action: structural racism as a fundamental driver of health disparities: a presidential advisory from the American Heart Association. Circulation 142, e454–e468 (2020).

Cohen, M. G. et al. Racial and ethnic differences in the treatment of acute myocardial infarction: findings from the Get With The Guidelines–Coronary Artery Disease Program. Circulation 121, 2294–2301 (2010).

Crafting your value proposition. In: MaRS [website]. Toronto: MaRS Discovery District; 2012 (https://www.marsdd.com/ mars-library/crafting-your-value-proposition/, accessed 21 March 2016).

Crenshaw, K. Demarginalizing the intersection of race and sex: a black feminist critique of anti-discrimination doctrine, feminist theory and anti-racist politics. Univ. Chic. Leg. Forum 140, 139 (1989).

Creswell JW. Research design: qualitative, quantitative and mixed methods approaches, second edition. SAGE Publications; 2003.

Curioso, W. H. Building capacity and training for digital health: challenges and opportunities in Latin America. J. Med. Internet Res. 21, e16513 (2019).

Damschroder, L. J. et al. Fostering implementation of health services research findings into practice: a consolidated framework for advancing implementation science. Implement. Sci. 4, 50 (2009).

Dattakumar A, Gray K, Henderson KB, Maeder A, Chenery H. We are not educating the future clinical health professional workforce adequately for e-health competence: findings of an Australian study. Stud Health Technol Inform. 2012;178:33-38.

DeFilippis, E. M. et al. Improving enrollment of underrepresented racial and ethnic populations in heart failure trials: a call to action from the Heart Failure Collaboratory. JAMA Cardiol. 7, 540–548 (2022).

Deguchi, N. et al. Sex-specific factors associated with acceptance of smartwatches among urban older adults: the Itabashi Longitudinal Study on Aging. Front. Public. Health 12, 1261275 (2024).

Dove, E. S. The EU General Data Protection Regulation: implications for international scientific research in the digital era. J. Law. Med. Ethics 46, 1013–1030 (2018).

Edirippulige S, Gong S, Hathurusinghe M, et al. Medical students' perceptions and expectations regarding digital health education and training: a qualitative study. J Telemed Telecare. 2022;28(4):258-265.

Egbert N, Thye J, Hackl WO, Müller-Staub M, Ammenwerth E, Hübner U. Competencies for nursing in a digital world. Methodology, results, and use of the DACH-recommendations for nursing informatics core competency areas in Austria, Germany, and Switzerland. Inform Health Soc Care. 2019;44(4):351-375.

Egbert N, Thye J, Schulte G, et al. An iterative methodology for developing national recommendations for nursing informatics curricula. Stud Health Technol Inform. 2016;228:660-664.

Englander R, Cameron T, Ballard AJ, Dodge J, Bull J, Aschenbrener CA. Toward a common taxonomy of competency domains for the health professions and competencies for physicians. Acad Med. 2013;88(8):1088-1094.

Eslava-Schmalbach, J. et al. Conceptual framework of equity-focused implementation research for health programs (EquIR). Int. J. Equity Health 18, 80 (2019).

Essien, U. R. et al. Association of race and ethnicity with oral anticoagulation and associated outcomes in patients with atrial fibrillation: findings from the Get With The Guidelines–Atrial Fibrillation Registry. JAMA Cardiol. 7, 1207–1217 (2022).

Fitch K, Bernstein SJ, Aguilar MD, et al. The RAND/UCLA appropriateness method user's manual. Published 2001. Accessed November 20, 2024.

Forman, R. et al. Technical dissonance in home blood pressure monitoring after stroke: having the machine, but not using correctly. Am. J. Hypertens. 36, 195–200 (2023).

Friedman, S. & Mottiar, S. A rewarding engagement? The Treatment Action Campaign and the politics of HIV/AIDS. Polit. Soc. 33, 511–565 (2005).

Functional suitability. In: ISO 25000 software product quality [website]. ISO 25000; 2015 (http://iso25000.com/index. php/en/iso-25000-standards/iso-25010/58-functional-suitability, accessed 9 May 2016).

Gawałko, M. et al. Changes in healthcare utilisation during implementation of remote atrial fibrillation management: TeleCheck-AF project. Neth. Heart J. 32, 130–139 (2024).

General Medical Council. Outcomes for graduates 2018. Accessed November 20, 2024.

Gill P, Stewart K, Treasure E, Chadwick B. Methods of data collection in qualitative research: interviews and focus groups. Br Dent J. 2008;204(6):291–5.

Gilmore, A. B. et al. Defining and conceptualising the commercial determinants of health. Lancet 401, 1194–1213 (2023).

Goergen, J. A. et al. Comparison of data quality and monitoring completion rates between clinic and self-applied ECG patches. Heart Rhythm. 20, 407–413 (2023).

Goldsack, Jennifer C., Andrea Coravos, Jessie P. Bakker, Brinnae Bent, Ariel V. Dowling, Cheryl FitzerAttas, Alan Godfrey, et al. "Verification, Analytical Validation, and Clinical Validation (V3): The Foundation of Determining Fit-for-Purpose for Biometric Monitoring Technologies (BioMeTs)." Npj Digital Medicine 3,

Gomez, S. E. et al. Racial, ethnic, and sex disparities in atrial fibrillation management: rate and rhythm control. J. Interv. Card. Electrophysiol. 66, 1279–1290 (2022).

Gonzalo JD, Dekhtyar M, Starr SR, et al. Health systems science curricula in undergraduate medical education: identifying and defining a potential curricular framework. Acad Med. 2017;92(1):123-131.

Greene, J. A. & Lea, A. S. Digital futures past – the long arc of big data in medicine. N. Engl. J. Med. 381, 480–485 (2019).

Grimes DA, Schulz KF. Descriptive studies: what they can and cannot do. Lancet. 2002;359(9301):145-9.

Groom, L. L., Schoenthaler, A. M., Mann, D. M. & Brody, A. A. Construction of the digital health equity-focused implementation research conceptual model – bridging the divide between equity-focused digital health and implementation research. PLOS Digit. Health 3, e0000509 (2024).

Group MSOW. Learning objectives for medical student education–guidelines for medical schools: report I of the medical school objectives project. Acad Med. 1999;74(1):13-18.

Haarmann, L. et al. Comprehensive systematic review and meta-analysis on physical health conditions in lesbian- and bisexual-identified women compared with heterosexual-identified women. Women's Health 19, 17455057231219610 (2023).

Hagan D, Uggowitzer S. Information and communication technologies for women's and children's health: a planning workbook for multi-stakeholder action. Geneva: The Partnership for Maternal, Newborn & Child Health (PMNCH); 2014. (http://www.who.int/pmnch/knowledge/publications/ict_mhealth.pdf, accessed 2 September 2015).

Harden RM, Laidlaw JM. Essential skills for a medical teacher: an introduction to teaching and learning in medicine. Elsevier Health Sciences; 2020.

Hautz SC, Hoffmann M, Exadaktylos AK, Hautz WE, Sauter TC. Digital competencies in medical education in Switzerland: an overview of the current situation. GMS J Med Educ. 2020;37(6):Doc62.

Health in Africa. Nat Commun 15, 967 (2024).

Health Information Technology Competencies. 2020. Accessed December 11, 2023.

Heckbert, S. R. et al. Differences by race/ethnicity in the prevalence of clinically detected and monitor-detected atrial fibrillation: MESA. Circ. Arrhythm. Electrophysiol. 13, e007698 (2020).

Hilty DM, Crawford A, Teshima J, et al. A framework for telepsychiatric training and e-health: competency-based education, evaluation and implications. Int Rev Psychiatry. 2015;27(6):569-592.

Holmes, D. R. Jr., Mack, M. J., Alkhouli, M. & Vemulapalli, S. Racial disparities and democratization of health care: a focus on TAVR in the United States. Am. Heart J. 224, 166–170 (2020).

Honeyman M, Maguire D, Evans H, Davies A. Digital technology and health inequalities: a scoping review (Wales). Health Inequalities. Published 2020. Accessed November 20, 2024.

Horne, M., Tierney, S., Henderson, S., Wearden, A. & Skelton, D. A. A systematic review of interventions to increase physical activity among South Asian adults. Public. Health 162, 71–81 (2018).

Hübner U, Thye J, Shaw T, et al. Towards the TIGER international framework for recommendations of core competencies in health informatics 2.0: extending the scope and the roles. Stud Health Technol Inform. 2019;264:1218-1222.

Husain, L., Greenhalgh, T., Hughes, G., Finlay, T. & Wherton, J. Desperately seeking intersectionality in digital health disparity research: narrative review to inform a richer theorization of multiple disadvantage. J. Med. Internet Res. 24, e42358 (2022).

IMI Association. Recommendations of the International Medical Informatics Association (IMIA) on education in health and medical informatics. Methods Inf Med. 2000;39(3):267-277.

Israel BA, Schulz AJ, Parker EA, Becker AB, Allen AJ, III, Guzman RJ. Community-based participatory research for health: from processes to outcomes (Chapter 3). In: Minkler M, Wallerstein N, editors. Critical issues in developing and following CBPR principles, second edition. Wiley; 2010.

Javdan, M., Ghasemaghaei, M. & Abouzahra, M. Psychological barriers of using wearable devices by seniors: a mixed-methods study. Comput. Hum. Behav. 141, 107615 (2023).

Jidkov L, Alexander M, Bark P, et al. Health informatics competencies in postgraduate medical education and training in the UK: a mixed methods study. BMJ Open. 2019;9(3):e025460.

Johns Hopkins Medical. The Metaverse, 2015.

Jünger S, Payne SA, Brine J, Radbruch L, Brearley SG. Guidance on conducting and reporting Delphi studies (CREDES) in palliative care: recommendations based on a methodological systematic review. Palliat Med. 2017;31(8):684-706.

Karabekmez, M. E. Data ethics in digital health and genomics. N. Bioeth. 27, 320–333 (2021).

Kaufman DM, Jennett PA. Preparing our future physicians: integrating medical informatics into the undergraduate medical education curriculum. Stud Health Technol Inform. 1997;39:543-546.

Keesara, S., Jonas, A. & Schulman, K. Covid-19 and health care's digital revolution. N. Engl. J. Med. 382, e82 (2020).

Kessel, R. V. et al. Digital health reimbursement strategies of 8 European countries and Israel: scoping review and policy mapping. JMIR Mhealth Uhealth 11, e49003 (2023).

Khurana MP, Raaschou-Pedersen DE, Kurtzhals J, Bardram JE, Ostrowski SR, Bundgaard JS. Digital health competencies in medical school education: a scoping review and Delphi method study. BMC Med Educ. 2022;22(1):129.

Kickbusch, I. et al. The Lancet and Financial Times commission on governing health futures 2030: growing up in a digital world. Lancet 398, 1727–1776 (2021).

Kim K, Shin S, Kim S, Lee E. The relation between eHealth literacy and health-related behaviors: systematic review and meta-analysis. J Med Internet Res. 2023;25:e40778.

Krijthe, B. P. et al. Projections on the number of individuals with atrial fibrillation in the European Union, from 2000 to 2060. Eur. Heart J. 34, 2746–2751 (2013).

Krittanawong, C. et al. Integration of novel monitoring devices with machine learning technology for scalable cardiovascular management. Nat. Rev. Cardiol. 18, 75–91 (2021).

Kuek A, Hakkennes S. Healthcare staff digital literacy levels and their attitudes towards information systems. Health Informatics J. 2020;26(1):592-612.

Kuhn S, Jungmann F. Medicine in the digital age: Telemedicine in medical school education. Article in German. Radiologe. 2018;58(3):236-240.

Kulkarni, K. et al. Ambulatory monitoring promises equitable personalized healthcare delivery in underrepresented patients. Eur. Heart J. Digit. Health 2, 494–510 (2021).

Kumar, A. A. et al. Mobile health for tuberculosis management in South India: is video-based directly observed treatment an acceptable alternative? JMIR Mhealth Uhealth 7, e11687 (2019).

Kyaw, M. Y. et al. Sociodigital determinants of eHealth literacy and related impact on health outcomes and eHealth use in Korean older adults: community-based cross-sectional survey. JMIR Aging 7, e56061 (2024).

Lance P, Guilkey D, Hattori A, Angeles G. How do we know if a program made a difference? A guide to statistical methods for program impact evaluation.

Chapel Hill (NC): MEASURE Evaluation; 2014 (http://www.cpc.unc.edu/measure/resources/publications/ms-14-87-en, accessed 2 May 2016).

Lee SA, Bates OB, Cecilie Perez E, Swift CP, Stanistreet D. Integrating planetary health into the medical curriculum. Centre for Global Education. Published 2022. Accessed November 20, 2024.

Liu Z, Ren L, Xiao C, Zhang K, Demian P. Virtual Reality Aided Therapy towards Health 4.0: A Two-Decade Bibliometric Analysis. Int J Environ Res Public Health, 2022; 19(3): 1525. doi: 10.3390/ijerph19031525. PMID: 35162546; PMCID: PMC8834834.

Lubitz, S. A. et al. Detection of atrial fibrillation in a large population using wearable devices: the Fitbit Heart Study. Circulation 146, 1415–1424 (2022).

Lyles, C. R., Wachter, R. M. & Sarkar, U. Focusing on digital health equity. JAMA 326, 1795–1796 (2021).

Ma M, Li Y, Gao L, et al. The need for digital health education among next-generation health workers in China: a cross-sectional survey on digital health education. BMC Med Educ. 2023;23(1):541.

Ma, X. Internet use and income gaps between rural and urban residents in China. J. Asia Pac. Econ. 29, 789–809 (2024).

MacDorman, M. F., Thoma, M., Declcerq, E. & Howell, E. A. Racial and ethnic disparities in maternal mortality in the United States using enhanced vital records, 2016–2017. Am. J. Public. Health 111, 1673–1681 (2021).

Machleid F, Kaczmarczyk R, Johann D, et al. Perceptions of digital health education among European medical students: mixed methods survey. J Med Internet Res. 2020;22(8):e19827.

Mack N, Woodsong C, MacQueen KM, Guest G, Namey E. Qualitative research methods: a data collector's field guide. Research Triangle Park (NC): Family Health International; 2005 (https://www.fhi360.org/resource/qualitative-researchmethods-data-collectors-field-guide, accessed 6 May 2016).

MacLure K, Stewart D. A qualitative case study of ehealth and digital literacy experiences of pharmacy staff. Res Social Adm Pharm. 2018;14(6):555-563.

Manninger, M. et al. Current perspectives on wearable rhythm recordings for clinical decision-making: the wEHRAbles 2 survey. Europace 23, 1106–1113 (2021).

Mantas J, Ammenwerth E, Demiris G, et al; IMIA Recommendations on Education Task Force. Recommendations of the International Medical Informatics Association (IMIA) on education in biomedical and health informatics. first revision. Methods Inf Med. 2010;49(2):105-120.

Masterson Creber, R. et al. Telehealth and health equity in older adults with heart failure: a scientific statement from the American Heart Association. Circ. Cardiovasc. Qual. Outcomes 16, e000123 (2023).

Mbunge, E., Muchemwa, B. & Batani, J. Are we there yet? Unbundling the potential adoption and integration of telemedicine to improve virtual healthcare services in African health systems. Sens. Int. 3, 100152 (2022).

McGowan JJ, Passiment M, Hoffman HM. Educating medical students as competent users of health information technologies: the MSOP data. Stud Health Technol Inform. 2007;129(Pt 2):1414-1418.

Meadows KA. So you want to do research? 3. An introduction to qualitative methods. Br J Community Nurs. 2003;8(10):464–9.

MedBiquitous. Curriculum inventory standardized instructional and assessment methods and resource types. Published March 2016. Accessed November 20, 2024.

Mercier, M. R. et al. Differential utilization patterns of total ankle arthroplasty vs arthrodesis: a United States national ambulatory database analysis. Foot Ankle Orthop. 8, 24730114231218011 (2023).

Modesti, P. A. et al. Cardiovascular risk assessment in low-resource settings: a consensus document of the European Society of Hypertension Working Group on Hypertension and Cardiovascular Risk in Low Resource Settings. J. Hypertens. 32, 951–960 (2014).

Monaghesh E, Hajizadeh A. The role of telehealth during COVID-19 outbreak: a systematic review based on current evidence. BMC Public Health. 2020;20(1):1193.

Monitoring and evaluation frameworks (3 parts). In: Virtual Knowledge Centre to End Violence against Women and Girls [website]. UN Women; 2012 (http://www.endvawnow.org/en/articles/335-monitoring-and-evaluation-frameworks-3- parts.html, accessed 3 May 2016).

Monitoring and evaluation: some tools, methods, and approaches. Washington (DC): The International Bank for Reconstruction and Development/The World Bank; 2004.

Moorhead, J. B. et al. Internet access and cardiovascular death in the United States. Am. Heart J. 21, 100200 (2022).

Narayan, S. M., Kohli, N. & Martin, M. M. Addressing contemporary threats in anonymised healthcare data using privacy engineering. NPJ Digit. Med. 8, 145 (2025).

National Health Service. Preparing the healthcare workforce to deliver the digital future: an independent report on behalf of the Secretary of State for Health and Social Care. The Topol Review. February 2019. Accessed November 20, 2024.

Nazeha N, Pavagadhi D, Kyaw BM, Car J, Jimenez G, Tudor Car L. A digitally competent health workforce: scoping review of educational frameworks. J Med Internet Res. 2020;22(11):e22706.

Ngiam, N. H. W. et al. Building digital literacy in older adults of low socioeconomic status in Singapore (Project Wire Up): nonrandomized controlled trial. J. Med. Internet Res. 24, e40341 (2022).

Nissenbaum, H. A contextual approach to privacy online. Daedalus 4, 32–48 (2011).

Nutbeam D, Lloyd JE. Understanding and responding to health literacy as a social determinant of health. Annu Rev Public Health. 2021;42(1):159-173.

Obermeyer, Z., Powers, B., Vogeli, C. & Mullainathan, S. Dissecting racial bias in an algorithm used to manage the health of populations. Science 366, 447–453 (2019).

Ochi, A., Saidi, Y. & Labidi, M. A. Nonlinear threshold effect of governance quality on poverty reduction in South Asia and Sub-Saharan Africa: a dynamic panel threshold specification. J. Knowl. Econ. 15, 4239–4264 (2024).

Odipo, E. et al. The path to universal health coverage in five African and Asian countries: examining the association between insurance status and health-care use. Lancet Glob. Health 12, e123–e133 (2024).

Oliver CW, (ed); Academy of Medical Royal Colleges. eHealth competency framework: defining the role of the expert clinician. The University Edinburgh. Published 2011. Accessed December 11, 2023.

Olu, O. et al. How can digital health technologies contribute to sustainable attainment of universal health coverage in Africa? A perspective. Front. Public. Health 7, 341 (2019).

Otto A, Kushniruk A. Incorporation of medical informatics and information technology as core components of undergraduate medical education—time for change! Stud Health Technol Inform. 2009;143:62-67.

Palacholla, R. S. et al. Provider- and patient-related barriers to and facilitators of digital health technology adoption for hypertension management: scoping review. JMIR Cardio 3, e11951 (2019).

Pearson, T. A. et al. The science of precision prevention: research opportunities and clinical applications to reduce cardiovascular health disparities. JACC Adv. 3, 100759 (2024).

Pelikan JM, Ganahl K, Roethlin F. Health literacy as a determinant, mediator and/ or moderator of health: empirical models using the European Health Literacy Survey dataset. Glob Health Promot. Published online November 14, 2018.

Perez, M. V. et al. Large-scale assessment of a smartwatch to identify atrial fibrillation. N. Engl. J. Med. 381, 1909–1917 (2019).

Performance monitoring and evaluation TIPS: building a results framework. Washington (DC): United States Agency for International Development (USAID); 2010 (https://www.ndi.org/files/Performance%20Monitoring%20 and%20 Evaluation%20Tips%20Building%20a%20Results%20Framework.pdf, accessed 6 May 2016).

Perret, S. et al. Standardising the role of a digital navigator in behavioural health: a systematic review. Lancet Digit. Health 5, e925–e932 (2023).

Peter, J., Benjamin, P., LeFevre, A. E., Barron, P. & Pillay, Y. Taking digital health innovation to scale in South Africa: ten lessons from MomConnect. BMJ Glob. Health 3, e000592 (2018).

Peters D, Tran N, Adam T. Implementation research in health: a practical guide. Geneva: Alliance for Health Policy and Systems Research, World Health Organization; 2013.

Peters DH, Adam T, Alonge O, Agyepong IA, Tran N. Implementation research: what it is and how to do it. BMJ. 2013;347:f6753. doi:10.1136/bmj.f6753.

Peterson, E. & Yancy, C. W. Eliminating racial and ethnic disparities in cardiac care. N. Engl. J. Med. 360, 1172–1174 (2009).

Petretto, D. R. et al. Digital determinants of health as a way to address multilevel complex causal model in the promotion of digital health equity and the prevention of digital health inequities: a scoping review. J. Public. Health Res. 13, 22799036231220352 (2024).

Philips. Future health index 2019. Accessed November 20, 2024.

Poncette AS, Glauert DL, Mosch L, Braune K, Balzer F, Back DA. Undergraduate medical competencies in digital health and curricular module development: mixed methods study. J Med Internet Res. 2020;22(10):e22161.

Powell-Wiley, T. M. et al. Role of technology in promoting heart healthy behavior change to increase equity in optimal cardiovascular health: a scientific statement from the American Heart Association. Circulation 151, e972–e985 (2025).

Probability sampling. In: Research methods knowledge base [website]. William M.K. Trochim; 2006 (http://www.socialresearchmethods.net/kb/sampprob.php, accessed 6 May 2016).

Qualitative research: getting started [website]. Durham (NC): Duke University Libraries; 2015 (http://guides.library. duke.edu/qualitative-research, accessed 6 May 2016).

Qualitative versus quantitative research. Xavier University Library; 2012 (http://www.xavier.edu/library/students/ documents/qualitative_quantitative.pdf, accessed 6 May 2016).

Quaosar, G., Hoque, M. R. & Bao, Y. Investigating factors affecting elderly's intention to use m-health services: an empirical study. Telemed. J. E Health 24, 309–314 (2018).

Ramachandran, N. et al. Mobile phone usage and willingness to receive health-related information among patients attending a chronic disease clinic in rural Puducherry, India. J. Diabetes Sci. Technol. 9, 1350–1351 (2015).

Reeves JJ, Hollandsworth HM, Torriani FJ, et al. Rapid response to COVID-19: health informatics support for outbreak management in an academic health system. J Am Med Inform Assoc. 2020;27(6):853-859.

Reeves CA, Bednar DA. Defining quality: alternatives and implications. Acad Manag Rev. 1994;19(3):419–45 (http://www.jstor.org/stable/258934, accessed 11 April 2016).

Richardson S, Lawrence K, Schoenthaler AM, Mann D. A framework for digital health equity. NPJ Digit Med. 2022;5(1):119.

Richardson, S., Lawrence, K., Schoenthaler, A. M. & Mann, D. A framework for digital health equity. NPJ Digit. Med. 5, 119 (2022).

Rodriguez, J. A. et al. Digital healthcare equity in primary care: implementing an integrated digital health navigator. J. Am. Med. Inf. Assoc. 30, 965–970 (2023).

Rodriguez, J. A., Clark, C. R. & Bates, D. W. Digital health equity as a necessity in the 21st century Cures Act era. JAMA 323, 2381–2382 (2020).

Rodriguez, J. A., Shachar, C. & Bates, D. W. Digital inclusion as health care – supporting health care equity with digital-infrastructure initiatives. N. Engl. J. Med. 386, 1101–1103 (2022).

Rodriguez-Villa, E. & Torous, J. Regulating digital health technologies with transparency: the case for dynamic and multi-stakeholder evaluation. BMC Med. 17, 226 (2019).

Rychetnik L, Frommer M, Hawe P, Shiell A. Criteria for evaluating evidence on public health interventions. J Epidemiol Community Health. 2002;56(2):119–27.

Santana, G. O. et al. Economic evaluations and equity in the use of artificial intelligence in imaging exams for medical diagnosis in people with skin, neurological, and pulmonary diseases: protocol for a systematic review. JMIR Res. Protoc. 12, e48544 (2023).

Sarkar, U. et al. Usability of commercially available mobile applications for diverse patients. J. Gen. Intern. Med. 31, 1417–1426 (2016).

Schreiweis, B. et al. Barriers and facilitators to the implementation of eHealth services: systematic literature analysis. J. Med. Internet Res. 21, e14197 (2019).

Shachar, C., Cadario, R., Cohen, I. G. & Morewedge, C. K. HIPAA is a misunderstood and inadequate tool for protecting medical data. Nat. Med. 29, 1900–1902 (2023).

Shah, N. S. et al. Social determinants of cardiovascular health in Asian Americans: a scientific statement from the American Heart Association. Circulation 150, e296–e315 (2024).

Shaver J. The state of telehealth before and after the COVID-19 pandemic. Prim Care. 2022;49(4):517-530.

Shen, Y. C., Sarkar, N. & Hsia, R. Y. Differential treatment and outcomes for patients with heart attacks in advantaged and disadvantaged communities. J. Am. Heart Assoc. 12, e030506 (2023).

Sieck CJ, Sheon A, Ancker JS, Castek J, Callahan B, Siefer A. Digital inclusion as a social determinant of health. NPJ Digit Med. 2021;4(1):52.

Sieck, C. J. et al. Digital inclusion as a social determinant of health. NPJ Digit. Med. 4, 52 (2021).

Sim, I. Mobile devices and health. N. Engl. J. Med. 381, 956–968 (2019).

Simovic, S. et al. The use of remote monitoring of cardiac implantable devices during the COVID-19 pandemic: an EHRA physician survey. Europace 24, 473–480 (2022).

Smith B, Magnani JW. New technologies, new disparities: The intersection of electronic health and digital health literacy. Int J Cardiol. 2019;292:280-282.

Smith L, Rosenzweig L, Schmidt M. Best practices in the reporting of participatory action research: embracing both the forest and the trees. Counseling Psychologist. 2010;38(8):1115–38.

Song JW, Chung KC. Observational studies: cohort and case–control studies. Plast Reconstr Surg. 2010;126(6):2234–42.

Sors, T. G. et al. Reciprocal innovation: a new approach to equitable and mutually beneficial global health partnerships. Glob. Public. Health 18, 2102202 (2023).

Spector-Bagdady, K. et al. Principles for health information collection, sharing, and use: a policy statement from the American Heart Association. Circulation 148, 1061–1069 (2023).

Staggers N, Gassert CA, Curran C. A Delphi study to determine informatics competencies for nurses at four levels of practice. Nurs Res. 2002;51(6):383-390.

Stanford Medicine. Standford Medicine health trends report 2020. Accessed November 20, 2024.

Stevens, M., Kraaijeveld, S. R. & Sharon, T. Sphere transgressions: reflecting on the risks of big tech expansionism. Inf. Commun. Soc. 27, 2587–2599 (2024).

Stewart K, Gill P, Chadwick B, Treasure E. Qualitative research in dentistry. Br Dent J. 2008;204(5):235–9.

Svennberg, E. et al. The digital journey: 25 years of digital development in electrophysiology from an Europace perspective. Europace 25, euad176 (2023).

Teo, C. L. et al. COVID-19 awareness, knowledge and perception towards digital health in an urban multi-ethnic Asian population. Sci. Rep. 11, 10795 (2021).

The Association of Faculties of Medicine of Canada. eHealth Competencies for Undergraduate Medical Education. May 2014. Accessed December 11, 2023.

The MAPS Toolkit: mHealth Assessment and Planning for Scale. Geneva: World Health Organization; 2015.

The World Bank. World bank country and lending groups. Accessed November 20, 2024.

Thye J, Shaw T, Hüsers J, et al. What are inter-professional ehealth competencies? Stud Health Technol Inform. 2018;253:201-205.

Tromp, J. et al. World Heart Federation roadmap for digital health in cardiology. Glob. Heart 17, 61 (2022).

Troy, A. L., Xu, J. & Wadhera, R. K. Access to care and cardiovascular health in US counties with low versus higher broadband internet availability. Am. J. Cardiol. 209, 190–192 (2023).

Tu, S. S., Leadmon, C., Daval, C. J. R. & Kesselheim, A. S. Inequitable conduct and invalidation of patents related to Food and Drug Administration-regulated products. JAMA 330, 2119–2121 (2023).

Tudor Car L, Kyaw BM, Nannan Panday RS, et al. Digital health training programs for medical students: scoping review. JMIR Med Educ. 2021;7(3):e28275.

Usability. In: ISO 25000 software product quality [website]. ISO 25000; 2015 (http://iso25000.com/index.php/en/iso25000-standards/iso-25010?limit=3&start=3, accessed 9 May 2016).

Use cases. In: usability.gov [website]. Washington (DC): United States Department of Health and Human Services; 2016 (http://www.usability.gov/how-to-and-tools/methods/use-cases.html, accessed 11 April 2016).

van der Vaart R, Drossaert C. Development of the digital health literacy instrument: measuring a broad spectrum of health 1.0 and health 2.0 skills. J Med Internet Res. 2017;19(1):e27.

van Kessel R, Wong BLH, Clemens T, Brand H. Digital health literacy as a super determinant of health: more than simply the sum of its parts. Internet Interv. 2022;27:100500.

Vasey B, Nagendran M, Campbell B, et al; DECIDE-AI expert group. Reporting guideline for the early-stage clinical evaluation of decision support systems driven by artificial intelligence: DECIDE-AI. Nat Med. 2022;28(5):924-933.

Vayena, E. Value from health data: European opportunity to catalyse progress in digital health. Lancet 397, 652–653 (2021).

Victor, R. G. et al. A cluster-randomized trial of blood-pressure reduction in Black barbershops. N. Engl. J. Med. 378, 1291–1301 (2018).

Vivo, R. P. et al. Short- and long-term rehospitalization and mortality for heart failure in 4 racial/ethnic populations. J. Am. Heart Assoc. 3, e001134 (2014).

Vogel I. Review of the use of "Theory of Change" in international development. London: United Kingdom Department of International Development; 2012

Walpole S, Taylor P, Banerjee A. Health informatics in UK Medical Education: an online survey of current practice. JRSM Open. Published online December 1, 2016.

Wang, C. J. & Huang, D. J. The HIPAA conundrum in the era of mobile health and communications. JAMA 310, 1121–1122 (2013).

Wang, M. L., Gago, C. M. & Rodriguez, K. Digital redlining – the invisible structural determinant of health. JAMA 331, 1267–1268 (2024).

Waseh S, Dicker AP. Telemedicine training in undergraduate medical education: mixed-methods review. JMIR Med Educ. 2019;5(1):e12515.

Westra BL, Delaney CW. Informatics competencies for nursing and healthcare leaders. AMIA Annu Symp Proc. 2008;2008:804-808.

WHO evaluation practice handbook. Geneva: World Health Organization; 2013 (http://apps.who.int/iris/ bitstream/10665/96311/1/9789241548687_eng.pdf, accessed 5 May 2016).

Wireframing. In: usability.gov [website]. Washington (DC): United States Department of Health and Human Services; 2016 (http://www.usability.gov/how-to-and-tools/methods/wireframing.html, accessed 11 April 2016).

Wong, C. X. et al. Underuse and overuse of anticoagulation for atrial fibrillation: a study in indigenous and non-indigenous Australians. Int. J. Cardiol. 191, 20–24 (2015).

World Health Organization. Countries. Accessed April 21, 2024.

World Health Organization. Digital health in the WHO European Region: the ongoing journey to commitment and transformation. Published September 1, 2023. Accessed November 20, 2024.

World Health Organization. Seventy-second regional committee for Europe (Tel Aviv, 12–14 September 2022): draft resolution sponsored by Israel—Leveraging digital transformation for better health in Europe—Regional digital health action plan for the WHO European Region 2023-2030. Published 2022. Accessed November 20, 2024.

Yaghobian S, Ohannessian R, Iampetro T, et al. Knowledge, attitudes and practices of telemedicine education and training of French medical students and residents. J Telemed Telecare. 2022;28(4):248-257.

Yaghobian S, Ohannessian R, Mathieu-Fritz A, Moulin T. National survey of telemedicine education and training in medical schools in France. J Telemed Telecare. 2020;26(5):303-308.

Yang K, Hu Y, Qi H. Digital health literacy: bibliometric analysis. J Med Internet Res. 2022;24(7):e35816.

Yasmin, F. et al. Understanding patients' experience living with diabetes type 2 and effective disease management: a qualitative study following a mobile health intervention in Bangladesh. BMC Health Serv. Res. 20, 29 (2020).

Yong, C. M. et al. Association of insurance type with receipt of oral anticoagulation in insured patients with atrial fibrillation: a report from the American College of Cardiology NCDR PINNACLE registry. Am. Heart J. 195, 50–59 (2018).

Yong, C. M. et al. Temporal trends in transcatheter aortic valve replacement use and outcomes by race, ethnicity, and sex. Catheter. Cardiovasc. Interv. 99, 2092–2100 (2022).

Yoon J, Lee M, Ahn JS, et al. Development and validation of digital health technology literacy assessment questionnaire. J Med Syst. 2022;46(2):13.

Zainal H, Xiaohui X, Thumboo J, Kok Yong F. Digital competencies for Singapore's national medical school curriculum: a qualitative study. Med Educ Online. 2023;28(1):2211820.

Zehra T, Parwani A, Abdul-Ghafar J, Ahmad Z. A suggested way forward for adoption of AI-Enabled digital pathology in low resource organizations in the developing world. Diagn Pathol. 2023;18(1):68.

Zhang, D. T. et al. Social determinants of health and cardiologist involvement in the care of adults hospitalized for heart failure. JAMA Netw. Open. 6, e2344070 (2023).

Index